Lippincott's
Review Series

Pediatric Nursing

Lippincott's Review Series

Pediatric Nursing

Third Edition

Mary E. Muscari, RN, PhD, CRNP, CS
Associate Professor of Nursing
University of Scranton
Scranton, Pennsylvania

Private Consultant
Adolescent Health
Lake Ariel, Pennsylvania

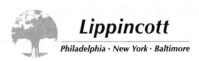

Lippincott
Philadelphia · New York · Baltimore

Sponsoring Editor: Jennifer Brogan
Developmental Editors: Danielle DiPalma, Sarah Kyle
Senior Project Editor: Sandra Cherrey Scheinin
Senior Production Manager: Helen Ewan
Production Coordinator: Pat McCloskey
Design Coordinator: Doug Smock
Cover Designer: Tom Jackson
Indexer: Lynne Mahan
Manufacturing Manager: William Alberti

3rd Edition

9 8 7 6 5 4 3

Library of Congress Cataloging in Publications Data
Pediatric nursing / [edited by] Mary E., Muscari.—3rd ed.
    p. ; cm.—(Lippincott's review series)
  Includes bibliographical references and index.
  ISBN 0-7817-2187-3 (alk. paper)
    1. Pediatric nursing—Examinations, questions, etc. 2. Pediatric nursing—Outlines, syllabi, etc. I. Muscari, Mary E. II. Series.
    [DNLM: 1. Pediatric Nursing—Examination Questions. 2. Pediatric Nursing—Outlines. WY 18.2 P3714 2000]
RJ245.L57 2000
610.73&28)76—dc21

                                                                    00-030162

Care has been taken to confirm the accuracy of the information presented and to describe generally accepted practices. However, the authors, editors, and publisher are not responsible for errors or omissions or for any consequences from application of the information in this book and make no warranty, express or implied, with respect to the contents of the publication.

The authors, editors and publisher have exerted every effort to ensure that drug selection and dosage set forth in this text are in accordance with current recommendations and practice at the time of publication. However, in view of ongoing research, changes in government regulations, and the constant flow of information relating to drug therapy and drug reactions, the reader is urged to check the package insert for each drug for any change in indications and dosage and for added warnings and precautions. This is particularly important when the recommended agent is a new or infrequently employed drug.

Some drugs and medical devices presented in this publication have Food and Drug Administration (FDA) clearance for limited use in restricted research settings. It is the responsibility of the health care provider to ascertain the FDA status of each drug or device planned for use in their clinical practice.

This book is dedicated to my parents, Joseph Nicholas and Mary Theresa Muscari, and to my grandfather, Charles Gruppe, LPN, who inspired my nursing career.

Reviewers

Jean Krajicek Bartek, PhD, ARNP
Associate Professor
College of Nursing and Medicine
University of Nebraska Medical Center
Omaha, Nebraska

Mary Emily Cameron, RN, PhD
Assistant Professor
Department of Nursing
Rutgers, The State University of New Jersey
Camden, New Jersey

Michelle A. Frey, RN, MS, AOCN
Administrative Director Children's Services
Duke University Medical Center
Durham, North Carolina

Mona Harris, RN, MS, EdS
Nurse Educator
Department of Nursing
Labotte Community College
Parsons, Kansas

Elizabeth Hobdell, CRNP, PhD
Nurse Practitioner
Child Neurology
Wayne, Pennsylvania

Kim Luciano, RN, NPC
Pediatric Nurse Practitioner
Pediatric Pulmonology
St. Joseph's Children's Hospital
Paterson, New Jersey

Sandra R. Mott, RN,C, PhD(c)
Associate Professor
School of Nursing
Boston College
Chestnut Hill, Massachusetts

Randa Sperling, RN,C, MSN
Standards Analyst
Performance Improvement
Deaconess Hospital, Inc.
Evansville, Indiana

Lori Steffani, RN, BSN, PNP
Nurse Consultant
Minnesota Colleagues in Caring
Roseville, Minnesota

Patty Stockert, RN, MS
Associate Professor
Saint Francis Medical Center College of
    Nursing
Peoria, Illinois

Donna Wilsker, RN, MSN
Assistant Professor
Department of Nursing
Lamar University
Beaumont, Texas

Introduction

Lippincott's Review Series is designed to help you in your study of the key subject areas in nursing. The series consists of six books, one in each core nursing subject area:

Medical-Surgical Nursing   Mental Health and Psychiatric Nursing
Pediatric Nursing   Pathophysiology
Maternal-Newborn Nursing   Fluids and Electrolytes

Lippincott's Review Series was planned and developed in response to your requests for comprehensive outline review books that address each major subject area and also contain a self-test mechanism. These books meet the need for strong and weak areas of knowledge. Each book is a complete source for review and self-assessment of a single core subject—all six together provide an excellent comprehensive review of entry-level nursing.

Each book is all-inclusive of the content addressed in major textbooks. The content outline review uses a consistent nursing process format throughout and addresses nursing care for well and ill clients. Also included, are necessary teaching and other concepts, such as growth and development; nutrition; pharmacology; and body structures, functions, and pathophysiology. Special features include the following:

- **Nursing process overview sections** review each step of the nursing process for the system or group of disorders in discussion. These reviews improve your ability to apply principles to practice by highlighting common assessment findings, diagnoses, goals, interventions, and outcomes.
- **Nursing process overview icons** remind you to refer back to the nursing process overview section for in-depth discussion of relevant nursing interventions.
- **Nursing Alerts** are fundamental guidelines you can follow to ensure safe and effective care.
- **Development boxes,** presented in each body systems chapter, highlight developmental changes from the fetal period through adolescence. These summaries of pertinent structure and function information allow you to focus on age-specific care.
- **Drug charts** provide quick reference for medications that are commonly used in treating the disorders discussed within a given chapter. The drug classification, indications, and selected nursing interventions are provided.
- **Child and family teaching boxes** detail health teaching information, which may be applied in the clinical setting.
- **Chapter study questions** help you chart your progress through each chapter. Answer keys are provided with rationales for correct and incorrect responses.
- **Comprehensive examination** mimics the NCLEX and allows you to assess your strengths and weaknesses. An answer key is provided with rationales for correct and incorrect responses.

- **Appendix A, Normal Laboratory Study Values,** is a handy quick reference guide containing normal pediatric laboratory study values. It is designed to enhance your understanding of nursing assessment for pediatric clients
- **Appendix B, Nursing Considerations for Laboratory and Diagnostic Studies,** contains helpful hints and vital tips to keep in mind while performing, or preparing your pediatric client for, common laboratory and diagnostic studies.
- **Accompanying CD-ROM** provides 200 additional NCLEX-style questions so you can practice computer adaptive test-taking skills. Answers are provided with rationales for correct and incorrect responses.

You can use the books in this series in several different ways. Overall, you can use them as subject reviews to augment general study throughout your basic nursing program and as a review to prepare for the National Council Licensure Examination (NCLEX-RN). How you use each book depends on your individual needs and preferences and on whether you review each chapter systematically or concentrate only on those chapters whose subject areas are particularly problematic or challenging. You may instead choose to use the comprehensive examination as a self-assessment opportunity to evaluate your knowledge base before you review the content outline. Likewise, you can use the study questions for pre- or post-testing after study, followed by the comprehensive examination as a means of evaluating your knowledge and competencies of an entire subject area. Regardless of how you use the books, one of the strengths of the series is the self-assessment opportunity it offers in addition to guidance in studying and reviewing content. The chapter study questions and comprehensive examination questions have been carefully developed to cover all topics in the outline review.

Unlike the NCLEX examination that tests the cumulative knowledge needed for safe practice by an entry-level nurse, these practice tests systematically evaluate the knowledge base that serves as the building block for the entire nursing educational process. In this way, you can prepare for the NCLEX examination throughout your course of study. Good study habits throughout your educational program are not only the best way to ensure ongoing success, but also will prove the most beneficial way to prepare for the licensing examination.

Keep in mind that these books are not intended to replace formal learning. They cannot substitute for textbook reading, discussion with instructors, or class attendance. Every effort has been made to provide accurate and current information, but class attendance and interaction with an instructor will provide invaluable information not found in books. Used correctly, these books will help you increase understanding, improve comprehension, evaluate strengths and weakness in areas of knowledge, increase productive study time, and, as a result, help you improve your grades.

MONEY-BACK GUARANTEE—Lippincott's Review Series will help you study more effectively during coursework throughout your educational program, and help you prepare for quizzes and tests, including the NCLEX exam. If you buy and use any of the six volumes in Lippincott's Review Series and fail the NCLEX exam, simply send us verification of your exam results and your copy of the review book to the address below. We will promptly send you a check for our suggested list price.

Lippincott's Review Series
Marketing Department
Lippincott Williams & Wilkins
530 Walnut Street
Philadelphia, PA 19106

Acknowledgments

The author wishes to thank the following people:

Jane Velker, Manager of Development; Danielle DiPalma, Managing Developmental Editor; Sarah Andrus Kyle, Freelance Developmental Editor; and Hilarie Surrena, Editorial Assistant, for their assistance in this project.

The reviewers for their time, patience, and expertise

The nursing students at the University of Scranton and all nursing students who use this book, for their ongoing support.

Contents

1 Pediatric Nursing Overview

I. Influences on pediatric health

A. Heredity and genetics

1. **Overview**
   a. **Heredity** is the process by which living organisms produce offspring like themselves. **Genetics** is the study of heredity.
   b. **Congenital** (present at birth) **defects** result from chromosomal abnormalities, monogenic (single-gene) mutations, or other intrauterine factors.
      (1) Alterations in a chromosome, part of a chromosome, or gene can cause a genetic disorder.
      (2) One or both biologic parents may pass such alterations to a child, or alterations may be new in the child.
      (3) Many common defects (congenital heart disease, pyloric stenosis, and central nervous system malformations) appear to be associated with multifactorial inheritance.
      (4) **Syndrome** is the term used for a recognizable pattern of malformations due to a single specific cause, such as fetal alcohol syndrome and Down syndrome.
      (5) **Association** is the term used for nonrandom patterns of malformations for which an etiology has not been determined. VATER (verbal defects, imperforate anus, tracheoesophageal fistula, and radial/renal defects) is an example of an association.
      (6) Certain problems, such as mental retardation, neural tube defects, and cleft lip or palate, can occur as part of a syndrome or an association and can have different etiologies, including single-gene or chromosome abnormalities, prenatal exposures (such as drugs or disease), or multifactorial causes.

2. **Chromosome disorders**
   a. Deviations in numbers of chromosomes (ie, gain or loss of a chromosome) are designated with the suffix **-somy**.
      (1) **Monosomy** refers to the loss of one chromosome from a pair. Monosomies are rare, and the fetus is usually nonviable. **Turner syndrome** (45, XO) is basically the only viable monosomy; however, 99% of these fetuses are spontaneously aborted.
      (2) **Trisomy** refers to an addition to a pair of chromosomes. Trisomies are relatively common. The most common include trisomy 12 (Patau syndrome), trisomy 18 (Edwards syndrome), and **trisomy 21 (Down syndrome)**. Down syndrome can also result from a translocation of chromosome 21.
   b. Cell division errors can occur during either meiosis (gamete formation) or mitosis (postzygotic cell division), resulting in unequal distribution of genetic material.

(1) Alterations in the number of sex chromosomes typically do not cause serious effects. **Klinefelter syndrome** (47, XXY) is the most common sex chromosome abnormality.

(2) Numeric and structural autosome anomalies account for a collection of syndromes that are usually characterized by mental deficiencies. These include the trisomies listed above, and classic deletions syndromes, such as **cri-du-chat**.

3. Monogenic (single-gene) disorders

a. Types of inheritance patterns include the following:

(1) **Autosomal dominant inheritance**. Children of a heterozygous parent have a 50% chance of possessing the defective gene. Children who do not inherit the defective gene will themselves have unaffected offspring.

(2) **Autosomal recessive inheritance**. Children of two heterozygous parents have a 25% chance of being affected. Unaffected children have a 66% chance of carrying the gene and possibly passing it to their offspring.

(3) **X-linked dominant inheritance.** Daughters of an affected father will probably be affected; sons will not. Half the daughters and half the sons of affected mothers will be affected. There are no carriers, and normal children will themselves have normal offspring.

(4) **X-linked recessive inheritance.** Males are usually affected; half the female children of affected fathers will be carriers and may pass the gene to their offspring.

b. Traditional inheritance patterns account for only one third of genetic disorders. Other disorders can be attributed to gene variation, nontraditional inheritance, and multifactorial disorders.

4. Nursing management

a. Obtain a comprehensive history that includes family history and a history of problems that may suggest genetic disorders such as congenital defects, growth abnormalities, hearing and vision problems, abnormal sexual development, metabolic disorders, and developmental disorders.

b. Construct a pedigree chart.

c. Encourage referral for genetic counseling, screening, and follow-up.

B. Family

1. Family functions include the following:

a. Childbearing and child-rearing

b. Providing basic needs (ie, food, safety, clothing, shelter, and health care)

c. Providing communication and emotional support

d. Enabling enculturation and socialization

e. Preparing children to become citizens

2. Family structures include the following:

a. A nuclear or conjugal family consists of a husband, wife, and children (natural or adopted) living in the same household.

b. A single-parent family consists of one parent who is responsible for the care of children as a result of death, divorce, desertion, birth outside of marriage, or adoption.

c. A reconstituted or stepfamily exists when one or both married adults have children from previous marriages.

d. An extended family is the nuclear family and grandparents, cousins, aunts, and uncles.

e. A same-sex family exists when two men or two women live in a common-law arrangement with or without children.

f. A two-career family exists when both adults in the family have jobs.

   g. A commuter family exists when the adults in a family live and work apart for professional or financial reasons.

   h. A return-to-nest family is created when adult children return home to live for financial, social, or cultural reasons.

   i. A binuclear family exists when the child is a member of two families (joint custody), and parenting is considered a joint venture.

   j. A communal family exists when a group of people lives together with most being unrelated by blood or marriage.

   k. A foster family is a temporary family for children who must be placed temporarily away from their parents in an effort to ensure their emotional and physical well-being.

3. Family reactions to a child's illness or hospitalization vary and may include:

   a. Possible impaired coping. Fears and anxieties about a child's illness or hospitalization may increase, compromising the family's ability to cope and their ability to help the child cope.

   b. **Loss of control.** A sense of helplessness may result from stressors such as seriousness of the illness, previous hospitalizations, medical procedures, lack of information, support systems, ego strengths, other family problems, cultural and religious beliefs, family communications, and previous coping abilities.

   c. **Possible parental displays of stress.** Examples include anxiety, denial, guilt, anger, fear, frustration, depression, and such defense mechanisms as displacement and projection.

4. Implications for the nursing process are as follows:

   a. Assess parents' energy levels, physical health, and developmental levels; how each parent was parented as a child, if appropriate; stressors; family support systems; cultural and religious beliefs; and education and experience in child-rearing.

   b. Develop nursing diagnoses based on assessment findings (eg, altered parenting, role performance, and family processes).

   c. Identify outcomes (eg, parenting role will be strengthened).

   d. Plan and carry out interventions.

     (1) Help the parents accept their child's individuality, and assist them in developing realistic goals.

     (2) Be supportive by allowing the parents to verbalize concerns, enlisting parental support from family members, and encouraging participation in support groups and community resources.

     (3) Keep the parents informed, but avoid making them dependent on the nurse.

     (4) Explain the child's growth and development; provide anticipatory guidance and explain the child's anticipated reactions.

   e. Evaluate outcomes (eg, parents can perform their parenting role).

C. Socioeconomic, cultural, and religious factors

1. Socioeconomic influences. Social class probably has the greatest influence due to differences in child-rearing practices and attitudes toward health. Children are raised differently by parents who vary in education, communication skills, occupation, and income.

   a. Low socioeconomic status has the greatest adverse influence on health. This is due to several factors:

     (1) Escalating health care costs and unaffordable health insurance premiums

     (2) Eating unbalanced meals and insufficient food

     (3) Forgoing health care related to lack of funds or lack of value in the importance of health, especially health promotion and disease prevention measures

(4) Inadequate housing that may result in overcrowding, poor sanitation, and thus, greater exposure to communicable diseases.

b. Homeless children have increased in numbers. These children face not only health problems, but also loss of the basics of growth and development, including friendship and schooling. Homeless children have more physical and psychiatric disorders than poor children with permanent residences.

c. Migrant children are one of the most disadvantaged groups. Schooling and health care are inadequate because the children are apt to live in a number of different places. Because their parents work in the fields most of the day, they have little supervision, leaving them susceptible to injuries.

2. Cultural and religious influences

a. Humans acquire culture early in life, and cultural understanding is usually established by 5 years of age.

b. Culture and religious beliefs influence choice of mate, postmarital residence, family kinships, household rules, household structure, family obligations, family–community interactions, dietary customs, communication patterns, interpersonal relationships, and health beliefs and practices.

c. Some groups consider folk healers as powerful.

d. Many cultures use home remedies. Some remedies are compatible with medical treatment, many have no scientific basis, and some actually may be harmful.

3. Nursing management

a. Understand your own beliefs and values, be sensitive to the beliefs and values of others, and avoid imposing personal beliefs and values on clients.

b. Perform a cultural assessment.

c. Consider clients' cultural and religious beliefs when developing and implementing plans of care.

D. Environment

1. Safety hazards in the home and community contribute to falls, burns, drownings, and motor vehicle and other accidents.

2. Passive smoking is a recognized health hazard for children and adolescents. Other pollution (eg, from radiation, chemicals, and water, air, or food contamination) poses significant health hazards as well.

3. Media influences include the following:

a. Children may identify with and mimic characters or criminals portrayed in the media (TV, videos, movies, magazines, newspapers), which may lead to violence and harm to self and others.

b. Excessive TV viewing has been linked to obesity and high blood cholesterol levels in children. (Researchers have not established how TV viewing affects weight and cholesterol levels; they have established only the relationship.)

4. Nursing management includes the following:

a. Assess the effects of environmental factors on children and families.

b. Contribute to community health by becoming involved in education and policy making.

E. Growth and development

1. Definitions

a. **Growth** refers to an increase in body size (ie, height and weight).

b. **Development** refers to an increasing capacity to function at more advanced levels.

2. Stages (approximate age ranges)

a. The **prenatal stage** extends from conception to birth.

b. The **infancy stage** extends from birth to about 12 months (neonatal, birth to 28 days; infancy, 29 days to about 12 months).

    c. The **early childhood stage** extends from 1 to 6 years (**toddlerhood**, 1–3 years; **preschool**, 3–6 years).

    d. The **middle childhood (school-age) stage** extends from 6 to 12 years.

    e. The **adolescent stage** extends from 12 to 18 (up to 21) years.

3. Patterns (trends) of growth and development

    a. These patterns are definite and predictable.

    b. Directional patterns include the following:

        (1) **Cephalocaudal** (head-to-tail) development occurs along the body's long axis. Control over the head, the mouth, and eye movement precedes control over the upper body, torso, and legs.

        (2) **Proximodistal** (midline-to-peripheral) development progresses from the center of the body to the extremities. The child develops arm movement before fine motor finger ability. Development is symmetrical, with each side developing in the same direction at the same time.

        (3) **Mass-to-specific** (differentiation) development occurs as a child masters simple operations before complex ones.

    c. Sequential patterns involve a predictable sequence of growth and development stages through which a child normally proceeds. Sequential patterns have been identified for motor skills, such as locomotion (eg, a child starts crawling before walking), and for behaviors, such as language and social skills (eg, first a child plays alone, then with others).

    d. Secular patterns are universal trends in the rate and age of maturation. In general, children mature earlier and grow larger than their counterparts in preceding generations.

4. Theories of growth and development. Theorists consider that emotional, social, cognitive, and moral skills develop in stages. Table 1-1 lists the stages defined by well-known theorists. Chapters 2 through 6 explain each of the theories as they apply to specific developmental stages.

    a. **Psychosocial**. Erik Erikson's theory of psychosocial development is most widely used. At each stage, children confront a crisis that requires the integration of per-

TABLE 1-1
Developmental Theories

STAGE	ERIKSON	FREUD	PIAGET	KOHLBERG
Infancy (birth to 1 year)	Trust vs mistrust	Oral	Sensorimotor (birth to 2 years)	
Toddlerhood (1–3 years)	Autonomy vs shame and doubt	Anal	Sensorimotor (1–2 years); preoperational (preconceptual) (2–4 years)	Preconventional
Preschool (3–6 years)	Initiative vs guilt	Phallic	Preoperational (preconceptual) (2–4 years); preoperational (intuitive) (4–7 years)	Preconventional
School-age (6–12 years)	Industry vs inferiority	Latency	Concrete operations (7–11 years)	Conventional
Adolescence (12–19 years)	Identity vs role diffusion (confusion)	Genital	Formal operations (11–15 years)	Postconventional

sonal needs and skills with social and cultural expectations. Each stage has two possible components, favorable and unfavorable.

    b. **Psychosexual**. Sigmund Freud considered sexual instincts to be significant in the development of personality. At each stage, regions of the body assume prominent psychologic significance as sources of pleasure.

    c. **Cognitive.** Jean Piaget proposed four major stages of development for logical thinking. Each stage arises from and builds on the previous stage in an orderly fashion.

    d. **Moral.** Lawrence Kohlberg's theory of moral development is based on cognitive development and consists of three major levels, each containing two stages.

5. Temperament involves the child's style of emotional and behavioral responses across situations.

    a. **Types of temperament** are the easy child, the difficult child, and the slow-to-warm-up child.

        (1) **Easy children** are even tempered, regular, and predictable; they approach new stimuli positively.

        (2) **Difficult children** are irritable, highly active, and intense; they react to new stimuli with negative withdrawal.

        (3) **Slow-to-warm-up** children are moody, inactive, and moderately irregular; they react with mild but passive resistance to new stimuli.

    b. **Attributes of temperament**

        (1) **Activity** refers to the level of motor movement and energy expenditure, such as sleeping, eating, playing, dressing, and bathing.

        (2) **Rhythmicity** is the regularity or predictability in the timing of physiologic functions such as hunger, sleep, and bowel movements.

        (3) **Approach-withdrawal** is the nature of initial responses to new stimuli, such as people, situations, places, foods, toys, and procedures. Approach responses are positive, displayed by activity or expression; withdrawal responses are negative expressions.

        (4) **Adaptability** is the ease or difficulty with which the child adapts or adjusts to a new situation.

        (5) **Threshold of responsiveness** is the amount of stimulation, such as sound or light, required to generate a response.

        (6) **Intensity of reaction** is the energy level of reactions, regardless of quality or direction; degree to which the child expresses himself or herself.

        (7) **Mood** is the amount of friendly, happy, pleasant behavior versus unfriendly, unhappy, behavior in various situations.

        (8) **Distractibility** is the ease with which external stimuli can divert attention or behavior.

        (9) **Attention span and persistence** is the length of time a child pursues a given activity (attention) and continues the activity despite obstacles (persistence).

    c. Temperament in infancy predicts the child's behavior in the preschool, school-age, and adolescent stages.

    d. Difficult temperament seems to be related to behavioral disorders; however, temperament alone is not a risk factor for maladjustment.

    e. The degree of fit between the infant's temperament and the parents' ability to respond and adapt determines if the parent–child relationship is at risk.

6. Nursing management includes the following:

    a. Understand that temperament and maturation patterns vary among individual children.

    b. Provide parents with information they need to promote normal growth and development of children.

    c. Provide health education for families within the constraints imposed by illness, disease, or disability.

    d. Assess development (physiologic, motor, cognitive, and psychosocial) using a systematic approach to ensure coverage of all significant areas.

II. Influences on pediatric mortality and morbidity

A. Leading causes of mortality (death) in children

    1. Congenital anomalies, sudden infant death syndrome (SIDS), disorders related to prematurity and low birth weight, and respiratory distress syndrome are the leading causes of death in children under age 1 year.

    2. Table 1-2 lists the leading causes of death for those aged 1 to 24 years.

    3. Unintentional injuries account for more death and disability in children than the combined causes of all other diseases.

B. Leading causes of morbidity in children

    1. Acute conditions that contribute to morbidity in children are respiratory illness (50%), with the common cold being the most prevalent; injuries (15%); and infections and parasitic diseases (11%).

    2. Factors that contribute to morbidity involve low birth weight, poverty, homelessness, chronic illness, foreign-born adoption, and day care.

    3. "Pediatric social illnesses" (also called the new morbidity) that adversely affect health include violence, aggression, noncompliance, school failures, and adjustment to divorce and bereavement.

III. Roles of pediatric nurses

A. Family advocate. Nurses assist in identifying the needs and goals of children and their families and in developing appropriate nursing interventions.

B. Health promoter. Nurses assist in promoting health and preventing disease by fostering growth and development, proper nutrition, immunizations, and early identification of health problems.

C. Health teacher. Nurses provide families with information on topics such as anticipatory guidance, parenting, and disease processes.

TABLE 1-2
Leading Causes of Death in Children 1 to 24 Years of Age

RANK	1–4 YEARS	5–14 YEARS	14–24 YEARS
1	Accidents	Accidents	Accidents
2	Congenital anomalies	Cancer	Homicide
3	Cancer	Homicide*	Suicide
4	Homicide	Congenital anomalies	Cancer
5	Heart disease	Heart disease	Heart disease

Incidence has increased since 1991.

Adapted from Anderson, R. N., Kochanek, K. D., & Murphy, S. L. (1995). Report of final mortality statistics.
Monthly Vital Statistics Report, 45(11 suppl 2), 23, 69. Hyattsville, MD: National Center for Health Statistics.

D. Counselor. Nurses support families through active listening. A therapeutic relationship between a nurse and the child and family includes caring as well as carefully defined boundaries.

E. Collaborator. As a key member of the interdependent health care team, nurses collaborate and coordinate nursing services with other health care professionals.

F. Researcher. Nurses use and contribute to research that enhances the nursing care of children and adolescents and their families.

Child health care settings

A. Ambulatory settings. Nurses provide direct care and teaching, and they perform triage.

B. School health. School nurses screen, teach, and monitor health status.

C. Home care. Nurses provide a range of nursing services in the home environment to decrease health care costs and maintain the integrity of the family.

D. Acute care settings. Nurses provide direct care and teaching in pediatric and adolescent units, emergency departments, intensive care units, and surgical units.

E. Other settings. Nurses also work with children in camps, rehabilitation facilities, hospices, and psychiatric settings.

V. Pediatric nursing health assessment

A. General considerations
 1. **Child considerations**
    a. Maintain eye contact (if culturally appropriate), bending to the child's level as needed.
    b. Use language appropriate for the child's cognitive level; involve the child in the assessment interview by asking appropriate questions.
    c. Remember that a child is aware of the caregiver's nonverbal communication and body language.
    d. Allow the child some "warm-up" time to become acquainted with the caregivers and the environment; introduce yourself and explain your purposes.
    e. Respect the child's responses and need for privacy as appropriate for age.
    f. Incorporate play into the assessment as appropriate.
 2. **Family considerations**
    a. Develop a family-oriented approach that encourages parents to participate.
    b. Choose a quiet environment for the assessment and for any teaching sessions.
    c. Ask open-ended questions to elicit responses other than "yes" or "no."
    d. Focus on the information needed or problem to be solved.
    e. Communicate the importance of parental roles with the health care team in planning and providing care for the child.
    f. Listen attentively, respect responses, and provide appropriate feedback. Use silence judiciously.
    g. Encourage parents to express concerns and ask questions.

B. Health history
 1. The purpose of the health history is to collect subjective data about the child's health status and to gain insight into actual or potential health problems.

2. Components of the health history include the following:

a. **Biographical data** include name, address, telephone number, parents' or guardians' names, date and place of birth, gender, race, religion, and nationality or cultural background.

b. **Chief complaint** is the child's or parent's (informant's) reason for seeking health care.

c. **Current health or illness status** refers to the sequence of events that led to the chief complaint and related information, including:

   (1) Symptom analysis of the chief complaint (ie, onset, timing, duration, character, severity, location, precipitating factors, associated symptoms, and alleviating factors)

   (2) Other current or recurrent illnesses or problems

   (3) Current medications

   (4) Any other health concerns

   (5) Allergies (identify and describe manifestations)

d. **Past health** refers to previous problems and health promotion activities, including:

   (1) Birth history (ie, pregnancy, labor and delivery, and perinatal history)

   (2) Previous illnesses, injuries, or surgeries

   (3) Allergies

   (4) Immunization status

   (5) Growth and developmental milestones

   (6) Habits

e. **Review of systems**

   (1) Ask about the child's **overall health status**.

   (2) **Integumentary system**. Ask about lesions, bruising, skin care habits, and problems with hair and nails.

   (3) **Head**. Ask about trauma and headaches.

   (4) **Eyes**. Ask about visual acuity, last eye examination, drainage, and infections.

   (5) **Ears**. Ask about hearing acuity, last hearing examination, drainage, and infections.

   (6) **Nose**. Ask about bleeding, congestion, discharge, and sinus infections.

   (7) **Mouth**. Ask about lesions, soreness, tooth eruption, patterns of dental care, and last dental examination.

   (8) **Throat**. Ask about sore throat frequency, hoarseness, and difficulty swallowing.

   (9) **Neck**. Ask about stiffness, tenderness, and adenopathy.

   (10) **Chest (respiratory)**. Ask about pain, cough, wheezing, shortness of breath, asthma, and infections.

   (11) **Breasts**. Ask about thelarche, lesions, discharge, and performance of breast self-examination (BSE).

   (12) **Cardiovascular system**. Ask about history of murmurs, exercise tolerance, dizziness, palpitations, and congenital defects.

   (13) **Gastrointestinal system**. Ask about appetite, bowel habits, food intolerances, nausea, vomiting, pain, and history of parasites.

   (14) **Genitourinary system**. Ask about urgency, frequency, discharge, urinary tract infections, sexually transmitted diseases, enuresis, sexual problems or dysfunctions (male), and performance of testicular self-examination (male).

   (15) **Gynecologic**. Ask about menarche, menstrual history, and sexual problems or dysfunctions (female).

   (16) **Musculoskeletal system**. Ask about pain, swelling, fractures, mobility problems, and scoliosis.

    (17) Neurologic system. Ask about ataxia, tremors, unusual movements, and seizures.

    (18) Lymphatic system. Ask about pain, swelling or tenderness, and enlargement of the spleen or liver.

    (19) Endocrine or metabolic system. Ask about growth patterns, polyuria, polydypsia, and polyphagia.

    (20) Psychiatric history. Ask about any psychiatric, developmental, substance abuse, or eating disorders.

  f. The family history should include any family genetic traits or diseases with familial tendencies, communicable diseases, psychiatric disorders, and substance abuse.

  g. **Nutritional history**

    (1) Quantity and kind of food or formula ingested daily (use 24-hour recall food diary for 3 days: 2 weekdays and 1 weekend day; or food-frequency record)

    (2) Problems with feeding

    (3) Use of vitamin supplements

    (4) Description of any special diets

    (5) Cultural or religious food practices, preferences, or restrictions

    (6) Dieting behaviors, including body image, types of diets, frequency of weighing, or use of self-induced vomiting, laxatives, and diuretics

  h. The **sleep history** should include time the child goes to bed and awakens, quality of sleep, nap history, and sleep aids (eg, blanket or toy).

  i. **Psychosocial history**

    (1) A home and family structure assessment should include composition of family members, occupation and education of members, culture, and religion.

    (2) A home and family function assessment should include communication patterns, family roles and relationships, pets, and financial status.

    (3) A school and work assessment should include grades, behavior, relationship with teachers and peers, type of part-time job, hours worked per week, and effect of job on schoolwork and socialization.

    (4) An activity assessment should include types of play; number of hours of TV viewing, video game playing, or both per day; amount of nonschool-related reading; hobbies; and chores.

    (5) A discipline assessment should include the type and frequency of discipline at home.

    (6) A sexual assessment should include the child's or adolescent's concerns, abuse history, sexual activity patterns, number of partners, use of condoms and contraceptives, and AIDS awareness.

    (7) A substance use assessment should include amount, frequency, and circumstances of use for tobacco, alcohol, prescribed or illicit drugs, steroids, and substances such as inhalants.

    (8) A violence assessment should include domestic violence, child abuse, self-abusive behaviors, suicidal ideation and attempts, violence perpetrated on others by child or adolescent, and access to guns and other weapons.

3. Age-related interview techniques

  a. **Infant**. Speak softly, allow the infant to identify you with a parent, and use touch.

  b. **Toddler**. Allow the toddler to stay close to parents and focus on a favorite toy or a unique characteristic about the child.

  c. **Preschooler**. Use simple questions and words without double meanings; allow the child to manipulate equipment; and use toys, puppets, and play.

  d. **Schoolager**. Offer explanations, teach about health, and provide demonstrations.

e. **Adolescent**. Maintain confidentiality, facilitate trust, ask to speak to the adolescent alone, encourage open and honest communication, be nonjudgmental, and use open-ended questions.

C. Developmental assessment

1. The purpose of developmental assessment is to identify any problems or possible concerns and to confirm normal achievement of growth and developmental milestones in the following areas:
   a. Gross motor skills
   b. Fine motor skills
   c. Language development
   d. Cognitive development
   e. Social and affective development

2. **Nursing management**
   a. Observe the child's behavior before structured interaction for spontaneous activity; observe the child's responses to the environment.
   b. Administer developmental tests as appropriate for age (eg, Denver Developmental Screening Test II, Developmental Profile II, Draw-A-Person: A Quantitative Scoring System [DAP], Home Observation for Measurement of the Environment [HOME], Early Screening Inventory [ESI]).

D. Physical assessment

1. The purpose of physical assessment is to obtain objective data on body systems functioning and overall health status.

2. **General guidelines**
   a. Complete less threatening and less intrusive procedures first to secure the child's trust.
   b. Explain what you will be doing and what the child can expect to feel; allow the child to manipulate the equipment before using it.

3. **Developmental approaches**
   a. **Infant**. Allow the infant to sit in the parent's lap, encourage parents to hold infant, use distraction, and enlist the parent's assistance.
   b. **Toddler**. Allow the toddler to sit on the parent's lap, enlist the parent's aid, use play, and praise cooperation.
   c. **Preschooler**. Use storytelling and doll and puppet play; offer choices when possible.
   d. **Schoolager**. Maintain privacy, provide a gown, explain procedures and equipment, and teach the child about his or her body.
   e. **Adolescent**. Provide privacy and confidentiality, provide the option of having parent present or not, emphasize normality, and include health teaching.

4. **Vital signs assessment**
   a. **Blood pressure**. Measure blood pressure annually in children 3 years and older. Select appropriate cuff width, so that cuff covers three fourths of the upper arm. Readings vary throughout childhood.
      (1) Normal systolic ranges
         (a) 1 to 7 years = age in years + 90
         (b) 8 to 18 years = (2 x age in years) + 83
      (2) Normal diastolic ranges
         (a) 1 to 5 years = 56
         (b) 6 to 18 years = age in years + 52
   b. **Pulse rate**. Take an apical pulse in children under age 2 years. Radial pulses may be taken in children over age 2 years. Count the pulse for a full minute in infants

and young children due to possible rhythm irregularities. Table 1-3 lists normal resting and awake rates for different age groups.

    c. **Respiratory rate**. Monitor infants by observing abdominal movements; monitor older children the same as adults. Table 1-4 lists normal respiratory rate ranges for different age groups.

    d. **Temperature**. Use a rectal, axillary, skin, or tympanic thermometer in children under age 4; do not use an oral thermometer until children are over age 4. Normal temperature ranges are the same as in adults.

5. Head-to-toe assessment. In most cases, physical assessment involves a head-to-toe examination that covers each body system.

    a. **Measurements**. Assess height and weight in all children and head circumference in children under 2 years of age.

    b. **General appearance**. Assess alertness and level of consciousness, physical appearance, nutritional state, hygiene, behavior, interactions with parents and nurse, and overall development and speech.

    c. **Skin**. Assess color, texture, turgor, temperature, lesions, scars, edema, and tattoos.

    d. **Hair**. Assess distribution, characteristics, and presence of lice.

    e. **Nails**. Assess texture, shape, color, and condition.

    f. **Lymph nodes**. Assess swelling, mobility, temperature, and tenderness.

    g. **Head**. Assess size, shape, symmetry, and condition of fontanelles.

    h. **Eyes**. Assess visual acuity; perform external and internal (ophthalmoscopic) examinations.

    i. **Ears**. Assess hearing acuity; perform external and internal (otoscopic) examinations.

    j. **Nose and sinuses**. Assess discharge, tenderness, and turbinates (color and swelling).

    k. **Mouth**. Assess tooth eruption and condition of gums, lips, teeth, palates, tonsils, tongue, and buccal mucosa.

    l. **Neck**. Assess suppleness and range of motion.

    m. **Chest**. Assess shape, breasts (sexual development stage), discharge, and lesions.

    n. **Lungs**. Assess breath sounds and adventitious sounds.

    o. **Heart**. Assess heart sounds, murmurs, and rubs.

    p. **Abdomen**. Assess appearance of umbilicus, shape, bowel sounds, hernias, liver, spleen, kidneys, masses, and tenderness.

    q. **Genitalia**

        (1) **Female**. Assess sexual developmental stage (pubic hair), vulva, meatus, external genitalia, discharge, and lesions.

        (2) **Male**. Assess sexual developmental stage (penis, scrotum, and pubic hair), penis, scrotum, testes, urinary meatus, discharge, and lesions.

TABLE 1-3
Normal Resting and Awake Pulse Rates

AGE GROUP	RATE
Newborn	100–180
1 week to 3 months	100–220
3 months to 2 years	80–150
2–10 years	70–110
10 years to adult	55–90

TABLE 1-4
Normal Respiratory Rate Ranges

AGE GROUP	RATE
Birth to 6 months	30–50
6 months to 2 years	20–30
3–10 years	20–28
10–18 years	12–20

r. **Anus**. Perform an external examination and assess for fissures, lesions, and bleeding.

s. **Musculoskeletal**. Assess muscle size and strength, posture and body alignment, symmetry, range of motion, gait, joints for movement, swelling, redness, tenderness, and warmth.

t. **Neurologic**. Assess cerebral function (language, memory, cognition), cranial nerve function, deep tendon and superficial reflexes, balance and coordination, sensory function, motor function, and infantile reflexes (Table 1-5).

 ## Overview of pediatric nursing procedures

A. General guidelines

1. Parents or legal guardians give informed consent in most cases. State laws vary on different aspects of informed consent, such as issues of treatment without parental consent and emancipated and mature minors.

2. Children require developmentally appropriate explanations for all procedures. Use play whenever possible.

3. Practice appropriate infection control measures when handling children in diapers.

TABLE 1-5
Infantile Reflexes

REFLEX	AGE AT DISAPPEARANCE	HOW TO ELICIT
Sucking	3–4 months	Touch infant's lips with finger.
Rooting	3–4 months	Stroke corner of mouth; observe infant move head toward stimulation.
Moro	Decreases 3–4 months Disappears 6 months	Make loud noise or brace infant's head and back and simulate falling. Infant extends then flexes arms and fingers.
Palmar grasp	Strongest 1–2 months Disappears 3–4 months	Place index fingers into infant's hand.
Tonic neck	Decreases 3–4 months Disappears 6 months	With infant supine, turn his head to one side. The upper and lower extremity on that side extend; the opposite extremities flex.
Stepping	Disappears before walking	Hold infant under axilla in standing position. Place feet on flat surface.

CHILD AND FAMILY TEACHING 1-1

Home Medications

- Review the name of the medication, why it was prescribed, what it does, how to take it, its side effects, and any dietary or activity restrictions.
- Teach how to use calibrated measuring device and ask for feedback demonstration.
- Instruct parents on proper storage, including keeping medication out of children's reach.

4. Crib rails should be up unless an adult is at the bedside.

5. Never use restraints for punishment or convenience.

B. Medications

1. Dosage calculations
   a. The calculation based on body surface area (BSA) is BSA of child (m²)/1.7 x adult dose = approximate dose.
   b. The calculation based on weight is usually mg/kg/day in divided doses or mg/kg/dose.

2. Two nurses are required to check dosages on several medications, including insulin, narcotics, digoxin, chemotherapy, and anticoagulants.

3. Special considerations for different types of medications (Child and Family Teaching 1-1)
   a. **Oral medications**
      (1) Check the child's gag reflex and ability to swallow before administering.
      (2) Use calibrated spoons, syringes, and cups. Once measured, medication may be administered in a nipple to infants.
      (3) If medication needs to be crushed, administer it in nonessential food.
      (4) Do not crush sustained-release capsules or tablets.
      (5) Verify placement by both aspiration and auscultation before administering medications via a feeding tube.
   b. **Injections**
      (1) Help the child realize that an injection is not punishment.
      (2) **EMLA** (eutectic mixture of local anesthetics). This cream numbs skin at a depth of 0.5 mm and is used before needlesticks. Apply it to intact skin only. EMLA is contraindicated in children with methemoglobinemia.
      (3) Do not flush the needle and hub because it may cause overdose. The air bubble technique is rarely used for this same reason.
      (4) The vastus lateralis is the site of choice for intramuscular injections. Use it for all children under 3 years of age.
   c. **Ophthalmic medications.** When administering ophthalmic medications, gently pull the lower lid down.
   d. **Otic medications.** When administering otic medications, pull the pinna up and back for children over age 3 years, and down and back for children younger than 3 years.

STUDY QUESTIONS

1. The parents of a child with an autosomal dominant genetic disorder ask the nurse, "What are the chances of our next child having this disorder?" Which of the following would be the nurse's **best** response?
   (1) "Each child has a 25% chance of being born with the disorder."
   (2) "Each child has a 50% chance of being born with the disorder."
   (3) "Your male children will be affected, but not your daughters."
   (4) "Females of the affected father will be affected, but not your sons."

2. When assessing a client from a culture different than nurse's own, which of the following should the nurse do **first**?
   (1) Be sensitive to the family's beliefs.
   (2) Understand his or her own beliefs.
   (3) Enact Western values on the family.
   (4) Modify family's cultural beliefs.

3. Which of the following factors plays the **greatest** role in adversely affecting a child's health?
   (1) Cultural background
   (2) Religious influences
   (3) Environmental influences
   (4) Socioeconomic status

4. Which of the following principles of development is being addressed when new parents are taught that infants are able to lift their heads before their trunks?
   (1) Cephalocaudal
   (2) Proximodistal direction
   (3) Simple to the complex
   (4) General to the specific

5. Which of the following is the **primary** cause of death and disability in children over the age of 1 year?
   (1) Cancer
   (2) Injuries
   (3) Acquired immunodeficiency syndrome (AIDS)
   (4) Anomalies

6. When assisting families in identifying their needs and goals, the nurse assumes which of the following roles?
   (1) Advocate
   (2) Health promoter
   (3) Health teacher
   (4) Counselor

7. The sequence of events that leads parents to seek health care for their child is called which of the following?
   (1) Chief complaint
   (2) Present illness (health)
   (3) Past history
   (4) Review of systems

8. When examining a 2-year-old, which of the following should the nurse do **first**?
   (1) Chest auscultation
   (2) Abdominal palpation
   (3) Otoscopic examination
   (4) Oral examination

9. When assessing family structure, which of the following would be inappropriate?
   (1) Composition of family and community environment
   (2) Occupation and education of family members
   (3) Cultural and religious background
   (4) Intrafamily communication patterns

10. When interviewing a 4-year-old, the nurse should do which of the following?
   (1) Ask detailed questions.
   (2) Maintain confidentiality.
   (3) Disallow the use of equipment.
   (4) Avoid words with double meaning.

ANSWER KEY

1. The answer is (2). Because the disorder is an autosomal dominant genetic disorder, children of a heterozygous parent have a 50% chance of possessing the defective gene. Children of two heterozygous parents have a 25% of being affected in autosomal recessive disorders. In X-linked dominant disorders, daughters of an affected father will probably be affected; sons will not. Half the daughters and half the sons of affected mothers will be affected. In X-linked recessive inheritance, males are usually affected.

2. The answer is (2). When dealing with a client from a different culture, nurses should first be aware of their own values and beliefs. This awareness is important to planning and developing a plan of care. Once this awareness is gained, additional actions include being sensitive to the family beliefs and values and never imposing the nurse's own values on clients. Nurses must modify health care to meet the client's beliefs.

3. The answer is (4). Socioeconomic status, but especially low socioeconomic status, has the most overwhelmingly adverse influence on health. Although culture and religious and environmental influences may impact a child's health, low socioeconomic status exerts the most adverse influence on health.

4. The answer is (1). Cephalocaudal development occurs along the body's long axis, in which control over the head precedes control over the upper body, torso, and legs. Proximodistal development progresses from the center of the body to the extremities. The child develops arm movement before fine finger ability. Mass to specific development occurs as the child learns to perform general, more simplified tasks before specific complex ones.

5. The answer is (2). Injuries cause more death and disability in this age group than all of the other combined causes. Cancer is a leading cause of disability, but it is not the leading cause of death in children over 1 year of age. The incidence of AIDS in children over 1 year of age is increasing and is becoming a leading cause of death. Congenital anomalies are the leading cause of death in children under 1 year of age.

6. The answer is (1). When assisting with identifying needs and goals, the nurse assumes the role of the advocate. In the role of health promoter, the nurse fosters health practices that facilitate positive growth and development. The health teacher provides information on topics such as anticipatory guidance, parenting, and disease processes. The counselor supports the family through active listening and the development of a therapeutic relationship.

7. The answer is (2). The sequence of the present illness (or present health) leads to the chief complaint. Components include symptom analysis of the chief complaint, other current or recurrent illnesses or problems, current medications, and any other health concerns. The chief complaint is the actual reason for seeking health care. The past history involves information regarding past health status, previous problems, and health promotion activities. The review of systems leads to identifying specific problems in each of the body systems.

8. The answer is (1). Chest auscultation is the least intrusive choice here, and the nurse should always proceed from least to most intrusive when examining a toddler. Abdominal palpation is somewhat intrusive and should be performed after chest auscultation. The otoscopic and oral examinations are very intrusive and should not be performed until the end of the examination.

9. The answer is (4). Evaluation of communication patterns among family members is part of the assessment of family function. Composition of family and community environment, occupation and education of family members, and cultural and religious background are components of family structure assessment.

10. The answer is (4). Preschoolers are prelogical and understand only one meaning of a word. Words with more than one meaning will create confusion and possible apprehension. The prelogical thought patterns are too immature to allow preschoolers to understand detailed questions. Although important, confidentiality is a more relevant concern for older children and adolescents. Nurses should encourage preschoolers to handle equipment. Doing so helps to alleviate fears that are common to the preschooler.

2 Infant Growth and Development (Birth to 1 Year of Age)

 Physical growth and development

A. General parameters

1. The best indicator of good overall health is steadily increasing size, specifically length, weight, and head and chest circumference, with normal fontanelle changes.

   a. **Length**
      (1) Between 0 and 6 months the infant grows 1 inch (2.5 cm) per month to an average size of 25.5 inches (63.8 cm).
      (2) Between 6 and 12 months the infant's birth length increases 50% to an average size at 12 months of 29 inches (72.5 cm).

   b. **Weight**
      (1) Between 0 and 6 months the infant gains 1.5 lb (682 g) per month. Birth weight doubles by 5 months. Average 6-month weight is 16 lb (727 g).
      (2) Between 6 and 12 months the infant gains 0.75 lb (341 g) per month. Birth weight triples by 12 months. Average 12-month weight is 21.5 lb (977 g).

   c. **Head circumference (HC) or occipital frontal circumference (OFC)**
      (1) Between 0 and 6 months HC increases 0.6 inch (1.32 cm) per month to an average size of 17 inches (37.4 cm).
      (2) Between 6 and 12 months HC increases 0.2 inch (0.44 cm) per month to an average size of 18 inches (45 cm). By 12 months, HC increases by one-third and brain weight increases 2.5 times from birth.

   d. **Chest circumference**
      (1) It is normally about 1 inch (2 cm) less than the HC.
      (2) Measure chest circumference at the level of the nipples.

   e. **Fontanelle changes**
      (1) At birth, the diamond-shaped **anterior fontanelle** measures about 2 inches (4–5 cm) at its widest part; it closes at between 12 and 18 months of age.
      (2) At birth, the triangular **posterior fontanelle** measures about 0.5 inch (0.5–1 cm) at its widest part; it closes by 2 months of age.

2. Growth and development are monitored by plotting measurements on a standardized growth chart, specific for boys and girls, from birth to 3 years, and from 3 to 18 years.

3. The infant's most basic task is survival, which includes physical tasks such as breathing, sucking, eating, sleeping, and eliminating.

B. Nutrition

1. **Initial food sources**
   a. **Breast milk** is the most desirable complete food source for the first 6 months. It is nutritionally superior, bacteriologically safe, and least allergic. It also contains anti-infectious factors and immune cells.
   b. **Commercially prepared iron-fortified formula** is an acceptable alternative to breast milk. Formula intake varies per infant, but average intake is 4 oz six times per day at 1 month to 4.2 oz five times per day at 6 months when solid foods are introduced.
   c. **Weaning** from breast or bottle to a cup should be gradual. The infant's desire to imitate (between 8 and 9 months) increases the success of weaning.

2. **Fluid requirements**
   a. Milk (and later strained food) is the primary source of water for infants.
   b. Water requirements average 125 to 150 mL/kg/day from 0 to 6 months, and 120 to 135 mL/kg/day from 6 to 12 months.

3. **Solids are not recommended before 4 to 6 months** largely because of the protrusion or sucking reflexes and the immaturity of the gastrointestinal tract and immune system. Breast milk or formula remains the primary source of nutrition for 6 to 12 months, although solid foods should be added.
   a. Infant rice cereal is usually the infant's initial solid food. It is easy to digest, contains iron, and rarely causes an allergic reaction. The cereal is mixed with breast milk or formula.
   b. Additional foods usually include other cereals, then fruits and vegetables, and finally meats. Foods are introduced one at a time, usually over a period of 3 days, because of the possibility of food allergies.
   c. Finger foods (eg, teething crackers, raw fruit) are introduced at 8 or 9 months.
   d. Honey should be discouraged because it may be a source of infant botulism.

C. Sleep patterns (vary among infants)

1. Most infants sleep when not eating during the first month.
2. Most infants sleep 9 to 11 hours at night between ages 3 and 4 months.
3. Most infants take morning and afternoon naps by 12 months of age.
4. Bedtime rituals should begin in infancy to prepare the infant for sleep and to prevent future sleep problems.

D. Dental health

1. Children 6 months and older who are exclusively breast-fed, receive ready-to-feed formula, or live where the local water is inadequately fluoridated need fluoride supplements. They should receive fluoride supplements 20 minutes before feedings.
2. Primary tooth eruption usually begins by 6 months with the primary mandibular central incisors.
3. Parents should clean the infant's teeth with a damp cloth.
4. Breast and bottle feeding during sleep is discouraged to prevent dental caries that may result from prolonged contact with milk.

E. Elimination

1. Elimination patterns usually develop by the second week of life and are typically associated with the frequency and amount of feedings.
2. Stool color and consistency depend on what the infant eats. For all infants, these qualities change with the introduction of solids (Child and Family Teaching 2-1).
3. Urinary output averages 200 to 300 mL by the end of the first week of life with about 20 voidings per day. The average is 350 to 550 mL/day during infancy.

CHILD AND FAMILY TEACHING 2-1

Stool Color and Consistency

BREAST-FED INFANTS

- Stools are orange-yellow and have a soft, even consistency.
- Stools have a sour but clean odor.
- These babies may have several stools each day in the first 2 months, and up to 4 to 5 per day in later months before solids are introduced.

BOTTLE-FED INFANTS

- Color, consistency, and odor depend on the type of formula used.
  - Infants who receive milk-based formula have yellow to brown, soft or formed stools.
  - Infants who receive soy-based formula have green, soft stools with a distinctive odor
  - Infants who receive protein hydrolysate formula have yellow-green soft to loose stools with some mucus.
- These infants have an average of 2 to 4 stools per day.

II. Motor development

A. Gross motor

1. The newborn can turn the head from side to side from a prone position unless the surface is very soft, which may lead to suffocation.
2. The infant exhibits almost no head lag at about 3 months.
3. The infant rolls from front to back at about 5 months. Rolling may be a bit delayed in some infants due to their sleeping in the supine position to reduce the chance of sudden infant death syndrome (SIDS).
4. The infant sits leaning forward at 7 months.
5. The infant sits unsupported at 8 months.
6. The infant pulls up to stand at 9 months.
7. The infant cruises (ie, walking while holding on to objects such as side of table or crib rails) at 10 months.
8. The infant walks holding someone's hand at about 12 months.

B. Fine motor

1. The infant has a strong grasp at about 1 month.
2. The infant's grasp reflex fades and she can actively hold a rattle at about 3 months.
3. The infant can grasp voluntarily at 5 months.
4. The infant can make a hand-to-hand transfer at about 5 months.
5. The infant can grasp with thumb and finger at 7.5 to 8.5 months.
6. The infant develops a pincer grasp at about 9 to 10 months.
7. The infant attempts to build a two-block tower at about 12 months.

C. Related safety concerns

1. **Accidental injuries** are a major cause of death during infancy; they include the following:
   a. Falling off beds and down stairs
   b. Aspiration of small objects

    c. Poisoning from overdose of medication or ingestion of toxic household substances

    d. Suffocation caused by inadvertently covered nose and mouth, pressure on the throat or chest, prolonged lack of air (possibly in a closed, parked car), or strangulation (from crib rails or household cords)

    e. Burns from hot liquids, foods, scalding bath water, excessive sun exposure, or electrical injury

    f. Motor vehicle accidents, most commonly linked to improper use, or nonuse, of infant car seat

  2. Nursing management includes the following:

    a. Instruct parents to maintain a safe environment by placing breakable or sharp objects, hazardous cords, and harmful substances out of the infant's reach.

    b. Alert parents to age-specific potential injury sources and accident-prevention strategies.

    c. Encourage parents to avoid repetitive negative expressions ("No-no, don't touch") and to stress the positive aspects of the infant's behavior, such as playing with suitable toys.

    d. Teach the parents how to use car seats properly.

    e. Instruct the parents not to leave their child unattended on a bed or other high place, even briefly.

III. Psychosocial development

A. Overview (Erikson)

  1. Erikson terms the crisis of infancy as **"trust versus mistrust."**

  2. The sense of trust the infant develops in the first year forms the foundation for all future psychosocial tasks.

    a. The significant other in the process of building trust is the "caregiving" person, and the quality of the caregiver–child relationship is a crucial factor.

    b. Infants who receive attentive care learn that life is predictable and that their needs will be met promptly, which fosters trust.

    c. Infants whose needs are consistently unmet or who experience significant delays in having them met will develop a sense of uncertainty, leading to mistrust of caregivers and the environment.

B. Fears

  1. Infants exhibit a reflexive startle (Moro) response to loud noises, falls, and sudden movements in the environment (see Table 1-5).

  2. Stranger anxiety typically begins around age 6 months.

  3. A caregiver's cuddling and warmth can ease fears.

  4. An infant commonly seeks comfort from a security object (eg, a blanket or a favorite toy) during times of uncertainty or stress.

C. Socialization

  1. Attachment to significant others begins at birth and is increasingly evident after 6 months.

  2. Signs of socialization progress almost monthly.

    a. The infant displays a social smile at 2 months of age.

    b. The infant recognizes familiar faces at 3 months of age.

    c. The infant enjoys social interactions at 4 months of age.

    d. The infant smiles at mirror image at 5 months of age.

    e. The infant begins to fear strangers at 6 months of age.

f. The infant consistently manifests "stranger anxiety" at 8 months of age.

g. The infant shows emotions such as jealousy and affection at 12 months of age.

D. Play and toys

1. Play is the work of children. For the infant:
   a. Play reflects development and awareness of the environment.
   b. Play is basically solitary (noninteractive).
2. Infants develop sensory and motor skills by manipulating toys and other objects.
   a. Purposes of toys are as follows:
      (1) Stimulate psychological development
      (2) Offer diversion from boredom, pain, and discomfort
      (3) Provide a means of communicating and expressing feelings
      (4) Aid in developing sensorimotor skills
   b. Infant toys should be safe and age appropriate. Safety considerations are that toys should have no sharp parts or edges and no small or detachable parts. Age-appropriate toys suit the infant's short attention span and have such features as bright colors to provide stimulation. Examples of safe, age-appropriate infant toys are as follows:
      (1) Appropriate toys for 1- to 3-month-old infants include mobiles, mirrors, music boxes, stuffed animals without detachable parts, and rattles.
      (2) Appropriate toys for 4- to 6-month-old infants include squeeze toys, busy boxes, and play gyms.
      (3) Appropriate toys for 7- to 9-month-old infants include various cloth-textured toys, splashing bath toys, large blocks, and large balls.
      (4) Appropriate toys for 10- to 12-month-old infants include durable books with large pictures, large building blocks, nesting cups, and push-pull toys

E. Discipline

1. Spoiling an infant is difficult; meeting the infant's needs always takes precedence over promoting discipline (training that molds behavior).
2. An infant has no capacity to delay gratification; patience develops progressively after infancy.
3. Disciplinary actions for an infant may seem fruitless. Nevertheless, setting limits should begin in infancy, because the earlier effective disciplinary measures are started, the easier they are to continue.
   a. Effective disciplinary measures may include negative voice, stern eye contact, and timeout.
   b. Corporal punishment is not recommended.

Psychosexual development

A. Overview (Freud)

1. The **oral stage** of development extends from birth to 18 months.
2. The infant sucks for enjoyment as well as nourishment and also gains gratification by swallowing, chewing, and biting.

B. Manifestations

1. In this stage, the infant meets the world orally by crying, tasting, eating, and early vocalizing.
2. The infant uses biting to get a hold on the environment and to gain a greater sense of control.
3. The infant uses grasping and touching to explore variations in the environment.

Cognitive development

A. Overview (Piaget)

1. During the **sensorimotor stage** (between birth and 18 months), intellect develops and the infant gains knowledge of the environment through the senses. Development progresses from reflexive activity to purposeful acts in five substages:

   a. **Substage 1 (birth to 1 month).** This period is marked by the use of innate and predictable survival reflexes (eg, sucking and grasping).

   b. **Substage 2 (1–4 months).** Primary circular reactions are marked by stereotyped repetition and the infant's focus on his own body as the center of interest (eg, infant discovers own body parts).

   c. **Substage 3 (4–8 months).** Secondary circular reactions are characterized by acquired adaptation and a shifting of attention to objects and the environment (eg, infant searches for objects that fall).

   d. **Substage 4 (8–12 months).** Intentionality and consolidation and coordination of schemes mark coordination of secondary schemes (eg, infant actively searches for hidden object).

   e. **Substage 5 (12–18 months).** Tertiary circular reactions are characterized by interest in novelty, creativity, and discovery of new means through active experimentation. This substage is complete when the child achieves a sense of object permanence (ie, child senses self as separate from others and retains mental image of absent objects or persons).

2. An emerging sense of body image parallels sensorimotor development.

B. Language

1. The infant's first means of communication is crying. Parents usually can differentiate cries (eg, hunger versus fatigue).
2. The infant coos between 1 and 2 months.
3. The infant laughs, babbles, and makes consonant sounds between 3 and 4 months.
4. The infant makes imitative sounds by 6 months.
5. The infant pronounces combined syllables (ma-ma) by 8 months.
6. The infant understands no-no by 9 months.
7. The infant says and understands ma-ma and da-da in correct context by 10 months.
8. The infant says between 4 and 10 words in correct context by 12 months.

VI. Wellness promotion

A. General. Encourage families to follow recommendations for age-appropriate well child care visits, screening, immunizations, and safety (Table 2-1).

B. Nutrition. Discuss breast or bottle feeding, feeding schedules, avoidance of overfeeding, progression to solids, using a cup, and self-feeding at appropriate ages.

C. Sleep

1. Reinforce proper sleep positioning to prevent SIDS.
2. Discuss discontinuing bottle in bed and bottle propping, sleep patterns and rhythm, and night awakenings.

D. Growth and development

1. Promote the importance of sucking.
2. Encourage sensorimotor learning.
3. Foster language skills.
4. Discuss teething.

Table 2-1
Recommendations for Well Child Care—Infants

ASSESSMENT	BIRTH	2 WEEKS	2 MONTHS	4 MONTHS	6 MONTHS	9 MONTHS	12 MONTHS
History and physical exam	X	X	X	X	X	X	
Dentist							X
Screening:							
Development	X	X	X	X	X	X	X
Vision and hearing	By history and exam	By history and exam	By history and exam	By history and exam	By history and exam	By history and exam	By history and exam
Tests:							
Heredity and metabolic screen	X						
Hemoglobin	At risk				X...	...	...X
Lead						X...	...X
Sickle cell	State required	...	X...	...X			
TB test							X
Immunizations	HEP B 1...	...	...X Hep B 2... HIB DTaP Polio	...X HIB DTaP Polio	Hep B 3 HIB(O) DTaP Polio		MMR... VZV...
Counseling and anticipatory guidance	X	X	X	X	X	X	X

X, recommended by leading authorities; O, recommended by some leading authorities; X....X, demonstrates age range; Hep B, hepatitis B; HIB, Hemophilus influenza type B conjugate; DPT, diphtheria, pertussis, tetanus; MMR, measles, mumps, rubella; VZV, varicella zoster virus (chicken pox).

Adapted from: American Academy of Family Physicians, Committee on Public Health and Scientific Affairs. (1993). Age charts and periodic health exams. Kansas City, MO: Authors.

American Academy of Pediatrics, Committee on Practice and Ambulatory Care. (1991). Recommendations for preventive health care. American Academy of Pediatrics News, 7, 19.

Centers for Disease Control and Prevention. (1999). Rotavirus vaccine for the prevention of rotavirus gastroenteritis among children. Morbidity and Mortality Weekly Report, 48 (RR-2), 1–22.

E. Family

1. Foster attachment and bonding.

2. Discuss parental roles and assist the family in developing support systems.

F. Health

1. Discuss spitting-up versus regurgitation versus vomiting, colic, elimination problems, upper respiratory infections, and rashes.

2. Encourage parents to take a course on infant and child cardiopulmonary resuscitation (CPR).

G. Anticipatory guidance. Prepare parents for separation anxiety, use of babysitters, and expectations for toddlerhood.

VII.   Illness and hospitalization

A. Reactions to illness

1. There are no general findings regarding the response of preverbal children to illness or fear of bodily injury.

2. Younger infants respond to pain with generalized body responses including, loud crying and some facial gestures.

3. Older infants respond with generalized body responses and deliberate withdrawal of the stimulated area, loud crying, facial gestures and anger, and physical resistance.

B. Reactions to hospitalization

1. Infants under age 3 months tolerate short-term hospitalization well if provided with a nurturing person who meets their physical needs consistently.

2. Between 4 and 6 months infants begin to recognize mother and father as separate from self (known as "stranger anxiety"); therefore, infants at this age may also experience separation anxiety when hospitalized.

C. Nursing management

1. Provide general interventions.

a. Spend time with parents within the infant's sight so the baby identifies you as a safe person.

 b. **Allow the parents to provide as much of the care as possible.**

c. Follow the infant's home schedule (eg, feeding times and bedtime) as closely as possible.

d. Provide sensorimotor stimulation.

2. Provide physical comfort and safety interventions.

a. Keep the infant warm and dry.

b. Meet hunger needs consistently.

(1) Follow the infant's home schedule as closely as possible.

(2) Encourage breast-feeding, if possible.

(3) Use the type and amount of formula used at home.

(4) Let parents feed the infant when possible and give guidance on feeding position as needed.

(5) Schedule treatments so as not to interfere with feeding.

c. Ensure safety.

(1) Keep crib side rails up.

(2) Provide safe crib toys, bumper pads, and play areas.

3. Provide cognitive interventions
   a. Provide a variety of stimulating toys (eg, mobiles, music boxes, busy boxes, and rattles).
   b. Promote language development (eg, make sounds and talk to the infant).
   c. Encourage learning through sensorimotor experience (eg, allow repetition of acts and a variety of toys and textures for manipulation).

4. Provide psychosocial and emotional interventions.
   a. Maintain a good relationship with parents of children in all age groups, encouraging them to give care, hold the child, play with the child, and room in with the child as appropriate.
   b. Maintain consistent staffing.
   c. Promote a sense of security (eg, handle gently, cuddle, talk, and respond to cues).

STUDY QUESTIONS

1. When assessing the weight of a 5-month-old, which of the following indicates healthy growth?
   (1) Doubling of birth weight
   (2) Tripling of birth weight
   (3) Quadrupling of birth weight
   (4) Stabilizing of birth weight

2. While performing physical assessment of a 12-month-old, the nurse notes that the infant's anterior fontanelle is still slightly open. Which of the following is the nurse's **most** appropriate action?
   (1) Notify the physician immediately because there is a problem.
   (2) Perform an intensive neurologic examination.
   (3) Perform an intensive developmental examination.
   (4) Do nothing because this is a normal finding for the age.

3. When teaching a mother about introducing solid foods to her child, which of the following indicates the earliest age at which this should be done?
   (1) 1 month
   (2) 2 months
   (3) 3 months
   (4) 4 months

4. When assessing a 4-month-old, which of the following sounds would the nurse expect to find as being **most** recently developed?
   (1) Cooing sounds
   (2) Babbling sounds
   (3) Imitated sounds
   (4) Combined syllables

5. The infant of a substance-abusing mother is at risk for developing a sense of which of the following?
   (1) Mistrust
   (2) Shame
   (3) Guilt
   (4) Inferiority

6. Which of the following toys should the nurse recommend for a 5-month-old?
   (1) A big red balloon
   (2) A teddy bear with button eyes
   (3) A push-pull wooden truck
   (4) A colorful busy box

7. The mother of a 2-month-old is concerned that she may be spoiling her baby by picking her up when she cries. Which of the following would be the nurse's **best** response?
   (1) "Let her cry for a while before picking her up, so you don't spoil her."
   (2) "Babies need to be held and cuddled; you won't spoil her this way."
   (3) "Crying at this age means the baby is hungry; give her a bottle."
   (4) "If you leave her alone she will learn how to cry herself to sleep."

8. Which of the following is the **primary** nursing intervention used to help a 1-month-old infant tolerate hospitalization?
   (1) Using consistent caregivers
   (2) Providing sensorimotor stimulation
   (3) Following the home schedule as possible
   (4) Keeping the infant warm and dry

9. Which of the following types of play would the nurse expect to see when assessing a 10-month-old infant?
   (1) Parallel
   (2) Solitary
   (3) Associative
   (4) Cooperative

10. Which of the following signs of socialization would the nurse expect to see when assessing a 5-month-old infant?
    (1) Displaying of a social smile
    (2) Enjoying social interactions
    (3) Smiling at a mirror image
    (4) Exhibiting fear of strangers

ANSWER KEY

1. The answer is (1). By the time an infant is 5 months old, his body weight typically doubles. It triples by the age of 1 year and quadruples by the age of 4 years. Infancy is a period of rapid growth exhibited by rapid weight gain.

2. The answer is (4). The anterior fontanelle typically closes anywhere between 12 and 18 months of age. Thus, assessing the anterior fontanelle as still being slightly open is a normal finding requiring no further action. Because it is a normal finding for this age, notifying the physician or performing additional examinations are inappropriate.

3. The answer is (4). Solid foods are not recommended before age 4 to 6 months because of the sucking reflex and the immaturity of the gastrointestinal tract and immune system. Therefore, the earliest age at which to introduce foods is 4 months. Any time earlier would be inappropriate.

4. The answer is (2). Laughing and babbling sounds appear by age 4 months. The infant coos by 1 to 2 months, produces imitated sounds by 6 months, and utters combined syllables by 8 months.

5. The answer is (1). According to Erikson, infants need to have their needs met consistently and effectively to develop a sense of trust. An infant whose needs are consistently unmet or who experiences significant delays in having them met, such as in the case of the infant of a substance-abusing mother, will develop a sense of uncertainty, leading to mistrust of caregivers and the environment. Toddlers develop a sense of shame when their autonomy needs are not met consistently. Preschoolers develop a sense of guilt when their sense of initiative is thwarted. Schoolagers develop a sense of inferiority when they do not develop a sense of industry.

6. The answer is (4). A busy box facilitates the fine motor development that occurs between 4 and 6 months. Balloons are contraindicated because small children may aspirate balloons. Because the button eyes of a teddy bear may detach and be aspirated, this toy is unsafe for children younger than 3 years. A 5-month-old is too young to use a push-pull toy.

7. The answer is (2). Infants need to have their security needs met by being held and cuddled. At 2 months of age, they are unable to make the connection between crying and attention. This association does not occur until late infancy or early toddlerhood. Letting the infant cry for a time before picking up the infant or leaving the infant alone to cry herself to sleep interferes with meeting the infant's need for security at this very young age. Infants cry for many reasons. Assuming that the child is hungry may cause overfeeding problems such as obesity.

8. The answer is (1). An infant who is 1 month of age needs consistency in meeting her needs to foster the development of trust. Therefore, using consistent caregivers is the primary method for meeting the infant's security needs at this age. Providing sensorimotor stimulation promotes cognitive growth, but it will not necessarily aid in helping the infant tolerate the hospitalization. Following the home schedule and keeping the child warm and dry help in maintaining security needs, but they are supplementary to using consistent caregivers.

9. The answer is (2). Infants from the age of 1 month to 1 year typically engage in solitary play. That is, the infant's play is noninteractive. Toddlers typically engage in parallel play (playing alongside others, but not with others); preschoolers engage in associative play (playing interactively and cooperatively with others).

10. The answer is (3). A 5-month-old infant would smile at a mirror image. A social smile is evident by 2 months of age; enjoyment with social interactions occurs at 4 months of age; and fear of strangers begins at 6 months of age with stranger anxiety occurring consistently by 8 months of age.

3 Toddler Growth and Development (1–3 Years of Age)

I. Physical growth and development

A. General parameters

1. Size increases in steplike rather than linear patterns, reflecting the growth spurts and lags characteristic of toddlerhood.
   a. **Height**
      (1) The average toddler grows about 3 inches (7.5 cm) per year.
      (2) The average 2-year-old is about 34 inches (86.6 cm) tall. Height at 2 years is about half the expected adult height.
   b. **Weight**
      (1) The average toddler gains from 4 to 6 lb (1.8–2.7 kg) per year.
      (2) The average 2-year-old weighs 27 lb (12.3 kg).
      (3) Birth weight quadruples by 2.5 years.
   c. **Head circumference (HC)**
      (1) From 1 to 2 years, HC equals chest circumference.
      (2) The total increase in HC in the second year is 1 inch (2.5 cm), then the rate of increase slows to 0.5 inch per year until 5 years.
2. A toddler's characteristic protruding abdomen results from underdeveloped abdominal muscles.
3. Bowleggedness typically persists through toddlerhood because the leg muscles must bear the weight of the relatively large trunk.

B. Nutrition

1. **Nutritional requirements**
   a. Growth rate slows dramatically, thereby decreasing the child's need for calories, protein, and fluid.
   b. Calorie requirements are 102 kcal/kg/d.
   c. Protein requirements are 1.2 g/kg/d.
   d. Milk should be limited to no more than 1 qt (about 1 liter) daily to help ensure intake of iron-enriched foods. Hematocrit should be used to screen for anemia.
   e. Toddlers on vegetarian diets may not receive sufficient plant proteins. They should be referred to a nutritionist.
2. **Food preferences and patterns**
   a. By 12 months, most toddlers eat the same foods as the rest of the family.
   b. At 18 months, many toddlers experience physiologic anorexia and become picky eaters, experiencing food jags (wanting a specific food item, such as peanut butter and jelly sandwiches for a period of days), and eating large amounts one day and very little the next.

    c. Toddlers prefer to feed themselves and prefer small portions of appetizing foods.

    d. Toddlers prefer single foods instead of mixtures of foods. A variety of foods should be offered, but the same foods should be repeated often enough to allow the toddler to recognize them.

    e. Parents should encourage the use of utensils but be aware that toddlers prefer to use fingers.

  3. Child and family teaching

    a. Frequent nutritious snacks can replace a meal; however, instruct parents not to offer snacks within an hour of meals to avoid decreasing toddlers' appetites.

    b. Toddlers are at risk for aspirating small food items such as peanuts. They can also choke on raw carrots, celery, and hot dogs.

    c. Remind parents not to use food as a reward or a punishment.

C. Sleep patterns

  1. Total sleep requirements decrease during the second year to an average of about 12 hours daily.

  2. Most toddlers nap once a day until the end of the second or third year.

  3. Sleep problems are common and may result from fears of separation.

  4. Bedtime rituals and transitional objects that represent security, such as blankets or stuffed toys, are helpful.

D. Dental health

  1. Primary dentition (20 deciduous teeth) is completed by 2.5 years.

  2. The first dental visit should occur before the toddler is 2.5 years old.

  3. Parents should clean the toddler's teeth with a soft toothbrush and water, and then floss the teeth. They should not use toothpaste because toddlers dislike its foaminess. Fluoridated toothpaste is dangerous if swallowed.

  4. Toddlers require fluoride supplementation if the water in their area is not fluoridated.

  5. Diet should be low in cariogenic foods, such as table sugar, which promote dental caries.

E. Elimination

  1. Stool appearance changes with additions to diet. Highly colored foods (eg, gelatin, beets, colored drinks, and blueberries) may color stool.

  2. Average urinary output during childhood is 500 to 1000 mL/day.

II. Motor development

A. Gross motor. The major gross motor skill of toddlerhood is locomotion.

  1. The toddler walks without help at 15 months.

  2. The toddler walks upstairs with one hand held at 18 months.

  3. The toddler walks up and down stairs one step at a time at 24 months.

  4. The toddler jumps with both feet at 30 months.

B. Fine motor

  1. The toddler builds a two-block tower and scribbles spontaneously at 15 months.

  2. The toddler builds a three- to four-block tower at 18 months.

  3. The toddler imitates vertical stroke at 24 months.

  4. The toddler builds an eight-block tower and copies a cross at 30 months.

C. Related safety concerns

  1. Toddlers are prone to the same injuries as infants are, including falls, aspiration, poisoning, suffocation, burns, and motor vehicle and other accidental injuries.

2. Nursing management includes the following:

    a. **Falls**. Instruct parents to keep crib rails up, place gates across stairways, secure screens on all open windows, and supervise the toddler at play.

    b. **Aspiration and poisoning**

        (1) Urge parents to lock all toxic substances away from the child's reach (child can now climb and open), secure safety caps on medications, and remove all small, easily aspirated objects from the child's environment.

        (2) Instruct parents to keep the telephone number of the poison control center by the telephone at all times.

    c. **Suffocation**

        (1) Encourage parents to teach the toddler water safety to help prevent accidental drowning in bathtubs and pools.

        (2) Instruct families to avoid storing plastic bags and balloons within the toddler's reach.

    d. **Burns**. Advise parents to avoid using tablecloths (a curious toddler may pull the cloth to see what is on the table, possibly spilling hot foods or liquids on himself). It also is important to teach the toddler what "hot" means, to store matches and lighters in locked cabinets out of reach, and to secure safety plugs in all unused electrical outlets.

    e. **Motor vehicle and other accidents**

        (1) Instruct parents to continue properly using an appropriate-sized car seat at all times.

        (2) Advise parents to lock cabinets and drawers that contain hazardous items, such as knives, firearms, and ammunition.

        (3) Encourage parents to teach the toddler how to cross a street safely, by holding parents' hand, and to not play in the street.

        (4) Urge parents to supervise tricycle riding and outdoor play.

III. Psychosocial development

A. Overview (Erikson)

    1. Erikson terms the psychosocial crisis the child faces between ages 1 and 3 as **"autonomy versus shame and doubt."**

        a. The psychosocial theme is to "hold on; to let go."

        b. The toddler has developed a sense of trust and is ready to give up dependence to assert her budding sense of control and autonomy. Parents who encourage the toddler to do so promote the toddler's independence.

        c. The toddler can develop a sense of shame and doubt if parents keep her dependent in areas where the toddler can use newly acquired skills or make the toddler feel inadequate when attempting these skills.

    2. The toddler begins to master social skills.

        a. Individuation (differentiation of self from others)

        b. Separation from parent(s)

        c. Control over bodily functions

        d. Communication with words

        e. Socially acceptable behavior

            (1) The toddler begins to learn that his own behavior has a predictable, reliable effect on others.

            (2) The toddler learns to wait longer to gratify needs.

    f. Egocentric interactions with others. (The toddler may not master some interactive skills until adolescence when she revisits uncomplicated tasks associated with early periods of development. Erikson refers to this as the "psychosocial moratorium.")

3. The toddler often uses "no" even when she means "yes," to assert independence (negativistic behavior).

4. A toddler often continues to seek a familiar security object, such as a blanket, during times of uncertainty and stress.

B. Fears

1. Common fears of toddlers include the following:
    a. Loss of parents (known as separation anxiety)
    b. Stranger anxiety
    c. Loud noises (eg, vacuum cleaner)
    d. Going to sleep
    e. Large animals

2. Emotional support, comfort, and simple explanations may allay a toddler's fears.

C. Socialization

1. Ritualism, negativism, and independence dominate the toddler's interactions.

2. Separation anxiety peaks as toddlers differentiate themselves from significant others. Transitional objects are important, especially during periods of separation, such as a nap.

3. Toddlers may use tantrums to assert independence. Caregivers can best deal with them by "extinction" (ignoring them).

4. Negativism is also common. The best way to decrease the number of "no's" is to decrease the number of questions that can lead to a "no" response.

D. Play and toys

1. Toddlers engage in parallel play, which is play alongside, not with, others. Imitation is one of the most common forms of play.

2. A short attention span causes toddlers to change toys frequently.
    a. Purposes of toys in toddlerhood are to enhance locomotion skills (push-pull toys) and to encourage imitation, language development, and gross and fine motor skills.
    b. Toys should be safe (still no detachable or small parts). Examples of safe, age-appropriate toys are as follows:
        (1) Dolls and housekeeping toys
        (2) Play phones and cloth books
        (3) Appropriate rocking horses and "riding" trucks, finger paints, play clay, large-piece wooden or plastic puzzles, and large blocks

E. Discipline

1. Unrestricted freedom is a threat to a toddler's security despite limit testing.

2. Discipline measures should be:
    a. Consistent
    b. Initiated after misbehavior
    c. Planned in advance
    d. Oriented to behavior, not the child
    e. Private and not shame-inducing

3. Timeouts are effective discipline measures.
    a. Parents should carry them out in a safe, nonstimulating area.
    b. Duration should be 1 minute per year of age. Parents can use an audible timer to monitor duration.

Psychosexual development

A. **Overview (Freud)**

  1. The **anal stage** of development extends from age 8 months to 4 years.

  2. The erogenous zone consists of the anus and buttocks, and sexual activity centers on the expulsion and retention of body waste.

    a. The child's focus shifts from the oral to the anal area, with emphasis on bowel control as she gains neuromuscular control over the anal sphincter.

    b. The toddler experiences both satisfaction and frustration as she gains control over withholding and expelling, containing and releasing.

    c. The conflict between "holding on" and "letting go" gradually resolves as bowel training progresses; resolution occurs once control is firmly established.

B. **Manifestations**

  1. Sexuality begins to develop.

    a. Masturbation can result from body exploration.

    b. Learned words may be associated with anatomy and elimination.

    c. Sex differences become evident.

  2. Toilet training is a major task of toddlerhood.

    a. Readiness is unusual before 18 (up to 24) months (Child and Family Teaching 3-1).

    b. Bowel training is accomplished before bladder; complete night bladder training usually does not occur until age 4 or 5.

    c. The training "potty" should offer security; the toddler's feet should reach the floor (needed for defecation).

 Cognitive development

A. **Overview (Piaget)**

  1. Sensorimotor stage. This stage, which lasts between ages 12 and 24 months, involves two substages.

    a. **Substage 1 (12–18 months)**. Tertiary circular reactions involve trial-and-error experimentation and relentless exploration. (This stage overlaps with substage 5 in infancy.)

CHILD AND FAMILY TEACHING 3-1

Signs of the Toddler's Readiness for Toilet Training

The toddler:
- Stays dry for 2 hours, with regular bowel movements
- Can sit, walk, and squat
- Can verbalize the desire to void or defecate
- Exhibits a willingness to please parents
- Wants to have soiled diapers changed immediately

Note: Toilet training should not be initiated during times of stress, such as a new baby, a move, a divorce, or a vacation.

    b. **Substage 2 (18–24 months)**. Mental combinations appear allowing the toddler to devise new means for accomplishing tasks.

  2. Preconceptual substage of the preoperational phase. In this stage, which extends between age 2 and age 4, the child uses representational thought to recall the past, represent the present, and anticipate the future. During this phase, the child:

    a. Forms concepts that are not as complete or as logical as adult concepts

    b. Makes simple classifications

    c. Associates one event with a simultaneous event (transductive reasoning)

    d. Exhibits egocentric thinking

B. Language

  1. The toddler uses expressive jargon (ie, toddler's own "words" for expression) at 15 months.

  2. The toddler says about 300 words, uses two- to three-word phrases, and uses pronouns at 2 years.

  3. The toddler gives first and last name and uses plurals at 2.5 years.

Moral development

A. Overview (Kohlberg)

  1. A toddler is typically at the first substage of the **preconventional stage**, which is oriented toward punishment and obedience. The toddler bases judgments on avoiding punishment or obtaining a reward.

  2. Discipline patterns affect a toddler's moral development.

    a. Physical punishment and withholding privileges tend to give the toddler a negative view of morals.

    b. Withholding love and affection as a form of punishment leads to feelings of guilt.

B. Appropriate discipline measures include providing simple explanations why certain behaviors are unacceptable, praising appropriate behavior, and using distraction to avoid unacceptable behaviors.

VII.   Wellness promotion

A. General. Encourage families to follow recommendations for well child care visits, screening, immunizations, and safety (Table 3-1).

B. Nutrition. Discuss appetite changes, food preferences, and appropriate portions, as well as food ritual behavior. Food rituals can include separating food types on the dish or cutting food in a specific manner.

C. Sleep. Discuss bedtime rituals, the need for transitional objects, and consistency.

D. Growth and development

  1. Discuss negativity and tantrums, and teach parents effective ways to manage them.

  2. Teach toilet training techniques and positive discipline.

  3. Encourage gross motor skills.

E. Family

  1. Foster learning social skills.

  2. Discuss sibling rivalry.

  3. Encourage parents to set example for child.

TABLE 3-1
Recommendations for Well Child Care—Toddlers

ASSESSMENT	15 MONTHS	18 MONTHS	24 MONTHS
History and physical exam	X	X	X
Dentist			X
Screening:			
Development	X	X	X
Vision	By history and	By history and	By history and
Hearing	physical exam	physical exam	physical exam
Tests:			
Hemoglobin	X...	...	...X
Lead			X
Immunizations	...Hep B	...Hep B	
	...HIB	...DTaP	
	DTaP...	...VZV	
	...MMR		
	...VZV		
Counseling and anticipatory guidance	X	X	X

X, recommended by leading authorities; O, recommended by some leading authorities; X... ...X, demonstrates age range; Hep B, hepatitis B; HIB, Hemophilus influenza type B conjugate; DPT, diphtheria, pertussis, tetanus; MMR, measles, mumps, rubella; VZV, varicella zoster virus (chicken pox).

Adapted from: American Academy of Family Physicians, Committee on Public Health and Scientific Affairs (1993). Age charts and periodic health exams. Kansas City, MO: Author.

American Academy of Pediatrics, Committee on Practice and Ambulatory Care. (1991). Recommendations for preventive health care. American Academy of Pediatrics News, 7, 19.

F. Health
   1. Stress importance of dental care.
   2. Teach basic first aid or encourage the parents to take a basic course in the subject.

G. Anticipatory guidance
   1. Discuss the establishment of a family routine.
   2. Inform the parents that parental interest will guide the child through upcoming "magic years" of preschool (3–6 years).

 VIII. Illness and hospitalization

A. Reactions to illness
   1. The concept of body image, especially body boundaries, is poorly defined in toddlers. Therefore, intrusive procedures are extremely anxiety-producing.
   2. Toddlers react to pain similarly to infants, and previous experiences may affect toddlers as well. They may also get upset if they only perceive that they will experience pain.

B. Reactions to hospitalization
   1. In response to stressful events, such as hospitalization, the toddler's primary defense mechanism is regression.

2. The toddler may also sense a loss of control related to physical restriction, a loss of routine and rituals, dependency, and fear of bodily injury or pain.

3. Separation affects most toddlers, who view it as abandonment (18 months is the peak age for separation anxiety). Hospitalization may promote separation anxiety, which has three distinct phases:

    a. **Protest**. The toddler verbally cries for parents, verbally or physically attacks others, attempts to find parents, clings to parents, and is inconsolable.

    b. **Despair**. The toddler is disinterested in the environment and play and shows passivity, depression, and loss of appetite.

    c. **Detachment (denial)**. The toddler makes a superficial adjustment and shows apparent interest, but remains detached. This phase usually occurs after prolonged separation and is rarely seen in hospitalized children.

C. Nursing management

  1. Provide general interventions.

    a. Allow protest and rooming in.

    b. Encourage the use of transitional or parental objects (things the child associates with the parents) that can be left with the child.

    c. Instruct the parents never to sneak out of the room or away from the hospital while the child is asleep.

    d. Be honest about the time of the parents' return.

    e. Find out and use the words that the child uses (for transitional object, toileting, and so forth).

    f. Continue home routines as much as possible.

  2. Provide physical comfort and safety interventions.

    a. Explore the toddler's already developed muscle skills (assess prehospital abilities), then give manipulable toys; provide supervised activities; use playroom.

    b. After assessing the child's level of function, promote self-care (in all age groups), for example self-feeding, toileting as at home, dressing (with assistance as needed), and hygiene (washing face and hands, brushing teeth).

  3. Provide cognitive interventions.

    a. Promote sensorimotor learning through imitation.

    b. Enhance language skills (assess vocabulary, avoid speaking for child, reinforce mastered words, use activities that use language).

    c. Provide simple explanation for procedures (use equipment).

  4. Provide psychosocial and emotional interventions.

    a. Promote the toddler's sense of autonomy by encouraging self-care, participation in bedtime rituals, and some control (eg, give the toddler "okay" choices).

    b. Support the toddler as he learns to separate from parents (assist family with coping with separation, encourage visiting, use primary nurse, and encourage pictures of parents).

    c. Promote social adaptation (reinforce socially acceptable behaviors, encourage parallel play).

    d. Maintain usual routines and rituals (assess usual routines, especially bedtime; identify preferences; maintain as many of the home rituals as possible).

STUDY QUESTIONS

1. When assessing an 18-month-old, the nurse notes a characteristic protruding abdomen. Which of the following would explain the rationale for this finding?
   (1) Increased food intake owing to age
   (2) Underdeveloped abdominal muscles
   (3) Bowlegged posture
   (4) Linear growth curve

2. If parents keep a toddler dependent in areas where he is capable of using skills, the toddler will develop a sense of which of the following?
   (1) Mistrust
   (2) Shame
   (3) Guilt
   (4) Inferiority

3. Which of the following fears would the nurse typically associate with toddlerhood?
   (1) Mutilation
   (2) The dark
   (3) Ghosts
   (4) Going to sleep

4. A 2-year-old's mother has just left the hospital to check on her other children. Which of the following would best help the 2-year-old who is now crying inconsolably?
   (1) Taking a nap
   (2) Peer play group
   (3) Large cuddly dog
   (4) Favorite blanket

5. Which of the following is an appropriate toy for an 18-month-old?
   (1) Multiple-piece puzzle
   (2) Miniature cars
   (3) Finger paints
   (4) Comic book

6. When responding to a mother who is concerned that her 1-year-old is not yet walking, the nurse's response would be based on the knowledge that the age when most children should be able to walk is which of the following?

   (1) 12 months
   (2) 15 months
   (3) 18 months
   (4) 24 months

7. When teaching parents about the child's readiness for toilet training, which of the following signs should the nurse instruct them to watch for in the toddler?
   (1) Demonstrates dryness for 4 hours
   (2) Demonstrates ability to sit and walk
   (3) Has a new sibling for stimulation
   (4) Verbalizes desire to go to the bathroom

8. The mother of a 20-month-old boy asks the nurse why her son has temper tantrums. Which of the following would be the nurse's best response?
   (1) "It is the only way he can get attention from his mother."
   (2) "He is probably spoiled and needs discipline."
   (3) "He cannot express his feelings or frustrations verbally."
   (4) "He is expressing his need for identity."

9. A 30-month-old girl always puts her teddy bear on the left side of her bed immediately after her mother reads a bedtime story. Which of the following describes the purpose of this repeated behavior?
   (1) Manipulation of the adults in the child's environment
   (2) Establishment of learning behaviors
   (3) Provision of a sense of security
   (4) Establishment of a sense of identity

10. When teaching parents about typical toddler eating patterns, which of the following should be included?
    (1) Food "jags"
    (2) Preference to eat alone
    (3) Consistent table manners
    (4) Increase in appetite

ANSWER KEY

1. The answer is (2). Underdeveloped abdominal musculature gives the toddler a characteristically protruding abdomen. During toddlerhood, food intake decreases, not increases. Toddlers are characteristically bowlegged because the leg muscles must bear the weight of the relatively large trunk. Toddler growth patterns occur in a steplike, not linear pattern.

2. The answer is (2). According to Erikson, toddlers experience a sense of shame when they are not allowed to develop appropriate independence and autonomy. Infants develop mistrust when their needs are not consistently gratified. Preschoolers develop guilt when their initiative needs are not met while schoolagers develop a sense of inferiority when their industry needs are not met.

3. The answer is (4). During toddlerhood, typical fears include going to sleep, loss of parents, stranger anxiety, loud noises, and large animals. Fear of mutilation, the dark, and ghosts are fears commonly associated with preschoolers.

4. The answer is (4). The mother's departure has triggered the protest stage of separation anxiety in this child. Therefore, a favorite blanket or other transitional object (representation of parent) will help best ease separation fears. A nap may actually increase separation fears. A 2-year-old is too young to interact with peers, other than in parallel play. Toddlers are usually fearful of large dogs.

5. The answer is (3). Young toddlers are still sensorimotor learners and they enjoy the experience of feeling different textures. Thus, finger paints would be an appropriate toy choice. Multiple-piece toys, such as puzzles, are too difficult to manipulate and may be hazardous if the pieces are small enough to be aspirated. Miniature cars also have a high potential for aspiration. Comic books are on too high a level for toddlers. Although they may enjoy looking at some of the pictures, toddlers are more likely to rip a comic book apart.

6. The answer is (2). Normal neuromuscular development should allow most children to walk without help by the age of 15 months. Many children walk by age 1 year, but a child is not considered abnormal if she is not walking by this age. By 18 months, the child is usually able to walk upstairs with one hand held; by 24 months, the child walks up and down stairs one step at a time.

7. The answer is (4). The child must be able to state the need to go to the bathroom to initiate toilet training. Usually, a child needs to be dry for only 2 hours, not 4 hours. The child also must be able to sit, walk, and squat. A new sibling would most likely hinder toilet training.

8. The answer is (3). Temper tantrums are a means for the toddler to exert independence because the child is unable to express his feelings or frustrations verbally. Temper tantrums usually decrease when a child learns words to express himself. Stating that tantrums are the only way to get attention is inappropriate because toddlers use many methods to get their parents' attention. Telling a parent that the child is spoiled is an inappropriate response. Identity is not an issue for toddlers; separation and individuation are.

9. The answer is (3). The child is demonstrating ritualistic behavior. For toddlers, rituals provide a sense of security so that they may achieve autonomy. A toddler's cognitive development is not at a level that would allow her to manipulate the environment. No evidence exists that rituals support learning. Independence, not identity, is the issue for toddlers.

10. The answer is (1). Toddlers become picky eaters, experiencing food jags and eating large amounts one day and very little the next. A toddler's food jags express a preference for the ritualism of eating one type of food for several days at a time. Toddlers typically enjoy socialization and imitating others at meal time. Toddlers prefer to feed themselves and thus are too young to have table manners. A toddler's appetite and need for calories, protein, and fluid decrease due to the dramatic slowing of growth rate.

4 Preschool Growth and Development (3–6 Years of Age)

Physical growth and development

A. General parameters. A healthy preschooler is slender, graceful, and agile and has good posture.

1. **Height**
   a. Average growth is 2.5 to 3 inches (6.25–7.5 cm) per year.
   b. The average 4-year-old is 40.5 inches (101.25 cm).
2. **Weight**
   a. Average weight gain is 5 lb (2.3 kg) per year.
   b. The average 4-year-old weighs 37 lb (16.8 kg).

B. Nutrition

1. **Nutritional requirements**
   a. The preschooler's requirements are similar to those of the toddler, although the calorie requirement decreases to 90 kcal/kg/day.
   b. Protein requirement remains 1.2 g/kg/day.
   c. Fluid requirement is 100 mL/kg/day, depending on the child's activity level.
2. **Food preferences and patterns**
   a. Preschoolers may reject vegetables, mixed dishes, and liver.
   b. Favorite foods include cereals, meat, baked potatoes, fruits, and sweets.
   c. Many 3- and 4-year-olds are still restless or fussy during meals with the family, and they may still struggle with utensils.
   d. Food habits of others influence the 5-year-old.
      (1) She tends to focus on "social" aspects of eating, including table conversation, manners, and willingness to try new foods, and help with meal preparation and clean up.
      (2) The older preschooler can manage a spoon and fork.

C. Sleep patterns

1. The average preschooler sleeps 11 to 13 hours a day.
2. Most preschoolers need an afternoon nap until age 5 when most begin kindergarten. The daytime nap may be eliminated if it seems to interfere with nighttime sleep. If the child still needs a nap, 30 to 60 minutes is all that is necessary.
3. Reassuring bedtime rituals and relaxation before bedtime should help the child settle down. Rituals may take 30 minutes or longer.
4. Sleep problems are common and include the following:
   a. Nightmares
   b. Night terrors
   c. Difficulty settling down after a busy day

d. Extending bedtime rituals to delay sleep

e. Nighttime awakening

5. For many preschoolers, a security object and a nightlight continue to provide help with sleep.

D. Dental health

1. All 20 deciduous teeth should be in by age 3.

2. The preschooler's fine motor development enables him to use a toothbrush properly; the child should brush twice a day.

3. Parents should supervise the child's brushing and should perform flossing.

4. The child should avoid cariogenic foods to help prevent dental caries.

E. Elimination

1. Most children are capable of independent toilet training by the end of the preschool period. Some may still have "accidents." Most forget to wash their hands and to flush.

2. Children void an average of 500 to 1000 mL/day.

II.   Motor development

A. Gross motor. Gross motor skills improve. The preschooler can hop, skip, and run more smoothly. She can develop athletic abilities, such as skating and swimming.

1. A preschooler can ride a tricycle, go upstairs using alternate feet, stand on one foot for a few seconds, and broad jump at age 3.

2. The child can skip, hop on one foot, catch a ball, and go downstairs using alternate feet at age 4.

3. The child can skip on alternate feet, throw and catch a ball, jump rope, and balance on alternate feet with eyes closed at age 5.

B. Fine motor. Fine motor skills show major development as demonstrated by an improved ability to draw.

1. The child can build a 9- or 10-block tower, construct a 3-block bridge, copy a circle, and draw a cross at age 3.

2. The child can lace shoes, copy a square, trace a diamond, and add three parts to a stick figure at age 4.

3. The child can tie shoelaces, use scissors well, copy a diamond and a triangle, add seven to nine parts to a stick figure, and print a few letters and numbers and her first name at age 5.

C. Related safety concerns

1. Although preschoolers are somewhat less accident prone than toddlers, they are still at risk for the same type of injuries (eg, falls, aspiration, and burns) and require many of the same safety precautions.

2. Parents and other adults should emphasize safety measures; preschoolers listen to adults and can understand and heed precautions.

3. Because preschoolers are keen observers and imitate others, adults need to "practice what they preach" regarding safety.

4. When a child weighs 40 lb and is 40 inches tall, he can use a safety belt instead of a car seat.

III. ## Psychosocial development

A. Overview (Erikson)

1. Erikson terms the crisis that children face between ages 3 and 6 as **"initiative versus guilt."**
   a. The preschooler's significant other is the family.
   b. The child has normally mastered a sense of autonomy. With parental encouragement of imagination and activity, the child moves on to master a sense of initiative.
   c. The child develops a sense of guilt when parents make the child feel that his imagination and activities are unacceptable. Anxiety and fear result when the child's thoughts and activities clash with parental expectations.
2. A preschooler is an energetic, enthusiastic, and intrusive learner with an active imagination. The child explores the physical world with all of his senses and powers.
3. Conscience (an inner voice that warns and threatens) begins to develop.
4. A preschooler begins to use simple reasoning and can tolerate longer periods of delayed gratification.

B. Fears

1. A child commonly experiences more fears during the preschool period than at any other time.
2. Common fears include the following:
   a. The dark
   b. Being left alone, especially at bedtime
   c. Animals, particularly large dogs
   d. Ghosts
   e. Body mutilation, pain, and objects and people associated with painful experiences
3. The preschooler is prone to induced fears that stem from parental remarks and actions. Parents are typically unaware that their behavior or words instill fear in the child.
4. Allowing preschoolers to have a nightlight and encouraging them to play out fears with dolls or other toys may help them develop a sense of control over the fear.
5. Exposing the child to a feared object in a controlled setting may provide an opportunity for desensitization and reduction of fear.

C. Socialization

1. The preschooler's radius of significant others expands beyond the parents to include grandparents, siblings, and preschool teachers.
2. The child needs regular interaction with peers to help develop social skills.
3. The primary purpose of preschool programs is to foster the child's social skills (Child and Family Teaching 4-1).

D. Play and toys

1. Typical preschoolers' play is associative (interactive and cooperative).
2. Preschoolers need contact with age mates.
3. Activities should promote growth and motor skills, such as jumping, running, and climbing. Parents can encourage toys and games that promote gross and fine motor development, including:
   a. Tricycle, big wheels, gym sets, wading pools, and sandboxes to enhance gross motor skills
   b. Large blocks, puzzles, crayons, paints, simple crafts, and age-appropriate electronic games to enhance fine motor skills
   c. Dress-up clothes and dolls, housekeeping toys, play tents, puppets, and doctor and nurse kits to enhance imitative play and imagination

CHILD AND FAMILY TEACHING 4-1

Selecting a Preschool Program

Criteria for parents to consider when selecting a preschool program include the following:
- Accreditation, licensing, and standards followed
- Daily schedule of activities and materials available
- Teacher's qualifications
- Environment, including safety, noise level, teacher/child ratio, and sanitary practices
- Recommendations of other parents
- Observations of the children at play and work and their interactions with the teachers
- Alternative plans offered when the child is ill and the parents work

4. Imitative, imaginative, and dramatic play is important. Preschool is the typical stage for imaginary playmates.

5. TV and video games should be only a part of the child's play and parents should monitor content and amount of time spent in use.

6. Curious and active preschoolers need adult supervision, especially near water, gym sets, and other potential hazards.

E. Discipline

1. Authority figures must apply discipline fairly, firmly, and consistently.

2. The child needs simple explanations of why certain behaviors are inappropriate.

3. In a situation involving conflict, a short timeout can help the child relieve intense feelings, regain control, and think about his behavior.

IV. Psychosexual development

A. Overview (Freud)

1. The **phallic stage** extends from about 3 to 5 years of age.

2. The child's pleasure centers on the genitalia and masturbation.

3. The child experiences what Freud termed the **Oedipal conflict**.

    a. This phase is marked by jealousy and rivalry toward the same-sex parent and love of the opposite-sex parent.

    b. The Oedipal stage typically resolves in the late preschool period with a strong identification with the same-sex parent.

B. Sexual development

1. Many preschoolers masturbate for physiologic pleasure.

2. Preschoolers form strong attachments to parents of the opposite sex but identify with the parent of the same sex.

3. As sexual identity develops, modesty may become a concern, as may castration fears.

4. Because preschoolers are keen observers but poor interpreters, they may recognize but not understand sexual activity.

    a. Before answering a child's questions about sex, adults should clarify what the child is really asking and what she already thinks about the specific subject.

    b. Adults should answer questions about sex simply and honestly, providing only the information that the child requests; additional details can come later.

Cognitive development

A. Overview (Piaget)

1. The **preoperational thought stage** of cognitive development, from ages 2 to 7 years, has two phases—preconceptual and intuitive.
   a. **Preconceptual phase (ages 2–4)**
      (1) The child forms concepts that are less complete and logical than adult concepts.
      (2) The child makes simple classifications.
      (3) The child associates one event with a simultaneous one (transductive reasoning).
      (4) The child exhibits egocentric thinking.
   b. **Intuitive phase (ages 4–7)**
      (1) The child becomes capable of classifying, quantifying, and relating objects but remains unaware of the principles behind these operations.
      (2) The child exhibits intuitive thought processes (she is aware that something is right but cannot say why).
      (3) The child is unable to see the viewpoint of others.
      (4) The child uses many words appropriately but lacks real knowledge of their meaning.

2. Preschoolers exhibit magical thinking and believe that their thoughts are all-powerful. They may feel guilty and responsible for "bad" thoughts, which sometimes coincide with a wished-for event (eg, wishing a sibling was dead and the sibling coincidentally becomes ill and is hospitalized).

B. Language

1. The average 3-year-old says 900 words, speaks three- to four-word sentences, and talks incessantly.
2. The average 4-year-old says 1500 words, tells exaggerated stories, and sings simple songs. Age 4 is the peak age for "why" questions.
3. The average 5-year-old says 2100 words, knows four or more colors, and can name the days of the week and the months.

 Moral development

A. Overview (Kohlberg). A preschooler is in the **preconventional stage** of moral development, which extends to age 10. In this phase, conscience emerges, and the emphasis is on external control.

B. Standards. The child's moral standards are those of others, and he observes them either to avoid punishment or to reap rewards.

 Wellness promotion

A. General. Encourage families to follow recommendations for well child care visits, screening (hearing and vision are added at this time), immunizations, and safety (Table 4-1).

B. Nutrition

1. Promote nutritious meals and discourage "grazing," an eating pattern by which the child eats small amounts of foods (usually nonnutritious foods) throughout the day instead of three meals.
2. Encourage trying new foods and learning socially acceptable table behavior.

TABLE 4-1
Recommendations for Well Child Care—Preschoolers

ASSESSMENT	3 YEARS	4 YEARS	5 YEARS
History and physical exam	X	X	X
Dentist	X	X	X
Screening:			
Development	X	X	X
Vision	X	X	X
Hearing	X	X	X
Tests:			
Hemoglobin	X...	...	...X
Lead	At risk	At risk	At risk
Cholesterol	At risk	At risk	At risk
Urinalysis		O	X
TB test			X
Immunizations		DTaP...	...DTaP
		Polio...	...Polio
		MMR...	...MMR
Counseling and anticipatory guidance	X	X	X

X, recommended by leading authorities; O, recommended by some leading authorities; X... ...X, demonstrates age range; DPT, diphtheria, pertussis, tetanus; MMR, measles, mumps, rubella.

Adapted from: American Academy of Family Physicians, Committee on Public Health and Scientific Affairs. (1993). Age charts and periodic health exams. Kansas City, MO: Author.

American Academy of Pediatrics, Committee on Practice and Ambulatory Care. (1991). Recommendations for preventive health care. American Academy of Pediatrics News, 7, 19.

C. Sleep

  1. Discus the management of nightmares and night terrors.

  2. Promote rituals and alleviation of fears.

D. Growth and development

  1. Discuss "magical thinking" and the importance of encouraging initiative.

  2. Foster imaginative play.

  3. Promote limited TV watching and foster reading.

  4. Encourage parents to start chores for child.

  5. Discuss sexual curiosity and masturbation.

E. Family. Encourage the family to allow the child to participate in important family rituals.

F. Health. Teach about hygiene (such as proper wiping for girls), communicable diseases, and infection control, especially for children in day care or preschool.

G. Anticipatory guidance. Prepare the family for preschool and kindergarten.

VIII. Illness and hospitalization

Preschoolers differentiate poorly between the self and the external world. They have a limited understanding of language and can see only one aspect of an object or situation at a time.

A. Reactions to illness

1. Preschoolers perceive unrelated concrete phenomena as causes of illness.
2. Magical thinking causes preschoolers to view illness as a punishment. Moreover, preschoolers are experiencing psychosexual conflicts and fears of mutilation, making them especially fearful of procedures such as rectal temperatures and urinary catheterizations.

B. Reactions to hospitalization

1. The primary defense mechanism of preschoolers is regression. They will react to separation by regression and refusal to cooperate.
2. Preschoolers sense a loss of control because they experience a loss of their own power.
3. Fear of bodily injury and pain lead to fear of mutilation and intrusive procedures.
4. Limited knowledge of the body enhances typical fears; for example, castration fears (evoked by enemas, rectal thermometers, and catheters) and fears that damage to the skin (eg, intravenous line and blood work procedures) will cause the insides of their body to leak out.
5. Preschoolers interpret hospitalization as punishment and parental separation as loss of love.

C. Nursing management

1. Provide general interventions.

 a. Use puppets and dolls to demonstrate procedures.
 b. Use terms that are appropriate for the child's age and level of understanding (eg, say "fix" rather than "cut out").
 c. Use adhesive bandages after giving injections.
 d. Stay with the child during procedures.
 e. Avoid performing invasive procedures, if possible.
 f. Give stars, badges, and other rewards.
 g. Play out the hospital experience (eg, improvise doctor and nurse kits).
 h. Reassure the preschooler that he is not responsible for illness.
 i. Assess for secondary gains.

2. Provide physical comfort and safety interventions.

 a. Allow the child to maintain control over body functions.
   (1) Allow normal patterns.
   (2) Reassure the child when accidents occur.
   (3) Praise success.
   (4) Provide motor stimulation.
 b. Promote self-care and allow the child to wear her own clothes.

3. Provide cognitive interventions.

 a. Protect from guilt.
   (1) Tell the child no one is to blame for illness or hospitalization.
   (2) Explain procedures.
 b. Protect from fears.
   (1) Use therapeutic play.
   (2) Do not talk beyond the child's level of understanding.

    c. Promote language.
        (1) Encourage questions.
        (2) Allow the child to tell stories.
        (3) Teach the child new words.

4. Provide psychosocial and emotional interventions.
    a. Encourage independence.
        (1) Permit self-care.
        (2) Allow the child to make some decisions.
        (3) Praise competence.
        (4) Respect suggestions.
    b. Allow the child to experience limits to feel secure.
        (1) Explain safety rules.
        (2) Define limits due to illness.
        (3) Follow home rules whenever possible.
    c. Allow rituals.
    d. Allow for separation without conflict.
        (1) Use primary nurse.
        (2) Encourage visiting.
        (3) Have the parents provide as much care as possible.
        (4) Encourage sibling and peer contact.
    e. Promote sexual identity.
        (1) Reassure child about the genitalia.
        (2) Use the child's hand when assessing genitalia.
        (3) Avoid intrusive procedures.

STUDY QUESTIONS

1. When providing health teaching for a 5-year-old, the nurse knows that the child is capable of which of the following?
   (1) Understanding another's point of view
   (2) Making simple classifications
   (3) Exhibiting intuitive thought
   (4) Seeing relationships in reverse

2. A preschooler who is made to feel that his imagination and activities are unacceptable is likely to develop a sense of which of the following?
   (1) Mistrust
   (2) Shame
   (3) Guilt
   (4) Inferiority

3. Which of the following suggestions should the nurse offer the parents of a 4-year-old boy who resists going to bed at night?
   (1) "Allow him to fall asleep in your room, then move him to his own bed."
   (2) "Tell him that you will lock him in his room if he gets out of bed one more time."
   (3) "Encourage active play at bedtime to tire him out so he will fall asleep faster."
   (4) "Read him a story and allow him to play quietly in his bed until he falls asleep."

4. When providing therapeutic play, which of the following toys would **best** promote imaginative play in a 4-year-old?
   (1) Large blocks
   (2) Dress-up clothes
   (3) Wooden puzzle
   (4) Big wheels

5. When assessing gross motor development in a 3-year-old, which of the following activities would the nurse expect to find?
   (1) Riding a tricycle
   (2) Hopping on one foot
   (3) Catching a ball
   (4) Skipping on alternate feet

6. Which of the following best describes preschool sexual identification?
   (1) Identification with same-sex parent; attachment to opposite-sex parent
   (2) Identification with opposite-sex parent; attachment to same-sex parent
   (3) Identification and attachment to same-sex parent
   (4) Identification and attachment to opposite-sex parent

7. Which of the following would the nurse identify as the underlying rationale for a 4-year-old who tells the nurse that his doll is in the hospital because it was bad?
   (1) Egocentrism
   (2) Past experience
   (3) Magical thinking
   (4) Oedipal conflict

8. When teaching a group of parents about seat belt use, when would the nurse state that a child be safely restrained in a regular automobile seat belt?
   (1) 30 lb and 30 inches tall
   (2) 35 lb and 3 years of age
   (3) 40 lb and 40 inches tall
   (4) 60 lb and 6 years of age

9. A preschooler typically views parents as which of the following?
   (1) Necessary evil
   (2) Persons who keep order
   (3) Omnipotent persons
   (4) Very rigid individuals

10. After administering an intramuscular injection to a preschooler, which of the following is the **primary** reason for the nurse to apply an adhesive bandage to the site?
    (1) Children will use them to get attention from their parents.
    (2) Children are afraid that they will leak from the "hole."
    (3) Bandages help to alleviate fear of strangers.
    (4) Children collect bandages to show their peers.

ANSWER KEY

1. The answer is (2). The preconceptual child, age 2 to 4 years, is capable of making simple classifications. Seeing another's point of view occurs during concrete operations, typically between the ages of 7 to 11 years. Intuitive thinking occurs during the intuitive phase, ages 4 to 7 years. Seeing relationships involving the reverse occurs in formal operations, ages 11 to 15 years.

2. The answer is (3). According to Erikson, preschoolers develop a sense of guilt when made to feel that their imagination and activities are wrong, thus disallowing the child to develop a sense of initiative. Mistrust develops when an infant's needs are consistently not met and the infant cannot develop a sense of trust. Shame develops when a toddler is not allowed to develop appropriate autonomy. Inferiority develops when a schoolager is not allowed to have a sense of industry.

3. The answer is (4). Preschoolers commonly have fears of the dark, being left alone especially at bedtime, and ghosts, which may affect the child's going to bed at night. Quiet play and time with parents is a positive bedtime routine that provides security and also readies the child for sleep. The child should sleep in his own bed. Telling the child about locking him in his room will viewed by the child as a threat. Additionally, a locked door is frightening and potentially hazardous. Vigorous activity at bedtime stirs up the child and makes it more difficult to fall asleep.

4. The answer is (2). Dress-up clothes enhance imaginative play and imagination, allowing preschoolers to engage in rich fantasy play. Building blocks and wooden puzzles are appropriate for encouraging fine motor development. Big wheels and tricylces encourage gross motor development

5. The answer is (1). A 3-year-old should have the gross motor ability to balance on and ride a tricycle. Hopping on one foot and the ability to catch a ball are accomplished by 4 years. Skipping on alternate feet is accomplished by 5 years.

6. The answer is (1). According to Freud, the preschooler experiences the Oedipal conflict, which typically resolves in a strong identification with the same-sex parent, but attaches to the parent of the opposite sex (Oedipal conflict). Alternate identifications and attachments are unusual in this age group.

7. The answer is (3). The fantasies of preschoolers can result in a sense of guilt. Because they cannot discern cause and effect, they see hospitalization as punishment for some real or fantasized misdoing. Magical thinking causes preschoolers to view illness as a punishment. Moreover, preschoolers are experiencing psychosexual conflicts and fears of mutilation, making them especially fearful of procedures such as rectal temperatures and urinary catheterizations. Egocentrism accounts for the preschooler's inability to see another's point of view. Past experience can affect the preschooler's reaction to hospitalization, but this is not the underlying rationale here. Oedipal conflicts do not directly affect hospitalization.

8. The answer is (3). When a child weighs 40 lb and is 40 inches tall, the child has sufficiently developed bone structure and muscle mass to use regular restraints. Any child under these parameters is too small to use a regular automobile seat belt. Use of a car seat can be discontinued before the child weighs 60 lbs and is 6 years of age.

9. The answer is (3). Typically, the preschooler believes that parents can do no wrong and enjoys their guidance. Thus the parents are viewed as omnipotent. The view of parents as a necessary evil is more typical of an adolescent. The preschooler has not yet developed the view of parents as those who keep order. Preschoolers are not bothered by rigidity. In fact, guidelines give them a sense of security.

10. The answer is (2). Preschoolers have poorly defined body boundary images. Therefore they are afraid that their body parts will come out of the injection site. Applying the bandage helps to control this fear. They may use the bandage for attention, but this is secondary. Fear of strangers is more apparent in toddlers. Schoolagers are more likely to collect things to show their peers.

5 School-Age Growth and Development (6–12 Years of Age)

Physical growth and development

A. General parameters

1. During this period, girls usually grow faster than boys and commonly surpass them in height and weight.
   a. **Height**
      (1) The average schoolager grows 2 inches (5 cm) per year.
      (2) The average 6-year-old is 45 inches (112.5 cm) tall.
      (3) The average 12-year-old is 59 inches (147.5 cm) tall.
   b. **Weight**
      (1) The average schoolager gains 4.5 to 6.5 lb (2–3 kg) per year.
      (2) The average 6-year-old weighs 46 lb (21 kg).
      (3) The average 12-year-old weighs 88 lb (40 kg).
2. During preadolescence, which extends from about ages 10 to 13, a child commonly experiences rapid growth.
3. The immune system becomes more efficient, allowing for more localization of infections and better antibody–antigen response.
   a. Schoolagers develop immunity to a wide number of organisms.
   b. Many schoolagers develop several infections in the first few years of school because of increased exposure to other children with germs.

B. Nutrition

1. **Nutritional requirements**
   a. A schoolager's daily caloric requirements diminish in relation to body size. Schoolagers require an average of 2400 calories per day.
   b. Caregivers should continue to stress the need for a balanced diet from the food pyramid; the body is storing resources for the increased growth needs of adolescence.
2. **Food patterns and preferences**
   a. The child is exposed to broader eating experiences in the school lunchroom; he may still be a "picky" eater but should be more willing to try new foods. Children may trade, sell, or throw away home-packed school lunches.
   b. At home the child should eat what the family eats; the patterns that develop now stay with the child into adulthood. The child's eating patterns should reflect family culture.
   c. Many schoolagers still dislike vegetables, casseroles, liver, and spicy foods. They may go on "food jags," eating only one type of food at a time, such as peanut butter and jelly sandwiches for lunch.

    d. Family members play an important role in the child's food preferences; however, peers and the media are also influences. Without adult supervision, schoolagers typically make poor food choices.

  3. Overweight and obesity. More than 90% of obese children are overweight due to overeating, with underactivity playing a significant role.

C. Sleep patterns

  1. Individual sleep requirements for schoolagers vary but typically range from 8 to 9.5 hours nightly. Because growth rate slows, schoolagers actually need less sleep than they will during adolescence.

  2. The child's bedtime can be later than during the preschool period but should be firmly established and adhered to on school nights.

  3. Reading before bedtime may facilitate sleep and set up a positive bedtime pattern.

  4. Children may be unaware of fatigue; if allowed to remain awake, they will be tired the next day.

D. Dental health

  1. Beginning around age 6, permanent teeth erupt and the child gradually loses the deciduous teeth.

  2. Regular dental visits are important, and fluoride supplements should continue when the water supply is insufficiently fluoridated.

  3. The child should brush her teeth after meals with a soft nylon toothbrush; because of the child's improved coordination, parental supervision and assistance usually are not necessary.

  4. Parents should floss the child's teeth until the child reaches age 8 or 9.

  5. Caries, malocclusion, and periodontal disease become evident in this age group.

E. Elimination

  1. By age 6 years, 85% of children have full bowel and bladder control.

  2. Elimination patterns are similar to adult patterns.

    a. Bowel movements occur on average 1 to 2 times per day.

    b. Urination occurs 6 to 8 times per day. The average urine volume in children is 500 to 1000 mL/day.

  3. Common problems include the following:

    a. Nocturnal **enuresis** (bed-wetting) occurs in 15% of 6-year-olds, 3% of 12-year-olds, and 1% of 18-year-olds (see Chap. 7).

    b. **Encopresis** (persistent stool leakage) occurs in up to 1.5% of second-grade children.

    c. Boys have more frequent problems with soiling and constipation than do girls. Such problems require referral to a primary health care provider.

II. Motor development

A. Gross motor

  1. Bicycling

  2. Roller skating, rollerblading, and skateboarding

  3. Progressively improved running and jumping

  4. Swimming

B. Fine motor

  1. Printing in early years; script in later years (by age 8)

  2. Greater dexterity for crafts and video games

  3. Computer competence (manual skills)

C. **Related safety concerns**

 1. Schoolagers learn to accept more responsibility for personal health care and injury prevention.
 2. Children's developing cognitive skills complement their own judgments and assist in helping them avoid many types of injuries.
 3. Schoolagers are still prone to accidents, mainly owing to increasing motor abilities and independence (eg, a bicycle can take a child farther from home independently).
    a. Major sources of injuries include bicycles, skateboards, and team sports. Learning proper techniques, using safe equipment, and, in the case of organized sports, good coaching and well-matched teams (playing with children of similar size) can reduce the risk of injury.
    b. Schoolagers who learn safe swimming and diving practices, fire safety, use of seat belts and bicycle helmets, and other safety practices are at reduced risk for injury.
 4. Parents should continue to provide guidance for new situations and threats to safety.
 5. School-age children should receive education about the use and abuse of alcohol, tobacco (including chew and snuff), and other drugs.

III. Psychosocial development

A. **Overview (Erikson)**

 1. Erikson terms the psychosocial crisis the child faces between ages 6 and 12 as **"industry versus inferiority."**
    a. The child's radius of significant others expands to include schoolmates and instructive adults.
    b. A school-age child normally has mastered the first three developmental tasks (trust, autonomy, and initiative) and now focuses on mastering industry.
    c. A sense of industry springs from a desire for achievement.
    d. A sense of inferiority can stem from unrealistic expectations or a sense of failing to meet standards others set for the child. When the child feels inadequate, his self-esteem declines.
 2. The schoolager engages in tasks and activities that he can carry through to completion.
 3. The schoolager learns rules, competition, and cooperation to achieve goals.
 4. Social relationships become increasingly important sources of support.

B. **Fears and stressors**

 1. During the school-age years, many fears of earlier childhood resolve or decrease; however, schoolagers may hide fears to avoid being labeled "chicken" or a "baby."
 2. Common fears
    a. Failure at school
    b. Bullies
    c. Intimidating teachers
    d. Something bad happening to parents
 3. Common stressors
    a. Stressors for young schoolagers are teasing, decision-making, need for approval, loneliness, independence, and the opposite sex.
    b. Stressors for older schoolagers are sexual maturation, shyness, health, competition, peer pressure, and temptation to use drugs.
 4. Parents and other caregivers can help reduce a child's fears by communicating empathy and concern without being overprotective.

    5. Children need to know that people will listen to them and that they will be understood.

C. Socialization

    1. The school-age years are a period of dynamic change and maturation as the child becomes increasingly involved in more complex activities, decision-making, and goal-directed activities.

    2. As a schoolager learns more about her body, social development centers on the body and its capabilities.

    3. Peer relationships gain new importance.

    4. Group activities, including team sports, typically consume much time and energy.

D. Play and toys

    1. Play becomes more competitive and complex during the school-age period.

    2. Characteristic activities include team sports, secret clubs, "gang" activities, scouting or other organizations, complex puzzles, collections, quiet board games, reading, and hero worship.

    3. Rules and rituals are important aspects of play and games.

    4. Toys, games, and activities that encourage growth and development include the following:

        a. Increasingly complex board and card games

        b. Books and crafts

        c. Music and art

        d. Athletic activities (eg, swimming)

        e. Team activities

        f. Video games (Encourage parental monitoring of content to avoid exposure to gratuitous violence and sexual situations.)

E. Discipline

    1. Schoolagers begin to internalize their own controls and need less outside direction. They do, however, need a parent or other trusted adult to answer questions and to provide guidance for decisions.

    2. Regular household responsibilities help schoolagers feel that they are an important part of the family and increase their sense of accomplishment.

    3. A weekly allowance, set in accordance with a schoolager's needs and duties, assists in teaching skills, values, and a sense of responsibility.

    4. When disciplining schoolagers, parents and other caregivers should set reasonable, concrete limits (and provide plausible explanations) and keep rules to a minimum.

IV. Psychosexual development

A. Overview (Freud)

    1. The **latency period**, which extends from about age 5 to 12 years, represents a stage of relative sexual indifference before puberty and adolescence.

    2. During this period, development of self-esteem is closely linked with a developing sense of industry to produce a concept of one's value and worth.

B. Sexual development

    1. Preadolescence begins near the end of the school-age years. At this time, discrepancies in growth and maturation between the genders becomes apparent.

    2. Schoolagers acquire much knowledge of and many attitudes toward sex at earlier stages. During the school-age years, they refine this knowledge and these attitudes.

    3. Questions about sex require honest answers based on the child's level of understanding.

Cognitive development

A. Overview (Piaget)

1. Between ages 7 and 11, a child is in the **concrete operations stage**, marked by inductive reasoning, logical operations, and reversible concrete thought.
2. Specific characteristics of this stage include the following:
   a. Transition from egocentric to objective thinking (ie, seeing another's point of view, seeking validation, and asking questions)
   b. Focus on immediate physical reality with inability to transcend the present
   c. Difficulty dealing with remote, future, or hypothetical matters
   d. Development of various mental classifying and ordering activities
   e. Development of the principle of conservation (ie, of volume, weight, mass, and numbers)
3. Typical activities of a child at this stage may include the following:
   a. Collecting and sorting objects (eg, baseball cards, dolls, and marbles)
   b. Ordering items according to size, shape, weight, and other criteria
   c. Considering options and variables when solving problems

B. Language

1. The child develops formal adult articulation patterns by ages 7 to 9.
2. The child learns that words can be arranged in terms of structure.
3. The ability to read is one of the most significant skills that the child develops.

 ## Moral development

According to Kohlberg, children arrive at the **conventional level of the role conformity stage**, generally, between ages 10 and 13. They have an increased desire to please others. They also observe and, to some extent, externalize the standards of others and want to be considered "good" by those persons whose opinions matter to them.

 ## Wellness promotion

A. General.
Encourage the family to follow guidelines for well child care visits, screening, immunizations, and safety (Table 5-1).

B. Nutrition

1. Encourage healthy eating patterns and help shape the child's food preferences positively.
2. Remind children and their caregivers to limit junk food.
3. Teach the basics of the food pyramid and help the child differentiate nutritious foods from junk foods.

C. Sleep.
Encourage the family to agree on a bedtime and allow flexibility on nonschool nights.

D. Growth and development

1. Foster a sense of industry by encouraging the child's skill development in school, sports, play, and other activities.
2. Counsel families about safety measures for latchkey children if needed (Child and Family Teaching 5-1).
3. Encourage parents to limit the family's TV watching.

TABLE 5-1
Recommendations for Well Child Care—School-Age

ASSESSMENT	6 YEARS	7 YEARS	8 YEARS	9 YEARS	10 YEARS	11 YEARS	12 YEARS
History and physical exam	X	X	X	X	X	X	X
Dentist	X	X	X	X	X	X	X
Screening:							
Development	X	X	X	X	X	X	X
Vision	X	X	X	X	X	X	X
Hearing	O	O	O	O	O	O	O
Tests:							
Hemoglobin	O	O	O	O	O	O	O
Cholesterol	At risk	At risk	At risk	At risk	At risk	At risk	At risk
TB test	At risk	At risk	At risk	At risk	At risk	At risk	At risk
Immunizations					MMR if not given at 4–6 years		
Counseling and anticipatory guidance	X	X	X	X	X	X	X

X, recommended by leading authorities; O, recommended by some leading authorities; MMR, measles, mumps, rubella.
Adapted from: American Academy of Family Physicians, Committee on Public Health and Scientific Affairs. (1993). Age charts and periodic health exams. Kansas City, MO: Authors.
American Academy of Pediatrics, Committee on Practice and Ambulatory Care. (1991). Recommendations for preventive health care. American Academy of Pediatrics News, 7, 19.

E. Family

1. Encourage open communication.
2. Foster responsibility with chores and adherence to family rules and schedules.
3. Encourage decision-making and individuality as the child learns to accept the consequences of his own actions.
4. Encourage parents to get to know the child's peer group. Peers are important, but the child will turn to family for support and approval.

F. Health

1. Promote self-care and hygiene, including flossing.
2. Monitor the child for behavior problems.

G. Anticipatory guidance. Teach the child about puberty and all its physical and emotional changes; drugs, alcohol, and tobacco; and sex education.

VIII. Illness and hospitalization

A. Overview

1. Stressors include immobilization, fear of mutilation and death, and concerns over modesty.
2. School-age children have difficulty with forced dependency. They may be unable to express themselves verbally and their self-consciousness may interfere with care.

CHILD AND FAMILY TEACHING 5-1

Safety Measures for Latchkey Children

- Post a list of emergency telephone numbers and make sure that the child knows how to use them.
- Instruct the child to tell callers that parents cannot come to the telephone because they are busy instead of saying that parents are not home.
- Teach the child first aid and basic safety (eg, fire, weather-related safety, and cooking) as appropriate.
- Establish an after school routine, and make sure that the child understands it.
- Instruct the child to lock the doors and to not display the key to others.
- Consider getting a pet to provide company for the child.
- Arrive home when planned. If a delay is necessary, telephone the child to alleviate anxiety.

B. Reactions to illness

1. School-age children perceive external forces as causes of illness.
2. They are aware of the significance of different illnesses. For example, they know that cancer is more serious than a "cold."

C. Reactions to hospitalization

1. The primary defense mechanism of school-age children is reaction formation, an unconscious defense mechanism in which the child assumes an attitude that is opposite of the impulse that they harbor. Typically, the child states he is brave when he is really frightened.
2. Schoolagers may react to separation by demonstrating loneliness, boredom, isolation, and depression. They may also show aggression, irritability, and inability to relate to siblings and peers.
3. The sensed loss of control is related to enforced dependency and altered family roles.
4. Fear of bodily injury and pain results from fear of illness, disability, and death.

D. Nursing management

1. **Provide general interventions.**
   a. Encourage verbalization.
   b. Encourage self-care.
   c. Encourage peer interactions.
   d. Inform schoolagers that it is "OK" to cry.
   e. Give factual information; use models to demonstrate concepts or procedures.
   f. Provide diversions.
2. **Provide physical comfort and safety interventions**.
   a. Allow the schoolager control over body functions.
   b. Assist in developing fine motor skills. Encourage the following:
      (1) Construction toys, such as Lego sets
      (2) Drawing
      (3) Computer games
      (4) Drawing body parts
      (5) "Taking notes" during patient education
   c. Allow schoolagers to participate in treatment.
3. **Provide cognitive interventions**.
   a. Assist in developing rational thinking (give scientific explanations, rationales, and rules) and provide for decision-making.

    b. Assist the child with mastering concepts of conservation, constancy and reversibility, classification, and categorization.

       (1) Allow the child to chart intake and output and vital signs.

       (2) Encourage the child to tell the nurse when procedures are due.

       (3) Help the child create a scrapbook.

       (4) Use concepts, such as cards and board games, in teaching and games.

       (5) Encourage the child to do schoolwork.

    c. Provide time for, and encourage, verbalization (talk time).

4. Provide psychosocial and emotional interventions.

    a. Provide the opportunity to channel drives.

       (1) Encourage peer interaction, group education, and limit setting.

       (2) Avoid coed rooms.

    b. Promote achievement of industry.

       (1) Praise cooperative play.

       (2) Assign tasks that the child can accomplish.

       (3) Involve the child in care.

STUDY QUESTIONS

1. Which of the following statements should the nurse stress when teaching parents to maintain a consistent bedtime schedule for their 9-year-old?
   (1) The child's need for sleep is greater now than in adolescence.
   (2) Nightmares and night terrors are common.
   (3) The child often is unaware of his own fatigue level.
   (4) Ten hours of sleep every night is the minimum requirement.

2. Which of the following activities, when voiced by the parents following a teaching session about the characteristics of school-age cognitive development would indicate the need for additional teaching?
   (1) Collecting baseball cards and marbles
   (2) Ordering dolls according to size
   (3) Considering simple problem-solving options
   (4) Developing plans for the future

3. The mother of a 5-year-old asks, "When do the deciduous teeth usually begin to fall out?" Which of the following is the nurse's **most** appropriate response?
   (1) Age 5 years
   (2) Age 6 years
   (3) Age 7 years
   (4) Age 8 years

4. Unrealistic expectations or a sense of failing to meet standards would cause a schoolager to develop a sense of which of the following?
   (1) Shame
   (2) Guilt
   (3) Inferiority
   (4) Role confusion

5. A hospitalized schoolager states: "I'm not afraid of this place, I'm not afraid of anything." This statement is most likely an example of which of the following?
   (1) Regression
   (2) Repression
   (3) Reaction formation
   (4) Rationalization

6. When assessing a schoolager, which of the following **best** describes typical annual growth?
   (1) The child grows an average of 2 inches (5 cm) per year.
   (2) The child gains an average of 3 lb (1.4 kg) per year.
   (3) Few differences are noted between age mates.
   (4) Increased fat pads give schoolagers a chubby appearance.

7. A home health nurse is teaching nutrition to the parents of an 8-year-old. Which of the following statements should the nurse include?
   (1) "The child should develop impeccable table manners."
   (2) "The child's preferences should reflect family culture."
   (3) "I recommend a rigid mealtime environment."
   (4) "High-energy activity requires high-calorie snacks."

8. After teaching a group of parents about accident prevention for schoolagers, which of the following statements by the group would indicate the need for more teaching?
   (1) "Schoolagers are more active and adventurous than are younger children."
   (2) "Schoolagers are more susceptible to home hazards than are younger children."
   (3) "Schoolagers are unable to understand potential dangers around them."
   (4) "Schoolagers are less subject to parental control than are younger children."

9. Which of the following skills is the **most** significant one learned during the school-age period?
   (1) Collecting
   (2) Ordering
   (3) Reading
   (4) Sorting

10. A child, age 7, was unable to receive the measles, mumps, and rubella (MMR) vaccine at the recommended scheduled time. When would the nurse expect to administer MMR vaccine?

(1) In a month from now
(2) In a year from now
(3) At age 10
(4) At age 13

ANSWER KEY

1. The answer is (3). Schoolagers are often unaware of their own fatigue. If allowed to remain awake, they will be tired the next day. Because of the slowing growth rate during this period, schoolagers require less sleep than adolescents do. Nightmares and night terrors are common during the preschool period. Although the requirements may vary, schoolagers typically require approximately 8 to 9.5 hours of sleep every night.

2. The answer is (4). The school-aged child is in the stage of concrete operations, marked by inductive reasoning, logical operations, and reversible concrete thought. The ability to consider the future requires formal thought operations, which are not developed until adolescence. Collecting baseball cards and marbles, ordering dolls by size, and simple problem-solving options are examples of the concrete operational thinking of the schoolager.

3. The answer is (2). The deciduous, or primary, teeth typically begin to fall out by age 6 years. Age 5 is too young, and age 7 or 8 is too old.

4. The answer is (3). According to Erikson, during the school-age period, feelings of inadequacy and a failure to develop a sense of industry result in a sense of inferiority. Failure to develop a sense of autonomy results in a sense of shame in the toddler. Failure to develop a sense of initiative results in a sense of guilt in the preschooler. Failure to develop a sense of identity results in a sense of role confusion in the adolescent.

5. The answer is (3). Reaction formation is the schoolager's typical defensive response when hospitalized. In reaction formation, expression of unacceptable thoughts or behaviors is prevented (or overridden) by the exaggerated expression of opposite thoughts or types of behaviors. Regression is seen in toddlers and preschoolers when they retreat or return to an earlier level of development. Repression refers to the involuntary blocking of unpleasant feelings and experiences from one's awareness. Rationalization is the attempt to make excuses to justify unacceptable feelings or behaviors.

6. The answer is (1). School-age children usually grow about 2 inches (5 cm) per year. Schoolagers normally gain about 4.5 to 6.5 lbs (2–3 kg) per year. Schoolagers grow at different rates with girls growing faster than boys do and commonly surpassing them in height and weight. Fat pads normally do not increase until adolescence.

7. The answer is (2). The family's cultural values determine the overriding value of nutrition and eating. Table manners are important, but peer pressure and society will help mold them in later life. Mealtime should be relaxed with conversation that includes the children and their interests. School-age children need nutritious snacks, not empty calories. A balanced diet is necessary because resources are being stored for the increased growth needs of adolescence.

8. The answer is (3). The schoolager's cognitive level is sufficiently developed to enable good understanding of and adherence to rules. Thus schoolagers should be able to understand the potential dangers around them. With growth comes greater freedom and children become more adventurous and daring. The school-aged child is also still prone to accidents and home hazards, especially because of increased motor abilities and independence. Plus the home hazards differ from other age groups. These hazards, which are potentially lethal but tempting, may include firearms, alcohol, and medications. School-age children begin to internalize their own controls and need less outside direction. Plus the child is away from home more often. Some parental or caregiver assistance is still needed to answer questions and provide guidance for decisions and responsibilities.

9. The answer is (3). The most significant skill learned during the school-age period is reading. During this time the child develops formal adult articulation patterns and learns that words can be arranged in structure. Collecting, ordering, and sorting, although important, are not the most significant skills learned.

10. The answer is (3). Based on the recommendations of the American Academy of Family Physicians and the American Academy of Pediatrics, the MMR vaccine should be given at the age of 10 if the child did not receive it between the ages of 4 to 6 years as recommended. Immunization for diphtheria and tetanus is required at age 13.

6 Adolescent Growth and Development (12–18 Years of Age)

Physical growth and development

A. **Puberty** is the period when primary and secondary sex characteristics develop and mature.

1. **Onset**
   a. In girls, puberty begins between ages 8 and 14 and usually ends within 3 years.
   b. In boys, puberty begins between the ages of 9 and 16 and ends by age 18 or 19.

2. **Gender differences**
   a. Girls experience increases in height, weight, breast development, and pelvic girth with expansion of uterine tissue. Menarche (onset of menstrual periods) typically occurs about 2.5 years after puberty's onset.
   b. Boys experience increases in height, weight, muscle mass, and penis and testicle size. Facial and body hair grows. The voice deepens. The onset of spontaneous nocturnal emissions of seminal fluid is an overt sign of puberty and is analogous to menarche in girls.

3. **Developmental changes resulting from hormonal influences**
   a. Body mass increases to adult size.
   b. Sebaceous glands are activated.
   c. Eccrine sweat glands become fully functional.
   d. Apocrine sweat glands undergo development, and there is hair growth in the axillae, breast areolae, and genital and anal regions.
   e. Body hair is distributed in a characteristic adult-like pattern, and it undergoes texture changes.

4. **Development of sex characteristics (Tanner's stages)**
   a. **Female breast development**
      (1) Stage 1 is the prepubertal stage.
      (2) Stage 2 is characterized by development of breast buds.
      (3) Stage 3 is characterized by further enlargement of the breasts and areolae with no separation of contours.
      (4) Stage 4 is characterized by projection of areolae and papillae to form secondary mounds.
      (5) Stage 5 is characterized by adult configuration.
   b. **Male genitalia development**
      (1) Stage 1 is the prepubertal stage
      (2) Stage 2 is characterized by enlargement of the scrotum and testes and ruggation and reddening of the scrotum.
      (3) Stage 3 is characterized by lengthening of the penis and further enlargement of the scrotum and testes.

(4) Stage 4 is characterized by an increase in the length and width of the penis, development of the glans, and darkening of the scrotum.

(5) Stage 5 is characterized by an adult configuration.

c. **Pubic hair (male and female) development**

(1) Stage 1 is the prepubertal stage.

(2) Stage 2 is characterized by sparse, long, straight downy hair.

(3) Stage 3 is characterized by darker, coarser, curly hair that is sparse over the entire pubis.

(4) Stage 4 is characterized by dark, curly, and abundant hair in the pubic area only.

(5) Stage 5 is characterized by an adult pattern.

B. General growth parameters

1. Height

a. Individuals achieve about 20% to 25% of adult height in adolescence.

b. Girls grow 2 to 8 inches (5–20 cm). Growth ceases at about age 16 or 17.

c. Boys grow 4 to 12 inches (10–30 cm). Growth ceases between ages 18 and 20.

2. Weight

a. Individuals gain about 30% to 50% of adult weight during adolescence.

b. On average, girls gain between 15 and 55 lb (6.8–25 kg).

c. On average, boys gain 15 to 65 lb (6.8–29.5 kg).

C. Nutrition

1. Nutritional requirements

a. An adolescent's daily intake should be balanced among the food groups (Fig. 6-1).

b. Average daily caloric intake requirements vary with gender and age.

(1) Girls between the ages of 11 and 14 require 48 kcal/kg/day.

(2) Girls between the ages of 15 and 18 require 38 kcal/kg/day.

(3) Boys between the ages of 11 and 14 require 60 kcal/kg/day.

(4) Boys between the ages of 15 and 18 require 42 kcal/kg/day.

c. Adolescents need milk (calcium) and protein in sufficient quantity for promotion of bone and muscle growth. High consumption of soft drinks can lead to inadequate milk intake, and thus inadequate calcium intake.

d. Common dietary deficiencies include iron, folate, and zinc. Iron needs for females vary according to menstrual blood loss.

2. Food patterns and preferences

a. Adolescents typically eat whenever they have a break in their activities; readily available nutritious snacks provide good insurance for a balanced diet.

b. Maintaining adequate quality and quantity of daily intake may be difficult because of such factors as a busy schedule, influence of peers, and easy availability of fast and fatty, empty-calorie foods.

c. At least 50% of adolescents skip one meal a day due to work schedules, peer activity, weight concern, or inadequate knowledge about nutritional needs.

d. Family eating patterns established during the school years continue to influence an adolescent's food selection.

e. Female adolescents are very prone to negative dieting behaviors. Anorexia nervosa, bulimia nervosa, and obesity are common in adolescents.

D. Sleep patterns

1. During adolescence, rapid growth, overexertion, and a tendency to stay up late commonly interfere with sleep and rest requirements.

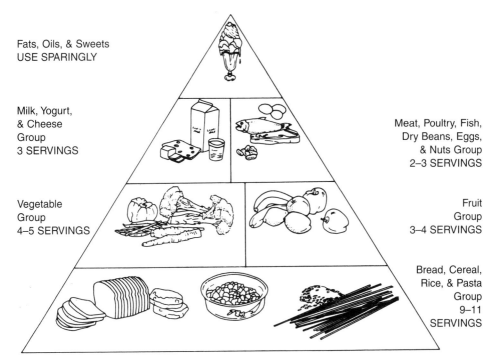

Fats, Oils, & Sweets
USE SPARINGLY

Milk, Yogurt,
& Cheese
Group
3 SERVINGS

Meat, Poultry, Fish,
Dry Beans, Eggs,
& Nuts Group
2–3 SERVINGS

Vegetable
Group
4–5 SERVINGS

Fruit
Group
3–4 SERVINGS

Bread, Cereal,
Rice, & Pasta
Group
9–11
SERVINGS

Smaller number of servings for Teen Girls—Larger number of servings for Teen Boys

FIGURE 6-1
Food guide pyramid adapted for adolescents. (From United States Department of Agriculture)

    2. In an attempt to "catch up" on missed sleep, many adolescents sleep late at every opportunity.

    3. Fatigue may be precipitated by faulty nutrition, overactivity, physical problems, or psychological disorders.

E. Dental health

    1. Regular and preventive dental check-ups should continue during adolescence.

    2. Many adolescents must wear orthodontic appliances, which may be sources of embarrassment.

    3. Adolescents must continue to pay special attention to careful brushing and care of the teeth.

F. Elimination

    1. Elimination patterns should be similar to adult patterns.

    2. Although constipation may be due to physiologic disorders, in adolescence it is typically due to improper nutrition or an eating disorder, such as anorexia nervosa.

    3. The average urinary volume during adolescence is 700 to 1400 mL/day.

II. Motor development

A. Gross motor development reaches adult levels.

B. Fine motor development continues to be refined.

C. Related safety concerns

1. Adolescents commonly feel that they are invulnerable. They are more likely to take risks and usually do not consider safety before action (Child and Family Teaching 6-1).

2. Adolescents contribute substantially to motor vehicle accidents through:
   a. Inexperience and poor judgment
   b. Reckless driving or speeding
   c. Driving under the influence of alcohol or other drugs
   d. Failure to use seat belts
   e. Unsafe driving practices in response to peer pressure

3. Similarly, adolescents also are prone to accidents from unsafe use of bicycles, skateboards, motorcycles, boats, all-terrain vehicles, and snowmobiles.

4. Accidental injury can result from improper use of firearms.

5. Adolescents are particularly prone to swimming and diving accidents as well.

III. Psychosocial development

A. Overview (Erikson)

1. Erikson terms the psychosocial crisis that adolescents face between ages 13 and 18 as **"identity versus role diffusion."**
   a. The radius of significant others is the peer group.
   b. Development of who they are and where they are going becomes a central focus for adolescents. They continue to redefine their self-concepts, and the roles that they can play, with certainty.
   c. According to Erikson, modern culture tends to make identity development challenging. Adolescents who cannot develop a sense of who they are and what they can become may experience role diffusion and an inability to solve core conflicts.

CHILD AND FAMILY TEACHING 6-1

Safety Instruction

Safety instruction for adolescents should include the following:
- Proper use and storage of firearms and other weapons, such as nonpowder arms (eg, BB guns)
- Swimming and diving safety
- Proper caution around gasoline, electricity, and fire
- Ways to avoid sports injuries (eg, avoiding overexertion and using proper equipment and techniques)
- Use of sunscreen during sun exposure
- Risks of tobacco, alcohol, and other drugs
- Problem-solving techniques to decrease use of physical violence as a coping mechanism
- Safe sex

2. As rapid physical changes occur, adolescents must reintegrate previous trust in their body, themselves, and how they appear to others.

B. Fears and stressors

1. Common fears and stressors of adolescents include the following:
   a. Relationships with persons of the opposite sex
   b. Homosexual tendencies or feelings
   c. Ability to assume adult roles
2. Listening to an adolescent's concerns and encouraging open communication help the adolescent develop increased confidence in his ability to cope.

C. Socialization

1. **Family influences**
   a. To free themselves from family domination, adolescents must define an identity apart from parental authority.
   b. Typical adolescent rebellion occurs at the final phase of childhood, called separation-individuation. This period of rebellion and uncertainty can resemble the toddler period in certain respects.
   c. Requisites for emancipation from home include acceptance by peers, a few close friends, and secure love from a supportive family.
   d. Relationships with parents change as the adolescent achieves competence and authority.
2. **Peers and peer relationships**
   a. Peers become all-important providers of advice and support.
   b. Being found attractive by peers is important to an adolescent's self-esteem.
   c. Heterosexual relationships typically begin with groups of teens spending time together, followed by group dating, paired dating in groups, and then a couple on a double-date or alone.
   d. The degree of sexual intimacy that an adolescent experiences depends in large part on peer-group codes and the adolescent's expectations and value system.
   e. Group parties and teams typically occupy much of an adolescent's social time.
   f. Movies and music provide enjoyable diversions for most adolescents.
3. **Roles and responsibilities**
   a. Older adolescents of both genders usually are interested in the independence and status represented by driving an automobile.
   b. Common early jobs for adolescents include baby sitting and lawn mowing. Starting at age 16, adolescents can obtain more formal jobs to earn money and learn responsibility.
   c. Adolescents typically spend money on dates, clothes, and other items important to them.

D. Age-appropriate activities and equipment

1. Sports, camping, fishing gear
2. Videos, video games, computer games, radios, and compact disc players
3. Personal telephones
4. Models and collectibles

E. Discipline

1. Firm but reasonable limit setting is still necessary and appreciated by most adolescents.
2. A supportive, yet noninterfering, family is essential.
3. An adolescent's privileges and responsibilities should be balanced in accordance with her maturity.

Psychosexual development

A. Overview (Freud)

1. In the **genital stage**, which extends from about age 12 to 20, adolescents focus on the genitals as an erogenous zone and engage in masturbation and sexual relations with others.
2. During this period of renewed sexual drive, adolescents experience conflict between their own needs for sexual satisfaction and society's expectations for control of sexual expression.
3. Core concerns of adolescents include body image development and acceptance by the opposite sex.

B. Sexual/sexuality development

1. Relationships with the opposite sex are important.
2. Adolescents engage in sexual activity for pleasure, to satisfy drives and curiosity, as a means of conquest or power, to express and receive affection, and in response to peer pressure.
3. Education about sexual function, begun during the school years, should expand to cover the physical, hormonal, and emotional changes of puberty.
4. An adolescent needs accurate, complete information on sexuality and cultural and moral values. Information must include the following:
   a. How pregnancy occurs
   b. Methods of preventing pregnancy, stressing that male and female partners both are responsible for contraception
   c. Transmission of, and protection against, sexually transmitted diseases (STDs), especially acquired immunodeficiency syndrome (AIDS)
   d. Proper condom usage
5. Adolescents may engage in homosexual activity or have homosexual feelings, but many do not become gay or lesbian adults. However, teens who question their sexual orientation should be referred for counseling; they should not be told it is just a phase. Nurses should acknowledge the possibility of homosexual and bisexual orientation and should use words like partner instead of boyfriend or girlfriend.

Cognitive development

A. Overview (Piaget)

1. In the stage called **formal operations**, which commonly occurs from age 11 to 15, the adolescent develops abstract reasoning.
2. Abstract reasoning includes inductive and deductive reasoning, the ability to connect separate events, and the ability to understand later consequences.

B. Formal thought

1. In formal thought, the adolescent thinks beyond the present and forms theories about everything, delighting especially in considerations of "that which is not."
2. The adolescent hypothesizes relationships as causal and analyzes them for their effects.
3. A systematic approach to problems replaces random cognitive behavior.
4. Manifestations of formal operational thought in adolescence include:
   a. **Idealism**—envisioning a perfect world
   b. **Egocentrism**—preoccupation with one's own power of thought (includes the imaginary audience ["everyone is watching me and is concerned about me"] and

the personal fable [thinks own thoughts and feelings are special; includes feelings of infallibility])

 VI. **Moral development**

According to Kohlberg, the **postconventional level of morality** occurs at about age 13. It is marked by the development of an individual conscience and a defined set of moral values. For the first time, the adolescent can acknowledge a conflict between two socially accepted standards and try to decide between them. Control of conduct is now internal, both in standards observed and in reasoning about right and wrong.

 VII. **Wellness promotion**

A. General. Encourage families to follow recommended guidelines regarding well child care, screening, immunizations, and safety (Table 6-1).

B. Nutrition
  1. Reinforce principles of proper nutrition and discuss ways that adolescents can incorporate these principles within their lifestyle.

TABLE 6-1
Recommendations for Well Child Care—Adolescents

ASSESSMENT	13 YEARS	14 YEARS	15 YEARS	16 YEARS	17 YEARS	18 YEARS
History and physical exam	X	X	X	X	X	X
Pelvic exam	SAF	SAF	SAF	SAF	SAF	SAF
Dentist	X	X	X	X	X	X
Screening:						
Development	X	X	X	X	X	X
Vision	X	X	X	X	X	X
Hearing	O	O	O	O	O	O
Tests:						
Hemoglobin	O	O	O	O	O	O
Cholesterol	At risk...	...	...	...	...	...At risk
Urinalysis			X			
TB test	At risk...	...	...	...	...	...At risk
STD screen	SA	SA	SA	SA	SA	SA
Immunizations	dt...	...	...	...	...	...dt
Counseling and anticipatory guidance	X	X	X	X	X	X

X, recommended by leading authorities; O, recommended by some leading authorities; SA, recommended for all sexually active adolescents; SAF, recommended for all sexually active females; DT, diphtheria and tetanus.

Adapted from: American Academy of Family Physicians, Committee on Public Health and Scientific Affairs. (1993). Age charts and periodic health exams. Kansas City, MO: Author.

American Academy of Pediatrics, Committee on Practice and Ambulatory Care. (1991). Recommendations for preventive health care. American Academy of Pediatrics News, 7, 19.

    2. Discuss the possibilities of supplementation when needed (eg, girls who may need iron supplements due to heavy menses).

    3. Encourage athletes and adolescents with eating disorders to receive proper nutritional counseling and follow-up.

C. Sleep

    1. Encourage adolescents to get adequate sleep and rest.

    2. Encourage them to discuss sleep problems and fatigue if needed.

D. Growth and development

    1. Stress importance of accident prevention, especially in regard to automobile safety, sports and recreational safety, and firearms.

    2. Encourage adolescents to take a first aid course.

    3. Discuss issues related to sex and sexuality, including contraception and prevention of STDs.

    4. Discuss the use of drugs, alcohol, and tobacco.

    5. Discuss issues of menstruation, masturbation, and nocturnal emissions.

    6. Discuss violence prevention, including measures to prevent date rape.

E. Family

    1. Reinforce the need for adequate and open family communication skills.

    2. Foster problem-solving and decision-making skills.

    3. Assist parents in understanding adolescent development and issues of individuality.

F. Health. Discuss the prevention and management of common adolescent health problems including acne, mononucleosis, and menstrual disorders.

G. Anticipatory guidance. Prepare the adolescent for college, independent living, the work force, serious relationships, marriage, parenting, and increasing community involvement.

VIII. Hospitalization

A. Overview. Hospitalized adolescents' concerns focus on:

    1. Alterations in body image

    2. Separation from peers

    3. Illness as punishment (12–14 years of age)

    4. Restricted independence (because of confinement)

B. Reactions to hospitalization

    1. Primary defense mechanisms include denial and displacement (shifting focus from undesired object or feeling to a more acceptable object or feeling).

    2. Loss of control is related to loss of identity and enforced dependence, possibly causing adolescents to react with rejection, uncooperativeness, self-assertion, anger, or frustration. They may withdraw, even from peers.

    3. Adolescents' fears of mutilation and sexual changes may be evidenced by their numerous questions, rejection of others, questioning adequacy of care, psychosomatic complaints, and sexual reactions.

    4. Separation, especially from the peer group, may result in further withdrawal, loneliness, and boredom.

C. Nursing management

    1. Provide general interventions.

        a. Relate to adolescents on their level.

        b. Be genuine.

   c. Allow adolescents to wear their own clothes.

   d. Allow adolescents to decorate their rooms.

   e. Provide a telephone whenever possible.

   f. **Respect adolescents' privacy.**

   g. Set limits.

   h. Do not flirt with adolescents.

   i. Do not assign adolescents to hospital rooms with small children.

2. Provide physical comfort and safety interventions.

   a. Provide nutritional information.

     (1) Use the skills of the dietitian.

     (2) Offer nutritious snacks.

   b. Provide counseling about issues related to puberty and health (eg, personal hygiene, breast self-examination, testicular self-examination, contraception, AIDS, and other STDs).

   c. Promote exercise and mobility.

     (1) Schedule activities.

     (2) Acknowledge the need for physical expression of frustration.

3. Provide cognitive interventions.

   a. Provide scientific explanations.

   b. **Encourage adolescents to participate in their own health management (include them as well as their parents in planning and instruction).**

   c. Support them in achieving academic and career goals.

     (1) Help them complete schoolwork.

     (2) Involve their teachers.

     (3) Reinforce realistic goals.

4. Provide psychosocial and emotional interventions.

   a. Assist adolescents to develop healthy attitudes about body image and sexuality.

     (1) Allow them to verbalize their fears and concerns.

     (2) Provide privacy.

     (3) Allow them to have their own belongings.

     (4) Assist with and promote grooming.

   b. Promote independence.

     (1) Compliment strengths.

     (2) Promote self-care.

     (3) Provide flexible limits.

     (4) Assist with setting of goals.

     (5) Support decision-making.

   c. Promote peer contact.

     (1) Allow visits and calls.

     (2) Sponsor group activities.

   d. Promote family support.

     (1) Encourage visiting.

     (2) Allow the family to discuss issues.

     (3) Support the family unit.

     (4) Assist with finding community resources.

STUDY QUESTIONS

1. Which of the following would the nurse use to respond to the mother of an 8-year-old girl who asks about when her child will begin puberty?
 (1) "It begins between ages 8 and 14 and ends within 3 years."
 (2) "It begins between ages 9 and 16 and ends by age 18 or 19."
 (3) "It begins between ages 8 and 14 and ends by age 18 or 19."
 (4) "It begins between ages 9 and 16 and ends within 3 years."

2. During assessment of a female adolescent, the nurse notes projection of the areola and papilla forming a secondary mound on the breast. The nurse would identify this adolescent as being in which of the following stages (Tanner's) of sexual development?
 (1) Stage 2
 (2) Stage 3
 (3) Stage 4
 (4) Stage 5

3. The adolescent's inability to develop a sense of who he is and what he can become results in a sense of which of the following?
 (1) Shame
 (2) Guilt
 (3) Inferiority
 (4) Role diffusion

4. The parents of a 13-year-old boy are concerned because he is exhibiting rebellious behavior. The nurse understands that typical adolescent rebellion occurs at which of the following?
 (1) Final separation-individuation phase
 (2) Start of aggressive behavior
 (3) Start of peer relationships
 (4) Final phase of relationships

5. When teaching about accident prevention to a group of high school juniors, the school nurse's **primary** focus would be on which of the following areas?
 (1) Falls
 (2) Motor vehicle accidents
 (3) Firearms
 (4) Diving accidents

6. After learning that he will need surgery to repair his knee, a 16-year-old throws a cup at the nurse. The nurse plans a course of action based on the knowledge that the adolescent is displaying which of the following?
 (1) Displacement
 (2) Reaction formation
 (3) Projection
 (4) Denial

7. According to Erikson, which of the following reasons explains why an adolescent may have difficulty mastering appropriate psychosocial tasks?
 (1) The basic focus is on mastery of sexual relationships.
 (2) Only a limited interaction occurs between culture and individual development.
 (3) Modern culture tends to make identity crisis the most challenging to resolve.
 (4) The adolescent commonly lacks positive role models.

8. Which of the following would be **most** appropriate for a nurse to use when describing menarche to a 13-year-old?
 (1) A female's first menstruation or menstrual "period"
 (2) The first year of menstruation or "periods"
 (3) The entire menstrual cycle or from one "period" to another
 (4) The onset of uterine maturation or peak growth

9. A 14-year-old boy has acne and, according to his parents, dominates the bathroom by using the mirror all the time. Which of the following remarks by the nurse would be **least** helpful in talking to the boy and his parents?
 (1) "This is probably the only concern he has about his body. So, don't worry about it or the time he spends on it."
 (2) "Teenagers are anxious about how their peers perceive them. So they spend a lot of time grooming."

(3) "A teen may develop a poor self-image when experiencing acne. Do you feel this way sometimes?"

(4) "You appear to be keeping your face well washed. Would you feel comfortable discussing your cleansing method?"

10. Which of the following characteristics would the nurse expect to see in an adolescent who has developed the capacity for formal thought?

(1) Ability to analyze relationships for their effects

(2) Use of random cognitive behavior to approach problems

(3) Ability to say that something is wrong but not why

(4) Focusing on immediate physical reality of here and now

ANSWER KEY

1. The answer is (1). In girls, puberty generally begins between ages 8 and 14 and generally ends within 3 years. In boys, puberty generally begins between ages 9 and 15 and ends by age 18 or 19.

2. The answer is (3). The papilla and areola project and form a secondary mound during stage 4. Breast budding occurs during stage 2. Further enlargement of the breasts and areolae with no separation of contours occurs during stage 3. Adult breast configuration occurs during stage 5.

3. The answer is (4). According to Erikson, role diffusion develops when the adolescent does not develop a sense of identity and a sense of where he fits in. Toddlers develop a sense of shame when they do not achieve autonomy. Preschoolers develop a sense of guilt when they do not develop a sense of initiative. School-age children develop a sense of inferiority when they do not develop a sense of industry.

4. The answer is (1). Rebellion against parents occurs during the last or final phase of separation-individuation phase. This assists the adolescent in developing a sense of identity. Typical adolescent rebellion is not a sign of an aggressive personality. Typically, peer relationships start in the school-age years. There is no final relationship phase.

5. The answer (2). Inexperience, poor judgment, use of drugs and alcohol, and peer pressure make motor vehicle accidents the leading cause of accidental injury in adolescents. Falls are more common in younger children. Although increasing, injuries caused by firearms are not yet the leading cause of accidental injury in adolescents. Diving accidents are a common cause of injuries, but not the leading cause.

6. The answer is (1). Displacement, the transferring of a feeling about or a response to one object onto another usually less threatening substitute object, is a common defense mechanism used by the hospitalized adolescent. Reaction formation involves the person acting in a way that is opposite of how he feels. Projection occurs when a person falsely attributes one's own unacceptable feelings, impulses, or thoughts to another. Denial involves ignoring unacceptable realities.

7. The answer is (3). According to Erikson, modern culture tends to make identity development challenging. An adolescent must resolve many choices and demands to master the task of identity. Adolescents who cannot develop a sense of who they are and what they can become may experience role diffusion and an inability to solve core conflicts. Mastery of sexual relationships is part of the young adult task of intimacy. Adolescents have several interactions with culture. Peers, teachers, parents, and extended family all serve as role models.

8. The answer is (1). Menarche refers to the onset of the first menstruation or menstrual period and refers only to the first cycle. Uterine growth and broadening of the pelvic girdle occurs before menarche.

9. The answer is (1). Stating that this is probably the only concern the adolescent has and telling the parents not to worry about it or the time he spends on it shuts off further investigation and is likely to make the adolescent and his parents feel defensive. The statement about peer acceptance and time spent in front of the mirror for the development of self-image provides information about the adolescent's needs to the parents and may help to gain trust with the adolescent. Asking the adolescent how he feels about the acne will encourage the adolescent to share his feelings. Discussing the cleansing method shows interest and concern for the adolescent and also can help to identify any patient-teaching needs for the adolescent regarding cleansing.

10. The answer is (1). With formal thought, the adolescent thinks beyond the present and forms theories about everything. Relationships are hypothesized as causal and are analyzed for effects that they bring. Random cognitive behavior of earlier stages is replaced by a systematic approach to problems. The ability to say that something is wrong but not the reason why it is wrong is characteristic of the intuitive phase of preoperational thought for the toddler. Focusing on the immediate physical reality of the here and now is characteristic of the concrete operations stage for the school-aged child.

7 Fluid and Electrolyte Balance and Imbalance

I. Fluid, electrolyte, and acid–base balance and imbalance

A. Fluids and electrolytes

1. Total body fluid is expressed as a percentage of body weight; this percentage varies with age.
   a. In infants, total body fluids constitute 80% of body weight.
   b. By age 3 years, total body fluids constitute about 65% of body weight.
   c. By age 15 years, total body fluids constitute 60% of body weight.

2. Total body fluids are composed of water and electrolytes and are distributed between the intracellular and extracellular fluid compartments. Intracellular fluids (ICF) include all fluids inside the cellular walls; potassium is the main electrolyte of ICF. Extracellular fluids (ECF) include all fluids outside of the cellular walls (ie, plasma, lymph, and cerebrospinal fluid); sodium is the main electrolyte of ECF.
   a. In the newborn, 50% of the total body fluids are ECF. This composition makes the newborn more susceptible to dehydration and fluid overload.
   b. By toddlerhood, 30% of the total body fluids are ECF.

3. Age-specific fluid requirements are as follows:
   a. Newborn requirements are 80 to 100 mL/kg/d.
   b. Infant requirements are 120 to 130 mL/kg/d.
   c. Two-year-old requirements are 115 to 125 mL/kg/d.
   d. Six-year-old requirements are 90 to 100 mL/kg/d.
   e. Fifteen-year-old requirements are 70 to 85 mL/kg/d.
   f. Eighteen-year-old requirements are 40 to 50 mL/kg/d.

4. Fluid and electrolyte disturbances (eg, caused by diarrhea, vomiting, fever, and burns) occur more frequently and develop more rapidly in infants and young children than in older children and adults.

5. Infants and very young children are more vulnerable to alterations in fluid and electrolyte balance because their bodies have:
   a. A higher proportion of water content and a greater surface area
   b. A greater proportion of fluid in the extracellular compartment
   c. A higher metabolic rate that increases the rate at which body water must be replenished (also called water turnover)
   d. Immature kidneys and an immature homeostatic regulation (buffer) system
   e. Greater insensible water loss
   f. An inability to shiver or sweat to control temperature

6. Fluid requirements change when infants and children have specific disorders.
   a. Requirements increase in fever, diarrhea, vomiting, diabetes insipidus, high-output renal failure, burns, shock, and tachypnea.

TABLE 7-1
Acid–Base Disturbances

DISTURBANCE	INITIAL METABOLIC CHANGE	EFFECT ON BLOOD pH	COMPENSATORY REACTION
Respiratory acidosis	Increased P_{CO_2}	Decreased	Increased HCO_3
Metabolic acidosis	Decreased HCO_3	Decreased	Decreased P_{CO_2}
Respiratory alkalosis	Decreased P_{CO_2}	Increased	Decreased HCO_3
Metabolic alkalosis	Decreased H^+; increased HCO_3	Increased	Increased P_{CO_2}

      b. Requirements decrease in congestive heart failure (CHF), oliguric renal failure, increased intracranial pressure (ICP), mechanical ventilation, syndrome of inappropriate antidiuretic hormone (SIADH), and postoperatively.

B. Acid–base imbalance

   1. Acid–base imbalances are common complications of diarrhea, vomiting, and febrile conditions in infants and young children. These disturbances also may occur as complications of respiratory, endocrine, renal, and metabolic disorders.

   2. Acid–base disturbances include acidosis, resulting from an accumulation of acid or a loss of base, and alkalosis, resulting from an accumulation of base or a loss of acid (Tables 7-1 and 7-2).

      a. **Respiratory acidosis** results from diminished or inadequate pulmonary ventilation, which leads to an elevated P_{CO_2} level and a decreased plasma pH.

      b. **Metabolic acidosis** results from a gain of nonvolatile acids, or the loss of base, and leads to decreased plasma pH and decreased plasma HCO_3 concentration.

      c. **Respiratory alkalosis** results from an increase in the rate and depth of pulmonary ventilation, which leads to a decreased P_{CO_2} level and an elevated plasma pH.

TABLE 7-2
Problems That Result in Acid–Base Disturbances

SYSTEM AFFECTED	ACIDOSIS	ALKALOSIS
Respiratory	Factors that depress respiratory center: head injury, narcotic drugs, CNS infections	Primary CNS stimulation from emotions, CNS infections, salicylate ingestion, mechanical respiration
	Lung disorders: cystic fibrosis, obstructive pulmonary disease, pneumonia, atelectasis	Reflex CNS stimulation from fever, CHF, anemia
	Factors that affect chest wall action: chest wall trauma, muscular dystrophy	Lung disease: irritant inhalation, pulmonary edema
Endocrine/Metabolic	Acid gain from salicylate ingestion, diabetic ketoacidosis, starvation, infection	Acid loss from vomiting, diuretic therapy
	Bicarbonate loss from diarrhea, renal tubular acidosis	Bicarbonate gain from (uncommon) bicarbonate ingestion

CHF, congestive heart failure; CNS, central nervous system.

    d. **Metabolic alkalosis**, produced by a gain in base or a loss of acid, results in elevated urine pH, elevated plasma pH, and elevated plasma HCO₃ concentrations.

  3. Compensatory mechanisms reflect the body's attempts to correct an acid–base imbalance through changes in the component of the acid–base equation that are not primarily affected.

  4. Interventions are necessary to sustain a child with an acid–base imbalance until the primary disorder resolves. These may include:
    a. Providing adequate hydration
    b. Replacing electrolytes
    c. Correcting the acid–base imbalance

II. Dehydration

A. Description

  1. Dehydration is the excessive loss of water from the body tissues. It is a common disturbance in infants and children whenever total fluid output exceeds total fluid intake.

  2. Dehydration can be classified by degree or type.
    a. **Degree**. Dehydration can be mild, moderate, or severe.
      (1) **Mild dehydration** is characterized by a loss of up to 5% of preillness weight.
      (2) **Moderate dehydration** is characterized by a loss of 5% to 10% of preillness weight.
      (3) **Severe dehydration** is characterized by a loss of more than 10% of preillness weight.
    b. **Type**. There are three types of dehydration—isotonic, hypertonic, and hypotonic.
      (1) **Isotonic dehydration** is characterized by electrolyte and water deficits occurring in approximately balanced proportions. It is the most common type of dehydration (accounting for about 70% of the dehydration cases linked to diarrhea in infants).
      (2) **Hypertonic dehydration** is characterized by water loss exceeding electrolyte loss. It accounts for about 20% of dehydration cases related to severe diarrhea in infants.
      (3) **Hypotonic dehydration** is characterized by electrolyte loss exceeding water loss. In infants, it accounts for 10% of dehydration cases resulting from severe diarrhea.

B. Etiology

  1. Dehydration may result from insensible water loss from the skin and respiratory tract, increased renal and gastrointestinal (GI) excretion of fluids, or decreased intake of fluids.

  2. Possible causes of dehydration include:
    a. Excessive vomiting and diarrhea
    b. Insufficient fluid intake
    c. Diabetic ketoacidosis
    d. Severe burns
    e. Prolonged high fever
    f. Hyperventilation

C. Pathophysiology depends on the type of dehydration.

  1. Isotonic dehydration
    a. The major fluid loss involves extracellular components and circulating blood volume, making the child susceptible to hypovolemic shock.

b. Serum sodium (Na^+) level decreases or remains within normal range; chloride (Cl^-) level decreases; and potassium (K^+) level stays normal or decreases.

2. Hypertonic dehydration

a. The excessive loss of water compared to electrolytes results in fluid shifts from the intracellular to the extracellular compartment, which can lead to neurologic disturbances such as seizures.

b. Serum sodium (Na^+) level increases; serum potassium (K^+) level varies; and chloride (Cl^-) level increases.

3. Hypotonic dehydration

a. In hypotonic dehydration, water shifts from the extracellular to the intracellular compartments in an attempt to establish osmotic equilibrium, which further increases loss of ECF and commonly results in hypovolemic shock.

b. Serum sodium (Na^+) level decreases; chloride (Cl^-) decreases; and potassium (K^+) level varies.

D. Nursing process for the child with dehydration

1. Assessment findings. Symptoms depend on the degree of dehydration (Table 7-3).

a. **Clinical manifestations**

(1) Thirst

(2) Fatigue

(3) Weight loss

(4) Dry mucous membranes

(5) Decrease or absence of tear production

(6) Poor skin turgor and increased capillary refill time

(7) Sunken eyes

(8) Depressed fontanelles

(9) Decreased urine output

(10) Tachycardia

(11) Tachypnea

(12) Decreased blood pressure

(13) Excessive thirst

b. **Laboratory and diagnostic study findings**

(1) Urinalysis will reveal concentrated urine with high specific gravity (>1.030) and high osmolarity.

TABLE 7-3

Clinical Findings According to Degree of Dehydration

	DEGREE OF DEHYDRATION		
SIGN	MILD	MODERATE	SEVERE
Fluid loss	<5%	5–9%	≥10%
Skin color	Pale	Gray	Mottled
Skin turgor	Decreased	Poor	Very poor
Mucous membranes	Dry	Very dry	Parched
Urine output	Decreased	Oliguria	Marked oliguria
Blood pressure	Normal	Normal or lowered	Lowered
Pulse rate	Normal or increased	Increased	Rapid and thready

Adapted from Wong, D. L. (1999). Whaley and Wong's Nursing Care of Infants and Children (6th ed., p. 1290). St. Louis: C.V. Mosby.

    (2) Complete blood count (CBC) will reveal elevated hematocrit.

    (3) Blood urea nitrogen (BUN) level is elevated.

    (4) **Electrolyte studies** will reveal decreased urine sodium concentration and altered serum electrolyte (eg, Na^+, K^+, Cl^-) values.

    (5) Arterial blood gases (ABGs) will indicate a low serum pH value (if the child is acidotic).

2. **Nursing diagnosis.** Fluid volume deficit

3. **Planning and outcome identification.** The child will attain and maintain adequate hydration status.

4. **Implementation. Restoring and maintaining adequate hydration are the primary goals of the nurse.**

    a. Obtain an accurate initial weight and monitor weight changes, indicating fluid gains and losses.

    b. Monitor and record an accurate fluid intake and output.

    c. Administer intravenous (IV) fluids. Replacement with IV fluids is required whenever a child is unable to meet daily losses, replace deficits, or replace ongoing losses.

        (1) Initial replacement consists of a bolus of an isotonic electrolyte solution given at a rate of 20 to 30 mL/kg. This phase is contraindicated in hypertonic dehydration due to the risk of water intoxication.

        (2) Subsequent therapy is used to replace fluid and electrolyte losses. The selected solution is usually a saline solution containing 5% dextrose. The selection is based on the probable type and cause of dehydration.

        (3) Sodium bicarbonate may be added to the IV solution to correct acidosis. Potassium is not added to the IV line until kidney function is ensured (the child voids).

        (4) Monitor IV replacement therapy and check the IV site frequently.

        (5) Teach parents how to position, move, and care for a child with an IV line.

    d. Administer oral rehydration therapy (ORT) and other fluids, as prescribed, to correct fluid balance. Offer oral fluids in small quantities (eg, 1–2 oz every hour).

    e. Withhold a full diet until the child is well hydrated and the underlying problem is under control.

    f. Gradually reintroduce the child to a regular diet, as prescribed, and monitor the child's response.

5. **Outcome evaluation.** The child attains and maintains adequate hydration status as evidenced by weight gain, normal skin color and tone, and normal electrolyte values.

III. Diarrhea

A. Description

1. Diarrhea is the frequent passage of loose, abnormally watery stools. Diarrhea may be mild, moderate, or severe; acute or chronic; inflammatory or noninflammatory. The disorder is a manifestation of abnormal water and electrolyte transport.

2. Acute diarrhea is differentiated from chronic diarrhea by the fact that it lasts fewer than 3 weeks in children or 4 weeks in infants.

3. Acute diarrhea is one of the most common problems in children younger than 5 years of age and is the leading cause of death in children of developing countries.

B. Etiology

1. **Acute diarrhea**

    a. Rotavirus is the most common cause of acute nonbacterial diarrhea (gastroenteritis).

  b. Bacterial causes of acute diarrhea include *Escherichia coli* and *Salmonella* and *Shigella* organisms. Diarrhea from *Clostridium difficile* toxin may follow antibiotic therapy.

  c. Other causes of acute diarrhea include other infections (eg, upper respiratory and urinary tract infections), overfeeding, antibiotics, ingested toxins, irritable bowel syndrome, enterocolitis, and lactose intolerance.

 2. Chronic diarrhea usually is associated with one or more of the following:

  a. Malabsorption syndromes

  b. Anatomic defects

  c. Allergic reactions

  d. Lactose intolerance

  e. Inflammatory response

  f. Immunodeficiency

  g. Motility disorders

  h. Endocrine disorders

  i. Parasites

  j. Chronic nonspecific diarrhea

 3. Predisposing factors of diarrhea include young age, malnutrition, chronic disease, use of antibiotics, contaminated water, poor sanitation or hygiene, improper food preparation and storage, and travel to underdeveloped areas.

C. Pathophysiology depends on the cause of diarrhea.

 1. Bacterial enterotoxins invade and destroy intestinal epithelial cells, stimulating fluid and electrolyte secretion from the mucosal crypt cell.

 2. Viral destruction of the mucosal cells of the villi results in a decreased capacity for fluid and electrolyte absorption due to a smaller intestinal surface area.

 3. The pathophysiology of chronic diarrhea depends on the underlying cause. See the section on celiac disease as an example of diarrhea caused by a malabsorption disorder.

D. Nursing process for the child with diarrhea

 1. Assessment findings

  a. **Associated findings**

   (1) History of possible exposure to infection, contaminated foods, or other causative agents

   (2) History of allergies

   (3) Recent travel (especially to developing countries)

   (4) Child's dietary habits, such as overfeeding

  b. **Clinical manifestations** are based on the severity of diarrhea.

   (1) Mild diarrhea is characterized by a few loose stools without other symptoms.

   (2) Moderate diarrhea is characterized by several loose or watery stools, elevated temperature, vomiting and irritability (possibly), no signs of dehydration (usually), and weight loss or failure to gain weight.

   (3) Severe diarrhea is characterized by numerous stools, signs of moderate to severe dehydration, drawn appearance, weak cry, irritability, purposeless movements, inappropriate responses, and, possibly, lethargic, moribund, or comatose appearance.

   (4) Associated symptoms may include fever, nausea, vomiting, and cough.

  c. **Laboratory and diagnostic study findings.** Extensive testing is unnecessary for uncomplicated diarrhea without dehydration.

   (1) Stool analysis may reveal:

    (a) Polymorphonuclear leukocytes, which differentiate bacterial infections from viral infections

(b) Stool culture positive for offending organisms (eg, *C. difficile* toxin, ova, parasites, and viruses)

(2) Enzyme-linked immunosorbent assay (ELISA) can confirm the presence of rotavirus in the stool

(3) Stool pH value under 6 and presence of **reducing substances** suggests carbohydrate malabsorption.

(4) Serum electrolytes and a urinalysis are performed to assess hydration status. See Section II.D.1.b. for dehydration discussion.

(5) ABGs may reveal metabolic acidosis.

2. Nursing diagnoses
a. Fluid volume deficit
b. Altered nutrition: less than body requirements
c. Risk for infection
d. Impaired skin integrity

3. Planning and outcome identification
a. The child will exhibit signs of rehydration.
b. The child will consume adequate nourishment.
c. The child does not exhibit signs of infection and does not transmit infection to others.
d. The child's skin remains intact.

4. Implementation
a. **Reinstate adequate hydration status.**
   (1) Administer ORT for moderate and severe diarrhea and dehydration.
   (2) Administer IV fluids for severe diarrhea and dehydration. A solution of 5% dextrose and normal saline is usually administered. An initial bolus of 20 to 30 mL/kg is given, and IV fluids are usually given for the first 24 hours.
   (3) Monitor fluid intake and output and daily weights.
b. **Ensure adequate nourishment.**
   (1) Observe and record the child's tolerance of feedings.
   (2) Administer ORT, followed by early reintroduction to nutrients. Breast-fed infants should continue breast-feeding.
   (3) Reintroduce nutrients early. Avoid a BRAT (bananas, rice cereal, apples, toast) diet. This type of diet is low in energy, electrolytes and protein, and high in carbohydrates.
c. **Prevent infection.**
   (1) Maintain enteric precautions.
   (2) Practice proper handwashing.
   (3) Teach the children and family proper handwashing.
   (4) Encourage parents of young infants to have them immunized with the rotavirus vaccine.
d. **Provide skin care.**
   (1) Expose the diaper area to air.
   (2) Change the diaper frequently.
   (3) Keep the area clean; avoid commercial wipes that may contain irritating chemicals.
   (4) Apply ointments as prescribed.

5. Outcome evaluation
a. The child is rehydrated.
b. The child is well nourished.
c. The child is infection free.
d. The child's skin remains intact.

IV. Burns

A. Description

1. Burns are tissue injuries caused by contact with dry heat (fire), moist heat (hot liquids or steam), chemicals, electricity, radiation, lightening, or extreme cold.
2. Burns are classified according to the following criteria:
   a. **Extent of injury** is measured by the percentage of total body surface area (TBSA) involved.
   b. **Depth of injury** is based on the extent of destruction as follows:
      (1) **Superficial partial-thickness** injury (first-degree burn)
      (2) **Partial-thickness** and **deep partial-thickness** injuries (second-degree burn)
      (3) **Full-thickness** injury (third-degree burn)
   c. **Severity of injury** is determined primarily by the extent and depth of injury, but also by location of the injury (eg, a burn to the genitals is always considered a major burn because of the potential for swelling and altered elimination). Based on these criteria, a burn is classified as major, moderate, or minor (Table 7-4). Where a burn is treated depends on whether it is a major, moderate, or minor injury.
      (1) Major injury requires treatment at a specialized burn unit.
      (2) Moderate injury can be treated in a hospital.
      (3) Minor injuries can be treated on an outpatient basis.
3. Children younger than 2 years old have a greater chance of sustaining burn injuries compared to older children.
4. Burn injuries and fatalities from house fires are highest among boys 2 to 5 years old. Common causes of house fires are children playing with matches and other ignition devices, cigarette smoking, and use of alternative heating devices.

B. Etiology

1. Most burns result from contact with thermal agents such as fire, hot surfaces, and hot liquids.
2. Electrical burns usually result from small children inserting a conductive object into electrical outlets or biting electrical cords. Serious electrical trauma results from a current passing through organs, muscle, and nerve or vascular pathways.
3. Chemical burns result from contact with agents such as acids, alkali, and organic compounds, which cause chemical disruption and alteration of the physical properties of the burned area. There is also a possibility of systemic toxicity.
4. Sunlight and medical therapies can result in radiation burns.
5. Child abuse is another source of burns in young children. Immersion burns (hot water) are most common, followed by contact burns (cigarettes).

TABLE 7-4
American Burn Association Grading of Burn Severity

BURN TYPE	MINOR	MODERATE	MAJOR
Second degree (partial thickness)	<15% TBSA, adult <10% TBSA, child	15–25% TBSA, adult 10–20% TBSA, child	>25% TBSA, adult >20% TBSA, child
Third degree (full thickness)	<2% TBSA, adult	2–10% TBSA, adult	>10% TBSA

TBSA, total body surface area.

American Burn Association (1976). American Burn Association Committee on Specific Optimal Criteria for Hospital Resources for Care of Patients with Burn Injury. *San Antonio, TX: Author.*

C. **Pathophysiology**. Local damage occurs with all burns, but systemic damage usually only occurs with severe burns.

   1. Local damage depends on the degree of the burn.

      a. **First-degree (superficial partial-thickness) burns** result in destruction of the epidermis. Physiologic functions remain intact and tissue damage is minimal. The damaged epithelium peels off in about 5 to 10 days without scarring.

      b. **Second-degree burns**

         (1) **Partial-thickness** injuries result in destruction of the epidermis and some of the dermis. Capillary damage occurs. This type of burn usually heals spontaneously in about 14 days through the generative capacity of the stratum germinativum and epithelial cells of the lining of the skin appendages. Scarring is minimal.

         (2) **Deep partial-thickness** injuries result in destruction of the epidermis and dermis. These heal more slowly by regeneration from the epithelial lining of skin appendages, sweat glands, and hair follicles. This type of burn may require months to heal and scarring is common. Edema can be significant in deep partial-thickness burns, resulting in **compartment syndrome** (a condition that compromises circulation and entraps nerves).

      c. **Third-degree (full-thickness) burns** result in destruction of the epidermis, dermis, and the underlying tissue, which may include fascia, muscle, tendon, and bone. These burns will not heal without treatment and require skin grafting. Autograft scarring can be minimized by early excision and grafting.

   2. Systemic damage. Severe burns cause systemic damage, including:

      a. **Respiratory compromise**. Inhalation injury leads to swelling in the tissues of the throat and upper airway within minutes of injury. The edema remains for 2 to 5 days.

      b. **Burn shock**. Hypovolemic shock can occur when burns affect more than 15% to 20% of TBSA. Its mechanisms are not well understood, but the sequence of major burn injury followed by massive capillary leakage into surrounding tissue is well recognized.

      c. **Growth retardation.** Growth hormone levels are suppressed after a major burn injury.

      d. **Accelerated metabolic rate.** Energy expenditure increases from 40% to 100% above basal levels. This is associated with increased catecholamine levels, hyperglycemia, and increased nutritional needs.

      e. **Local infection and sepsis.** Burns create moist, warm environments for bacteria, including the body's own flora. Gram-positive organisms, such as *Staphylococcus*, and gram-negative organisms, particularly *Pseudomonas aeruginosa*, colonize by the third day.

D. **Nursing process for the child with a burn**

   1. Assessment findings. Findings depend on the depth and severity of the burn.

      a. **Clinical manifestations**

         (1) **First-degree burns** (superficial partial-thickness burns) are characterized by:

            (a) Dry skin surface

            (b) Red skin color; skin that blanches on pressure and refills

            (c) Minimal to no edema

            (d) Blisters that appear after 24 hours

            (e) Pain and touch sensitivity

         (2) **Second-degree burns**

            (a) Partial-thickness injuries are characterized by:

               (i) Moist skin surface

        (ii) Red to pale ivory skin color

        (iii) Edema

        (iv) Blisters that form within minutes and are thin walled and fluid filled

        (v) Moderate pain

    (b) Deep partial-thickness injuries are characterized by:

        (i) Dry skin surface

        (ii) Mottled, waxy white skin color

        (iii) Edema

        (iv) Flat, dehydrated, and tissue paper-like blisters (common); fluid-filled blisters (possible)

        (v) Moderate pain with severe pain on exposure to air or water

  (3) **Third-degree (full-thickness) burns** are characterized by:

    (a) Dry, leathery skin surface

    (b) Cherry red, white or black skin color; skin that does not blanch on pressure

    (c) Edema

    (d) Blisters (rare, but may have dehydrated); skin that has a tissue paper-like appearance

    (e) No pain in burn area due to nerve ending destruction; very painful surrounding areas

  (4) **Severe burns** will cause systemic clinical manifestations, which include:

    (a) **Respiratory compromise and distress** is manifested by head bobbing with respiratory effort, nasal flaring, abdominal breathing, coughing, stridor, or wheezing.

    (b) **Burn (hypovolemic) shock** is manifested by hypotension, increased heart and respiratory rates, weak, thready, or absent peripheral pulses, prolonged capillary refill, and cool extremities.

    (c) **Fluid and electrolyte imbalance** is manifested by signs of fluid deficit (ie, increased pulse, decreased urine output, and restlessness).

    (d) **Growth retardation** can be exhibited by a growth lag that continues as long as 3 years in some children.

    (e) **Accelerated metabolic rate (hypermetabolism)** is characterized by increased core body temperature and increased nutritional needs.

    (f) **Signs of local infection and sepsis** include disorientation, temperature above 103°F (39.5°C), hypothermia, tachypnea, and abdominal distention or signs of ileus. Infection in a second-degree burn will convert the injury to a third-degree burn.

  b. **Laboratory and diagnostic study findings**

    (1) Fasting blood glucose is elevated due to altered glucose metabolism.

    (2) CBC reveals initial elevation of hematocrit from hemoconcentration.

    (3) Electrolyte studies will reveal hyponatremia (low sodium), which is caused by a sodium shift from the intravascular to the interstitial spaces, and hyperkalemia (elevated potassium), which is caused by cell lysis.

    (4) ABGs will indicate metabolic acidosis due to hypovolemia and cell damage.

2. Nursing diagnoses

  a. Altered tissue perfusion

  b. Risk for infection

  c. Impaired skin integrity

  d. Pain

  e. Risk for fluid volume deficit

  f. Risk for ineffective thermoregulation

g. Altered nutrition: less than body requirements
h. Impaired physical mobility
i. Body image disturbance
j. Altered family processes

3. **Planning and outcome identification**
   a. The child will retain optimal functioning, including good respiratory and metabolic status, and circulation to distal regions of affected extremities.
   b. The child will exhibit no evidence of infection.
   c. The child will exhibit wound healing and maintain integrity of the graft site.
   d. The child will experience a reduction in pain.
   e. The child will maintain an adequate hydration status.
   f. The child will maintain normal thermoregulation.
   g. The child will receive optimal nourishment.
   h. The child will achieve optimal physical functioning and minimal scarring.
   i. The child and family will receive adequate emotional support.
   j. The child and family will be prepared for discharge.

4. **Implementation.** The information below is related to care for major burns. See Child and Family Teaching 7-1 for minor burn care.
   a. **Assess for signs of respiratory distress, burn shock, fluid and electrolyte imbalance, altered metabolism, and infection** (as noted above). **Assess for signs of vascular heat loss** (coolness, acrocyanosis, and mottling).
   b. **Administer prescribed medications,** including:
      (1) Tetanus prophylaxis
      (2) Topical or IV antimicrobials and antibiotics (IV antibiotics are used for systemic sepsis; they are not used for localized infection because there is no blood supply to the wound to deliver the medication.)
      (3) Analgesics (to control the pain of both the burn and the painful procedures)
      (4) Antipruritics and soothing lotions (to control itching)
      (5) Vitamins A, B, and C and iron and zinc (to facilitate wound healing and epithelialzation)
      (6) Antipyretics (for fever control)
   c. **Promote optimal circulation to distal regions of the affected area.**
      (1) Monitor for signs of compression, which are numbness, tingling, color changes, and temperature changes.
      (2) Assess diminished pulses and prolonged capillary refill. Perform frequent Doppler ultrasonography checks.
      (3) Position extremity so that it is elevated above the level of the heart.
      (4) Avoid using restrictive dressings.

CHILD AND FAMILY TEACHING 7-1

Minor Burn Care

- Cleanse the wound with mild soap and tepid water.
- Cover the wound with antimicrobial ointment and a fine mesh dressing or an occlusive dressing (practitioner preference varies).
- Monitor for infection (child may be seen in ambulatory site for regular monitoring).
- Call health provider if child exhibits signs of wound infection or systemic reaction, such as fever.
- Continue with follow-up care as scheduled.

    d. **Prevent infection and promote wound healing.**
  (1) Maintain infection control precautions according to institutional policy.
  (2) Maintain careful handwashing.
  (3) Debride the eschar (slough produced by burn), crust, and blisters.
  (4) Avoid patient contact with infected persons.
  (5) Cover the wound according to protocol.
  (6) Obtain baseline and serial wound cultures.
  (7) Shave the hair around the wound.
  (8) Thoroughly cleanse the wound and surrounding area.
  (9) Keep the child from scratching.
  (10) Pad burned ears and wrap burned toes and fingers separately.

    e. **Maintain integrity of the skin graft.**
  (1) Position the child to minimize mechanical disturbance to the graft site.
  (2) Maintain splints and dressings.
  (3) Inspect grafts for evidence of hematoma or fluid accumulation.
  (4) Restrain the child, if necessary, to prevent the graft from being dislodged.

    f. **Reduce pain.**
  (1) Recognize that burn pain is overwhelming.
  (2) Position the child to minimize pain.
  (3) Anticipate the need for pain medication.
  (4) Use nonpharmacologic pain techniques, such as guided imagery.

    g. **Maintain an adequate hydration status**.
  (1) Administer replacement fluids.
  (2) Monitor daily weights and fluid intake and output.
  (3) Administer potassium-rich fluids if the child is hypokalemic or potassium-restricted fluids if the child is hyperkalemic.

    h. **Maintain normal thermoregulation.**
  (1) Avoid exposing the child to cold stress.
  (2) Minimize chilling and shivering.

    i. **Promote optimal nutrition.**
  (1) Encourage oral feeding and self-feeding.
  (2) Provide high-calorie, high-protein meals and snacks.
  (3) Make mealtime as pleasant as possible by using foods that the child likes, providing companionship during meals, and providing attractive surroundings.
  (4) Administer enteral feedings as needed.
  (5) Record the child's food intake.

    j. **Encourage optimal physical functioning and minimize scarring.**
  (1) Conduct range-of-motion exercises.
  (2) Encourage mobility whenever possible.
  (3) Ambulate the child as soon as possible.
  (4) Splint the joints in extension when sleeping to prevent contractures.
  (5) Encourage self-help.
  (6) Wrap healing tissue with elastic bandages or pressure dressings to minimize scarring.
  (7) Assist with physical therapy.

    k. **Provide emotional support to the child and family.**
  (1) Convey a positive attitude.
  (2) Encourage parents to participate in the care of the child.
  (3) Arrange for continued schooling.
  (4) Promote peer contact when possible.
  (5) Prepare the family, child, and peers for the child's appearance.

    (6) Encourage age-appropriate activities.

    (7) Encourage verbalization and discussion of feelings.

    (8) Discuss camouflaging aids (eg, wigs, clothing, and makeup).

    (9) Provide diversional activities.

  l. **Prepare the child and family for discharge.**

    (1) Teach about wound care.

    (2) Discuss diet, rest, and activity.

    (3) Discuss how the family will assist the child in reentry into the family.

    (4) Explore the family's concept of the child's abilities.

    (5) Help the family develop realistic goals.

    (6) Assist the family in acquiring the necessary equipment and supplies.

    (7) Reinforce the need for follow-up care.

    (8) Arrange for a referral to community agencies.

5. Outcome evaluation

  a. The child functions at an optimal level.

  b. The child is free of infection.

  c. The child's wounds heal and the graft site remains intact.

  d. The child experiences minimal, or no, pain.

  e. The child is hydrated.

  f. The child maintains normal thermoregulation.

  g. The child is nourished.

  h. The child has minimal scarring.

  i. The child and family receive adequate emotional support.

  j. The child and family understand home care.

STUDY QUESTIONS

1. When assessing the fluid and electrolyte balance in an infant, which of the following would be important to remember?
   (1) Infants can concentrate urine at an adult level.
   (2) The metabolic rate of an infant is slower than in adults.
   (3) Infants have more intracellular water than adults do.
   (4) Infants have greater body surface areas than adults.

2. When assessing a child who is admitted for an aspirin overdose, which of the following would be expected?
   (1) Metabolic alkalosis
   (2) Respiratory alkalosis
   (3) Metabolic acidosis
   (4) Respiratory acidosis

3. When planning care for an 8-month-old infant with dehydration, which of the following interventions would be the **most** accurate for monitoring hydration status?
   (1) Measuring fluid intake and output
   (2) Monitoring daily weight
   (3) Checking electrolyte values
   (4) Assessing skin turgor

4. Which of the following clinical assessments would be **most likely** exhibited by a child with a 12% fluid loss?
   (1) Pale skin color
   (2) Normal skin turgor
   (3) Marked oliguria
   (4) Normal blood pressure

5. A child with second-degree, deep partial-thickness burns to both legs becomes disoriented. The nurse recognizes this as one of the first signs of which of the following?
   (1) Sepsis
   (2) Burn shock
   (3) Hypermetabolism
   (4) Respiratory compromise

6. Which of the following statements by the parents of a child with a minor burn indicates that the nurse's teaching has been successful?
   (1) "We will cover the wound with antimicrobial ointment."
   (2) "We will wash the area with mild soap and cold water."
   (3) "We will leave the dressing in place until our follow-up visit."
   (4) "We will administer acetaminophen if the child develops a fever."

ANSWER KEY

1. The answer is (4). Infants have greater body surface areas than adults, increasing their predisposition to fluid and electrolyte imbalances. Also, infants are unable to concentrate urine at the adult level and their metabolic rate, also called water turnover, is two to three times higher than that for adults. Plus, infants have a greater proportion of fluid in the ECF spaces.

2. The answer is (3). Aspirin is an acid, specifically, acetylsalicylic acid. Therefore, the ingestion of aspirin in overdose results in an acid gain, which can lead to metabolic acidosis. Metabolic alkalosis results from a gain in base or a loss of acid and results in elevated urine pH, elevated plasma pH, and elevated plasma HCO_3 concentrations. Respiratory alkalosis results from an increase in the rate and depth of pulmonary ventilation, which leads to a decreased PCO_2 level and an elevated plasma pH. Respiratory acidosis results from diminished or inadequate pulmonary ventilation, which leads to an elevated PCO_2 level and a decreased plasma pH.

3. The answer is (2). Infants and very young children experience a greater insensible fluid loss. Therefore, obtaining daily weight is the most accurate way to measure a child's fluid loss or gain. Monitoring intake and output, checking electrolyte values, and assessing skin turgor are necessary interventions. However, none of these measures address or can account for insensible fluid losses.

4. The answer is (3). A fluid loss of 12% indicates severe dehydration (fluid loss of >10% of body weight). Therefore, the child would most likely exhibit marked oliguria with mottled skin color, very poor skin turgor, and low blood pressure. Pale skin color would be seen with mild dehydration (fluid loss of <5% of body weight). Normal skin turgor would not be present with any degree of dehydration. Normal blood pressure may be evident with mild or moderate dehydration (fluid loss of 5–9%).

5. The answer is (1). Disorientation is one of the first signs of overwhelming sepsis. Other signs of sepsis include temperature above 103°F (39.5°C) or hypothermia, tachypnea, abdominal distention or signs of ileus. Signs of burn shock include hypotension, increased heart and respiratory rates, weak thready or absent peripheral pulses, prolonged capillary refill, and cool extremities. An early sign of hypermetabolism is fever. Signs of respiratory compromise include head bobbing with respiratory effort, nasal flaring, abdominal breathing, coughing, stridor, or wheezing.

6. The answer is (1). Teaching has been successful when the parents state that they will cover the wound with an antimicrobial ointment. An antimicrobial ointment is used to prevent infection. Washing the area is correct but tepid, not cold, water is used for cleansing. Daily dressing changes and cleansing of the burn area are indicated to prevent infection, avoid scarring, and monitor site for infection. The health care provider should be notified if child develops a fever because the fever may be a sign of infection.

8 Common Psychosocial Problems

Attention deficit hyperactivity disorder (ADHD)

A. Description

1. ADHD is the latest terminology used to refer to a persistent pattern of inattention or hyperactivity with impulsivity. The hyperactivity pattern is pronounced and more frequent in children with ADHD than in other children at comparable development levels.
2. The disorder is classified according to three subtypes.
   a. **Combined type** (most common). The individual has six or more symptoms of inattention and six or more symptoms of hyperactivity and impulsivity.
   b. **Predominantly inattentive type**. The individual has six or more symptoms of inattention but fewer than six symptoms of hyperactivity with impulsivity.
   c. **Predominantly hyperactive and impulsive type**. The individual has six or more symptoms of hyperactivity and impulsivity but fewer than six symptoms of inattention.
3. For most children, the disorder stabilizes in early adolescence and, in most cases, symptoms subside between late adolescence and early adulthood. A few individuals experience the full range of ADHD symptoms into middle adulthood.
4. The estimated prevalence of ADHD is 2.0% to 6.3% of the population.

B. Etiology

1. The etiology is uncertain and may be related to any illness or trauma affecting the brain at any stage of development. Multiple causes are probably involved. Some experts think the disorder has a neurochemical etiology because many persons with ADHD respond to medications classified as central nervous system (CNS) stimulants.
2. Predisposing factors may include exposure to toxins, medications, chronic otitis media, head trauma, perinatal complications, neurologic infections, and mental disorders.
3. Genetic transmission is unknown.

C. Nursing process for the child with ADHD

1. Assessment findings

   a. The behaviors observed are not unusual aspects of typical childhood behavior; the difference is in the quality of motor activity and developmentally inappropriate inattention, impulsivity, and hyperactivity the child displays.
   b. Most behaviors are observed at an early age, but learning disabilities may not become apparent until the child is in school.
   c. The diagnosis of ADHD is based on the following groups of specific criteria proposed by the American Psychiatric Association in the *Diagnostic and Statistical Manual of Mental Disorders* (DSM IV) *(Note: Combined type is based on [1] and [2];*

predominantly inattentive type is based on [1]; and predominantly hyperactive and impulsive type is based on [2]):

(1) Six or more symptoms of **inattention** that have persisted for at least 6 months to a degree that it is maladaptive and inconsistent with the child's developmental level

    (a) The child fails to give close attention to details or makes careless mistakes; often has difficulty sustaining attention in tasks or play; often does not seem to listen when spoken to; and often does not follow through on instructions.

    (b) In addition, the child often has difficulty organizing; often avoids or dislikes tasks that require sustained mental effort; often loses things necessary for tasks; often is easily distracted; and often is forgetful of daily activities.

(2) Six or more symptoms of **hyperactivity** and **impulsivity** that have persisted for at least 6 months to a degree that it is maladaptive and inconsistent with the child's developmental level

    (a) Hyperactivity. The child often fidgets or squirms; often leaves his seat in the classroom; often runs or climbs excessively or during inappropriate times; often has difficulty playing quietly; often is "on the go"; and often talks excessively.

    (b) Impulsivity. The child often blurts out answers before questions are complete; often has difficulty waiting his turn; and often interrupts or intrudes on others.

(3) Some symptoms causing impairment were present before 7 years of age.

(4) Some impairment is present in two or more settings (eg, home and school).

(5) Clear evidence of social, academic, or occupational dysfunctioning.

(6) Symptoms do not occur during episodes of pervasive developmental disorder, schizophrenia, or other psychotic disorder and are not attributable to any other mental disorder.

2. **Nursing diagnosis**. Altered growth and development

3. **Planning and outcome identification.** The child will function at her fullest capacity both at home and at school.

4. **Implementation. Promote full capacity functioning.**

    a. Actively participate in all aspects of managing the child with ADHD.

    b. Serve as a liaison between other health care professionals and educators.

    c. Allow parents to vent their feelings.

    d. Assist parents in understanding the importance and longevity of treatment.

    e. Teach the parents and the child about the nature of the disorder; provide reading material and refer to support groups.

    f. Teach the parents about the treatment plan. Advise them that management usually involves a multiple approach including medication, such as methylphenidate (Ritalin), dextroamphetamine (Dexedrine), magnesium pemoline (Cylert), and tricyclic antidepressants; family counseling and education; behavioral and psychotherapy; proper classroom placement; and environmental manipulation.

    g. Provide education concerning prescribed medications (Child and Family Teaching 8-1).

    h. Evaluate the effectiveness of the medication by questioning parents, child, and teachers and by direct observation.

    i. Assist families in learning environmental manipulation, which consists of using organizational charts, decreasing distractions, and modeling positive behaviors. Encourage consistency both at home and at school.

Medications for ADHD

- Explain that some medications (eg, pemoline [Cylert]) require 2 to 3 weeks to achieve the desired effects; others begin at low dosages, which are increased until the desired effect is achieved.
- Inform parents about possible medication side effects, such as anorexia, blurred vision, and sleeplessness.
- If the child takes methylphenidate (Ritalin):
  - Suggest small frequent meals and finger-food snacks to help compensate for anorexia induced by medication.
  - Reduce sleeplessness by administering medication earlier in the day (before 6 PM).
  - Carefully monitor growth because methylphenidate may retard growth. As appropriate, the health care team may recommend medication "holidays and vacations" on weekends and during the summer or other nonschool periods.
  - Monitor outcomes of complete blood counts (CBC), including platelet counts. These laboratory and diagnostic studies should be performed when the child is on long-term therapy due to the incidence of leukopenia and thrombocytopenia.
  - Instruct parents to not crush time-release capsule forms of the drug.
  - Advise parents and child of side effects, which include nervousness, restlessness, dizziness, impaired thinking, headache, loss of appetite, and dry mouth.
  - Advise parents and child to avoid use of alcohol and over-the-counter (OTC) medications while taking methylphenidate because the combination can have dangerous effects.
- If the child takes tricyclic antidepressants, point out the importance of regular dental care because these medications cause increased dental caries. Meticulous dental care is needed.
- To prevent accidents, warn parents to keep these drugs out of children's reach.

     j. Encourage appropriate placement in classrooms equipped for special training.

     k. Encourage counseling for children and families who demonstrate anxiety or depression.

5. Outcome evaluation. The child functions at her fullest capacity both at home and at school as evidenced by the child's ability to perform self-care activities, cooperate, and participate in academics.

 School phobia

A. Description. School phobia is an abnormal, persistent fear of attending school.

B. Etiology

1. School phobia may be related to dreaded school situations, such as failing examinations; facing gangs, bullies, or overly critical teachers; or giving an oral recital.

2. The child may fear leaving home because of feelings of desertion.

3. A common cause is **separation anxiety**, which is based on a strong dependent relationship between the child and the mother. These children are afraid to leave home; they are not afraid to go to school.

4. Some children have unrealistic expectations of themselves and may feel threatened by challenges.

C. Nursing process for the child with school phobia

1. **Assessment findings. Clinical manifestations** include nausea, vomiting, headache, and stomachache. These symptoms tend to resolve when the child is allowed to stay home from school.
2. **Nursing diagnoses**
   a. Ineffective individual coping
   b. Fear
3. **Planning and outcome identification.** The child will attend school regularly without fear.
4. **Implementation. Foster the child's return to school.**
   a. Collaborate with the child's parents, teacher, and school counselor to determine the cause of the problem and identify possible solutions.
   b. Discuss the problem and possible causes and solutions with the child.
   c. Implement plans to return the child to school. The child should attend school even during resolution of the problem. Keeping the child out of school only reinforces feelings of worthlessness, dependency, and inability to cope.
5. **Outcome evaluation**. The child attends school regularly without fear and copes with underlying separation issues.

 ## Child abuse

A. Description

1. The term child abuse is used to describe acts of commission or omission by caregivers that prevent a child from actualizing his or her potential growth and development.
2. In 1995, child protective services (CPS) determined that more than 1 million children were the victims of abuse or neglect.
3. Different types of child abuse include:
   a. **Physical abuse** is the intentional infliction of injury to a child.
   b. **Munchausen syndrome by proxy (MSP)** is the fabrication or inducement of illness by one person onto another (usually mother to child).
   c. **Emotional abuse** is the deliberate attempt to destroy the child's self-esteem or competence.
   d. **Neglect** can be physical or emotional.
      (1) **Physical neglect** involves deprivation of necessities such as food and shelter.
      (2) **Emotional neglect** involves failure to meet the child's need for attention, affection, and emotional nurturing.
   e. **Sexual abuse** is contact or interaction between a child and an adult when the child is used for sexual stimulation of an adult.

B. Etiology

1. **Parental factors**
   a. Severe punishment of parents when they were children
   b. Poor impulse control
   c. Free expression of violence
   d. Social isolation
   e. Poor social–emotional support system
   f. Low self-esteem
   g. Substance abuse
   h. A history of cruelty to animals

2. Child factors
   a. Temperament ("misfit")
   b. Illness, disability, and developmental delay
   c. No other siblings abused
   d. Illegitimate or unwanted pregnancy
   e. Hyperkinesis
   f. Resemblance to someone the parent does not like
   g. Failure to bond
   h. Problem pregnancy and delivery, or prematurity
3. Environmental factors (all socioeconomic groups are affected)
   a. Chronic stress
   b. Poverty, poor housing, and unemployment
   c. Divorce
   d. Frequent relocation
4. Factors specific to sexual abuse
   a. Anyone can be the abuser, including siblings and mothers. But the abuser is typically a male whom the victim knows.
   b. Offenders come from all socioeconomic levels. Some hold prominent positions; some, especially in the case of pedophiles, have positions working closely with children.
   c. Father and stepfather–daughter incestuous relationships tend to be prolonged, and the daughter is usually reluctant to disclose the relationship. The eldest daughter is usually the victim.
   d. Incestuous abuse typically occurs at a later age than other forms of child abuse.
   e. Males are victims of both intrafamilial and extrafamilial abuse, but are less likely than females to report it. In addition, they suffer greater emotional harm from incest than female victims do.

C. Nursing process for the abused child

1. Assessment findings
   a. **Clinical manifestations** depend on the type of abuse.
      (1) **Physical abuse**
         (a) **Physical indicators** include cutaneous injuries (eg, different stages of bruises in odd locations, possibly shaped like the object responsible for the bruise); burns (eg, cigarette marks or "glove-stocking marks"); fractures (eg, femoral spiral fracture in an infant); head injuries (especially in a young child); eye injuries (eg, conjunctival hemorrhages seen in "shaken baby syndrome"); mouth injuries; poisonings; drownings; or repetitive accidents.
         (b) **Behavioral indicators** include wariness of adults, fear of parents, suffers pain without crying, afraid to go home, superficial relationships, overly friendly, reports injury by parents, or exhibits attention-seeking behaviors.
      (2) **MSP**
         (a) MSP is difficult to confirm.
         (b) **Indicators** include unexplained, prolonged, or extremely rare illnesses; discrepancies between history and clinical findings; illness that is unresponsive to treatment; symptoms that occur only when the parent is present; parent overly interested in health care team members; parent overly attentive to the child; or family members with similar symptoms.
         (c) **Common presentations** include (*Note: Most of the presentations below can be fabricated as well as actually induced.*):
            (i) Apnea, which may be due to suffocation, drugs, or poisons
            (ii) Seizures, which may be due to drugs, poisons, or asphyxiation

(iii) Bleeding, which may be caused by adding blood to urine and vomitus, or by opening an intravenous (IV) line

(iv) Fever and infection, which can be due to injection of feces, saliva, or contaminated water into the child

(v) Vomiting, which can be induced with poisons

(vi) Diarrhea, which can be induced by laxatives

(3) **Emotional abuse**

(a) **Physical indicators** include failure to thrive (FTT), developmental lags, feeding problems, enuresis, or sleep problems.

(b) **Behavioral indicators** include habit disorders (eg, rocking, biting, and hair pulling), withdrawal, unusual fearfulness, conduct problems, behavioral extremes (eg, very passive or very aggressive), age-inappropriate behaviors, or attempted suicide.

(4) **Neglect**

(a) **Physical indicators** include FTT, malnutrition, constant hunger, poor hygiene, inappropriate clothing, bald patches on infant, lack of adequate supervision, abandonment, or poor health care.

(b) **Behavioral indicators** include dull, inactive infant, begging or stealing food, school attendance problems (eg, arrives early and leaves late), drug and alcohol abuse, delinquency, or reports of no caretaker.

(5) **Sexual abuse**

(a) In many cases, there are no overt signs of sexual abuse.

(b) Possible **physical indicators** include difficulty walking or sitting; torn, stained, and bloody underclothes; gross evidence of trauma in the genital, oral, or anal regions; pain; itching; sexually transmitted diseases (STDs); genital discharge; pregnancy; weight loss; eating disorders; or vague somatic complaints.

(c) **Behavioral indicators**

(i) Indicators in children under 5 years old include regression, feeding or toileting disturbances, temper tantrums, requests for frequent underwear changes, and seductive behavior.

(ii) Indicators in children between 5 and 10 years old include school problems, night terrors, sleep problems, anxieties, withdrawal, refusal of physical activity, and inappropriate behaviors.

(iii) Indicators in adolescents include school problems, running away, delinquency, promiscuity, drug and alcohol abuse, eating disorders, depression, and other significant psychological problems (eg, suicide attempts).

2. **Nursing diagnoses**

a. Risk for injury

b. Fear

c. Anxiety

d. Risk for post-trauma syndrome

e. Altered parenting

3. **Planning and outcome identification**

a. The child will experience no further harm or neglect.

b. The child will experience a reduction in fear and anxiety.

c. The parents will exhibit positive interactions with the child.

4. Implementation

a. **Protect the child from further injury or neglect.**

(1) **Make sure that the child is free from further harm. Remove the child from an abusive environment.**

(2) **Report the incident(s) to the proper authorities.**

(3) Document assessment findings carefully and objectively.

(4) Collaborate with the multidisciplinary team concerning immediate and long-term therapies to prevent further abuse.

b. **Minimize the child's fear and anxiety.**

(1) Demonstrate acceptance of the child during the physical assessment.

(2) Carefully assess the child's emotional status and behavior.

(3) Provide a consistent person to whom the child can relate.

(4) Provide the child with positive attention and age-appropriate play and activities.

(5) Encourage the child to talk about fears and feelings.

(6) Encourage introduction to a foster family if the child is to be placed in one.

c. **Foster positive parenting.**

(1) Work with parents or caregivers on identifying and changing factors that led to the abuse.

(2) Maintain a positive and caring attitude when dealing with parents, and convey a sense of concern.

(3) Teach growth and development, child-rearing practices, and effective discipline.

(4) Encourage use of counseling and support systems.

(5) Promote attachment.

5. Outcome evaluation

a. The child remains free of harm and is not neglected.

b. The child experiences less fear and anxiety.

c. The parents demonstrate positive interactions with the child.

IV. Nonorganic failure to thrive (NFTT)

A. Description

1. In NFTT, the child's weight (and sometimes height) remains below the fifth percentile compared with children of the same age.

2. Failure to gain weight results from a definable cause that is not related to disease.

3. NFTT is seen most often in infants.

B. Etiology

1. NFTT may result from parental deprivation. If so, growth and development should improve with nurturing.

2. Other causes include a parental lack of nutritional knowledge and a disturbance in the parent–child attachment.

3. A disturbance in the child's ability to separate from the parents may cause NFTT if the child refuses food to gain attention.

C. Nursing process for the child with NFTT

1. Assessment findings

a. **Clinical manifestations**

(1) Growth below the fifth percentile, developmental retardation, and apathy

(2) History of difficult feeding, vomiting, sleep disturbance, and excessive irritability

(3) May exhibit "difficult" temperament pattern

(4) Poor hygiene, withdrawn behavior, and feeding problems

(5) No fear of strangers, eye contact avoidance, stiff or flaccid posture, and minimal smiling

(6) May be vigilant of people at a distance and then distressed when they come closer

(7) May be more interested in inanimate objects than people

b. **Laboratory and diagnostic study findings**. Tests are performed only to rule out organic problems.

2. **Nursing diagnoses**

a. Altered growth and development

b. Altered parenting

c. Altered nutrition: less than body requirements

3. **Planning and outcome identification**

a. The child will reach an appropriate developmental status.

b. The parents will exhibit appropriate parenting behaviors.

c. The child will gain appropriate weight.

4. **Implementation**

a. **Promote age-appropriate growth and development**.

(1) Assess the child's present developmental level.

(2) Provide adequate and age-appropriate developmental stimulation.

(3) Foster social interaction and touch.

b. **Foster appropriate parenting behaviors.**

(1) Observe parent–child interaction and temperament; observe parents' general behaviors.

(2) Provide appropriate developmental stimulation.

(3) Teach parents developmental norms.

(4) Encourage referrals for problems such as finances, impaired mental health, inadequate support, or isolation.

(5) Provide positive role models. Encourage participation in support groups.

c. **Provide adequate nutrition.**

(1) Monitor feeding patterns.

(2) Provide age appropriate foods. Supplements such as Polycose or medium-chain triglycerides (MCT) may be added slowly in 2-kcal increments to yield up to 28 or 30 kcal/oz.

(3) Administer vitamin and mineral supplements.

(4) Provide structure during feedings.

(a) Use primary core of staff to feed the child.

(b) Provide a quiet and pleasant atmosphere.

(c) Maintain calmness during the feeding.

(d) Be persistent.

(e) Maintain face-to-face posture.

(f) Introduce new foods slowly.

(g) Follow the child's rhythms.

5. **Outcome evaluation**

a. The child attains appropriate developmental level.

b. The parents demonstrate developmentally appropriate parenting behaviors.

c. The child gains weight as appropriate for age and length.

Adolescent pregnancy

A. **Description**

1. Adolescent pregnancy is a pregnancy that occurs before the age of 19. These pregnancies are usually unplanned and out of wedlock.
2. Mortality is declining, but morbidity remains high (although the incidence of adolescent pregnancy has declined since 1991).
3. Adolescent pregnancy is still viewed as socially, economically, psychologically, and educationally handicapping to the mother.
4. Seven percent of all births are to adolescents.

B. **Etiology**. Various theories explain the causes of adolescent pregnancy, such as earlier sexual activity and ignorance of reliable contraceptive methods.

C. **Complications**

1. Physical complications of teenage pregnancy include premature labor and low-birth-weight infants, high neonatal mortality, iron deficiency anemia, prolonged labor, and fetopelvic disproportion.
2. A pregnant adolescent commonly faces many psychological crises throughout the pregnancy:
   a. Recognizing the pregnancy and informing her partner and her parents
   b. Deciding whether to carry the fetus to term or seek an abortion
   c. Providing financial, medical, and nutritional needs
   d. Dealing with interpersonal relationships at home and at school
   e. Deciding whether to keep the infant or put it up for adoption
   f. Coping with body image changes
   g. Coping with bonding and parenting issues

D. **Nursing process for the pregnant adolescent**

1. **Assessment findings. Clinical manifestations** that indicate pregnancy include cessation of menstrual periods and breast enlargement. Because an adolescent commonly denies pregnancy, early recognition by a parent or health care provider may be crucial to timely initiation of prenatal care.
2. **Nursing diagnosis**. Altered growth and development
3. **Planning and outcome identification**. The adolescent will understand and follow a plan of care.
4. **Implementation**
   a. **Assess for complications of pregnancy**.
   b. **Implement a plan of care,** in collaboration with the pregnant adolescent and her support persons, that includes:
      (1) Prenatal health care
      (2) Proper nutritional intake
      (3) Exercise
      (4) Avoidance of alcohol, nonprescribed drugs, nicotine, and illicit drugs
      (5) Emotional support
      (6) Plans for delivery
      (7) Plans for infant care
      (8) Anticipatory guidance about birth control and future sexual conduct
5. **Outcome evaluation.** The adolescent understands and follows a plan of care that promotes optimal health for both the adolescent and the infant.

VI. Suicide

A. Description

1. Suicide is the term used for destructive, self-inflicted actions that result in actual or attempted self-harm or death; the intentional ending of one's life.

2. Suicide is the third leading cause of death in adolescents.

B. Etiology

1. The common stresses of adolescence, compounded by limited problem-solving abilities, sometimes lead to harmful, life-threatening behaviors. Adolescents who are depressed, psychotic, or substance abusers are at highest risk.

2. Common contributing factors

  a. **Past history factors** include previous suicide attempts, family member or friend who has made an attempt, child abuse, and death of a parent when the child was young.

  b. **Family factors** include conflict, parental rejection or hostility, divorce and separation, relocation, unrealistic parental expectations, and parental indifference.

  c. **Adolescent factors** include hopelessness, depression, substance abuse, impulsivity, difficulty tolerating frustration, feelings of self-loathing or guilt, thought disorder, physical or body image problems, gender identity concerns, and a perfectionist personality.

  d. **Socioenvironmental factors** include access to firearms; isolation; ineffective support system; incarceration; limited social, educational, or vocational opportunities; and exposure to suicides of others.

C. Nursing process for the child with a suicide risk

1. Assessment findings

  a. Depression usually precedes suicide; signs of depression may be overt or subtle.

  b. **Danger signs include:**

   (1) **Lethargy and malaise**

   (2) **Inability to sleep or early morning awakening**

   (3) **Loss of appetite or overeating**

   (4) **Excessive crying**

   (5) **Giving away cherished possessions**

   (6) **Preoccupation with death or death themes (eg, music, art, or movies with death themes)**

   (7) **Statement of intention to commit suicide**

2. Nursing diagnoses

  a. Ineffective individual coping

  b. Hopelessness

  c. Altered family processes

3. Planning and outcome identification

  a. An adolescent who has made suicide gestures or attempts will display improved self-esteem, positive behaviors, and more effective coping and problem-solving strategies.

  b. Family and friends of an adolescent who committed a completed suicide will work through their grief and resolve the loss over time.

4. Implementation

  a. **Assist the adolescent in alleviating feelings of helplessness and hopelessness.**

   (1) Provide information for teachers, parents, and adolescents about risk factors, counseling available to adolescents, and stress-reduction and problem-solving strategies.

(2) Provide crisis intervention for an adolescent who gestures or attempts suicide and plan for family follow-up care. Ensure that the adolescent understands that he or she must cease or not implement this destructive behavior.

(3) Arrange for counseling and hospitalization if necessary; refer the adolescent and the family to a professional therapist who will work with them through the crisis.

b. **Assist the family and friends in coping with loss**. After a completed suicide occurs, counsel the adolescent's family and friends to help them understand and work through their grief.

5. **Outcome evaluation**

a. The adolescent demonstrates improved self-esteem, positive behaviors, and more effective coping and problem-solving strategies.

b. If a completed suicide occurs, the family and friends work through their grief and resolve the loss over time.

Death and dying

A. **Developmental reactions**

1. **Infants and toddlers (0–3 years of age)**

a. Infants and toddlers have no concept of death.

b. Infants and toddlers react to separation and loss.

c. Infants and toddlers respond to changes in caregivers, routines, and caregiver emotions.

2. **Preschoolers (3–5 years of age)**

a. Children see death as temporary and reversible. They may attribute living qualities to the dead (eg, "What do dead hamsters eat?") or see death in degrees (eg, "Just a little bit dead.").

b. Children may believe that they have caused a death or that death is a punishment or a wish fulfillment.

c. Children fear separation and abandonment.

d. A strong possibility exists that children are aware of the seriousness of their illnesses at this age. They also may fear contagion of a terminal illness.

3. **Early schoolagers (6–8 years of age)**

a. Children begin to see death as real and irreversible.

b. Children may view death as destructive, frightening, and violent.

c. Children are often unable to comprehend their own mortality. They may believe that they can avoid death by being good.

d. Children may personify death (eg, "the boogie man").

4. **Older schoolagers (8–12 years of age)**

a. Children see death as final, irreversible, and universal.

b. Children are interested in the details of death and funerals.

c. Children may respond by feeling sad or lonely.

d. Death may be defied by daredevil behavior and jokes.

5. **Adolescents (13–18 years of age)**

a. Adolescents normally respond with grief and reactions. Typical adolescent reactions to death indicate an almost adult understanding and a search for meaning in death.

b. Adolescents are unable to prioritize their losses; therefore, the loss of a friend may be as debilitating as the loss of a mother.

c. Death may seem remote and adolescents typically test the boundaries between life and death with risk-taking behaviors.

B. Nursing process for the child facing his own or another's death

1. **Assessment findings**. When evaluating a child's psychosocial health in relation to death and dying, assessment findings usually focus on the following:

   a. Developmental level of the child

   b. Cultural and spiritual issues

   c. Socioeconomic implications

   d. Support network and family themes

   e. Grief symptoms

   f. "Unfinished business" between the parents and the child

2. **Nursing diagnoses**

   a. Anticipatory grieving

   b. Fear

   c. Anxiety

   d. Pain

3. **Planning and outcome identification**

   a. The child and family will receive adequate support.

   b. The child and family will experience minimal fear, anxiety, and pain.

4. **Implementation**

   a. **Provide support**.

      (1) Assist the family and child to understand the process of death and dying and to maintain a healthy grieving process.

      (2) Discuss the child's experiences with death and dying.

      (3) Use the child's and family's customs and rituals whenever possible; refer to clergy if needed.

      (4) Allow the child and the family to express feelings.

      (5) Determine the need for financial assistance and refer if assistance is needed.

      (6) Mobilize support systems.

      (7) Assist family in completing unfinished emotional business; refer to a specialist if needed.

   b. **Minimize fear, anxiety, and pain**.

      (1) Determine the child's comfort and security measures or objects.

      (2) Decrease anxiety by being honest, involving the parents in the child's care, and explaining all procedures. Provide for constant attendance for child whenever possible.

      (3) Avoid excessive light and noise.

      (4) Provide adequate pain control, which includes both pharmacologic and non-pharmacologic measures.

      (5) Minimize or avoid intrusive procedures.

5. **Outcome evaluation**

   a. The child and family receive adequate support.

   b. The child and family experience minimal fear, anxiety, and pain.

STUDY QUESTIONS

1. Which of the following statements would the nurse expect a 5-year-old boy to say whose pet gerbil has just died?
   (1) "He's not real dead."
   (2) "The boogie man got him."
   (3) "Did you hear the joke about...?"
   (4) "I'll be good so I won't die."

2. Which of the following nursing diagnoses is **most** appropriate for a child with non-organic failure to thrive (NFTT)?
   (1) Ineffective infant feeding pattern
   (2) Ineffective breathing pattern
   (3) Altered parenting
   (4) Risk for injury

3. Which of the following should the nurse suspect when noting that a 3-year-old is engaging in explicit sexual behavior during doll play?
   (1) The child is exhibiting normal pre-school curiosity.
   (2) The child is acting out personal experiences.
   (3) The child does not know how to play with dolls.
   (4) The child is probably developmentally delayed.

4. When assessing a family for potential child abuse risks, the nurse would observe for which of the following?
   (1) Periodic exposure to stress
   (2) Low socioeconomic status
   (3) High levels of self-esteem
   (4) Problematic pregnancies

5. Which of the following would the nurse suspect if a mother administers laxatives to her infant to deliberately induce diarrhea?
   (1) Nonorganic failure to thrive (FTT)
   (2) Munchausen syndrome by proxy (MSP)
   (3) Emotional child abuse
   (4) Medical child neglect

6. Which of the following statements by the parents of a child with school phobia would indicate the need for further teaching?
   (1) "We'll keep him at home until phobia subsides."
   (2) "We'll work with his teachers and counselors at school."
   (3) "We'll try to encourage him to talk about his problem."
   (4) "We'll discuss possible solutions with him and his counselor."

7. Which of the following would require careful monitoring in the child with attention deficit hyperactivity disorder (ADHD) who is receiving methylphenidate (Ritalin)?
   (1) Dental health
   (2) Mouth dryness
   (3) Height and weight
   (4) Excessive appetite

8. When developing a teaching plan for a group of high school students about teenage pregnancy, the nurse would keep in mind which the following?
   (1) The incidence of teenage pregnancies is increasing.
   (2) Most teenage pregnancies are planned.
   (3) Denial of the pregnancy is common early on.
   (4) The risk for complications during pregnancy is rare.

ANSWER KEY

1. The answer is (1). A 5-year-old views death in "degrees," so the child would most likely say that the pet is "not real dead." Personification of death, such as using the term "boogie man," occurs in ages 7 to 9 years. Denying death, such as with jokes, and attributing life qualities to the dead, such as the dead being able to eat, occurs during ages 3 to 5. Thinking that being good will avoid death occurs in children between ages 7 and 9.

2. The answer is (3). Commonly, NFTT is a result of parental deprivation, parents' inadequate nutritional information, or a disturbance in the parent–child attachment. Thus, altered parenting is the most appropriate nursing diagnosis. Implementation focuses on promoting normal growth and development and fostering appropriate parenting behaviors. Feeding problems may be seen as a result of NFTT, but these are related to the underlying problem of altered parenting. Because the cause is not related to a disease, ineffective breathing pattern is inappropriate. The child may be at risk for injury from altered nutrition, but again this is the result of the underlying altered parenting.

3. The answer is (2). Preschoolers should be developmentally incapable of demonstrating explicit sexual behavior. If a child does so, the child has been exposed to such behavior, and sexual abuse should be suspected. Explicit sexual behavior during doll play is not characteristic of preschool development nor symptomatic of developmental delay. Whether or not the child knows how to play with dolls is irrelevant.

4. The answer is (4). Typically some of the factors associated with the risk for child abuse include problematic pregnancies, chronic stress, and low levels of self-esteem. Child abuse occurs in families spanning across all socioeconomic levels.

5. The answer is (2). MSP is a syndrome by which one person (the mother or father) deliberately fabricates or causes illness in another (the child) to call attention to themselves. NFTT is a syndrome in which a child's growth falls below the fifth percentile for nonorganic reasons, such as parental deprivation. Emotional child abuse occurs when an adult deliberately attempts to destroy the self-esteem of a child. Medical neglect occurs when the responsible adult fails to procure needed medical care for the child.

6. The answer is (1). The parents need more teaching if they state that they will keep the child home until the phobia subsides. Doing so reinforces the child's feelings of worthlessness and dependency. The child should attend school even during resolution of the problem. Allowing the child to verbalize helps the child to ventilate feelings and may help to uncover causes and solutions. Collaboration with the teachers and counselors at school may lead to uncovering the cause of the phobia and to the development of solutions. The child should participate and play an active role in developing possible solutions.

7. The answer is (3). Methylphenidate (Ritalin) can suppress growth. Therefore, growth, including height and weight, must be carefully monitored. Dental caries and mouth dryness are associated with tricyclic antidepressant therapy. Ritalin is more likely to suppress appetite not increase it.

8. The answer is (3). The adolescent who becomes pregnant typically denies the pregnancy early on. Early recognition by a parent or health care provider may be crucial to timely initiation of prenatal care. The incidence of adolescent pregnancy has declined since 1991, yet morbidity remains high. Most teenage pregnancies are unplanned and occur out of wedlock. The pregnant adolescent is at high risk for physical complications including premature labor and low-birth-weight infants, high neonatal mortality, iron deficiency anemia, prolonged labor, and fetopelvic disproportion as well as numerous psychological crises.

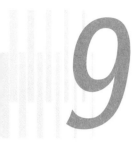

Immune System Disorders

 Immune system

A. Purpose

1. Essentially, the overall purpose of the immune system is to recognize "self" from "non-self" and initiate responses to eliminate "nonself" foreign matter known as **antigens**.
2. The immune system acts to neutralize, eliminate, or destroy microorganisms that invade the body's internal environment before the invaders can multiply or overwhelm the body's defense mechanisms.
3. The immune system must work against invaders (antigens) so as not to harm the host.
   a. Increased immune function (too much immune activity) may damage healthy tissue.
   b. Decreased immune system function (too little activity) increases the risk of infection.

B. Structure

1. All cells have specific cell surface markers called **major histocompatibility complex (MHC)** that are unique to that individual. Markers were first identified on leukocytes and were commonly referred to as human leukocyte antigens (HLAs).
2. The body consists of several complex, overlapping protective systems:
   a. Intact skin serves as the first line of protection.
   b. Secretions such as tears, saliva, and sweat contain chemicals that can kill several organisms.
   c. Stomach acid destroys organisms that adhere to mucous membranes.
   d. Coughing and sneezing eliminate organisms from the body.
   e. If any of these protective mechanisms are penetrated, cellular elements are mobilized.
3. The immune system includes two major components:
   a. The **primary lymphoid organs** include the thymus, bone marrow, and, probably, the liver. The bone marrow produces T lymphocytes (T cells) and B lymphocytes (B cells). B cells mature in the bone marrow and then enter the circulation; T cells move to the thymus where they mature into several different types that are capable of different functions.
   b. The **secondary lymphoid organs** include the spleen, lymph nodes, and gut-associated lymphoid tissue (GALT).

C. Function

1. **Nonspecific immune defenses** activate in a manner similar to any foreign substance.
   a. Offer immediate but short-term protection
   b. Generate symptoms (eg, redness, heat, swelling, and pain)

    c. Occur as a response to infection (eg, otitis media) or tissue injury (eg, sprain, incision, and blister)

    d. Mobilize leukocytes (ie, neutrophils, macrophages, eosinophils, and basophils) in a search-and-destroy type of action known as phagocytosis, whereby the phagocytic cells are exposed, attracted, and adhered to the invader. At this point they ingest and destroy the invader.

  2. Specific (adaptive) defenses recognize antigens and respond selectively (Table 9-1).

    a. **Humoral (antibody) immunity**

      (1) B lymphocytes become sensitized to specific proteins or antigens ("invaders") and produce antibodies directly against specific proteins as follows:

        (a) During antigen exposure, B cells divide and differentiate into plasma cells.

        (b) The plasma cells produce and excrete large quantities of antibodies that are antigen specific.

        (c) Antibodies are **IgA** (viral protection), **IgD** (function unknown), **IgE** (involved in allergy and parasitic infection), **IgG** (bacterial protection), and **IgM** (bacterial protection).

      (2) Initial exposure to an antigen creates the primary antibody response.

      (3) Subsequent exposure to the same antigen creates the secondary antibody response. Memory B cells allow the system to recognize the same antigens for months or years.

      (4) The antigen–antibody complex is formed when the antigen and antibody bind. This aids in phagocytosis by sensitizing it in a way to more readily destroy the antigen (oponization). Antibody activity also mobilizes complement, which is a group of proteins (C1 through C9) that cause a cascade of enzymatic actions that kill the identified antigens.

    b. **Cell-mediated (cellular) immunity (CMI)**

      (1) CMI occurs in the cells and is involved in several specific functions mediated by T lymphocytes.

TABLE 9-1
Development of the Immune System

AGE	STRUCTURE AND FUNCTION
Infant (0–1 year)	The immune system is immature but developing. Phagocytosis is mature, but the inflammatory process is inadequate and unable to localize infection. Antibody protection is chiefly from the mother after fetal life because antibody production ability is limited. Immune development depends on the infant's exposure to infectious agents and foreign bodies.
Toddler/Preschooler (1–6 years)	Antibodies have been developed to exposed organisms, but the child is still susceptible to new ones. Antibody IgG increases, IgA gradually increases, and IgM reaches a mature level. Lymph tissue enlarges.
Schoolager (6–12 years)	Adenoidal tissue reaches maximum size by 7 years of age, and enlarged adenoids and tonsils are normal. IgA and IgG reach adult levels and the immune system is mature by the late school-age period. The thymus reaches its peak mass before puberty.
Adolescent (12–21 years)	IgG reaches adult levels when the adolescent is between 10 and 15 years old. The number of Peyer patches exceeds the adult mean.

(2) T lymphocytes do not carry immunoglobulins, but they have several subsets, which include cytotoxic T cells, helper T lymphocytes, and suppressor T lymphocytes.

(3) T cells can be further differentiated by the distinct molecules on their surfaces, which are known as cluster designations (CDS).

(4) Once mature, they carry markers known as T2 (CD2), T3 (CD3), T5 (CD5), and T7 (CD7).

(5) Helper T cells carry a T4 (CD4) marker and a suppressor, whereas cytotoxic T cells carry a T8 (CD8) marker.

(6) Specific functions of CMI include:

  (a) Protection against most viral, fungal, and protozoal infections, and slow-growing bacterial infections, such as tuberculosis

  (b) Protection against rejection of histoincompatible grafts

  (c) Mediation of cutaneous delayed hypersensitivity reactions, such as the tuberculosis skin test

  (d) Probable immune surveillance for malignant cells

(7) CMI is initiated when a T lymphocyte is sensitized by an antigen.

(8) Once contact is made, the T cell releases humoral factors known as lymphokines that eventually cause the death of the antigen.

(9) Interferons are a group of proteins secreted by leukocytes and infected host cells. They nonspecifically inhibit viral replication, promote phagocytosis, and stimulate the killer activity of sensitized lymphocytes.

3. Types of hypersensitivity reactions

a. A **type I reaction** is an allergic or atopic reaction mediated by IgE. Anaphylaxis, allergic rhinitis, urticaria, and allergic asthma are type I hypersensitivity reactions.

b. **Type II reactions** are caused by activation of the complement system, especially protein fragments C3a and C5a. When aggravated by antigens, they trigger the release of mediators from basophils and mast cells, causing cell damage. Rh hemolytic disease is a type II reaction.

c. A **type III reaction** is an antigen–antibody reaction that affects the vascular endothelium. It is brought about by direct stimulation of basophils and mast cells by foreign agents. An example of a type III hypersensitivity reaction is serum sickness.

d. A **type IV reaction** is a T–cell-mediated hypersensitivity of a delayed type. Contact dermatitis is an example of a type IV hypersensitivity reaction.

  NURSING PROCESS OVERVIEW FOR
The immune system

A. Assessment

1. Health history

a. Elicit a description of symptoms, including onset, duration, location, and precipitation. **Cardinal symptoms** may include:

  (1) Chronic infections

  (2) Fever

  (3) Pruritus

  (4) Difficulty breathing

  (5) Joint pain

b. Explore prenatal, personal, and family history for **risk factors** for immune system disorders:

      (1) Prenatal history risk factors include maternal exposure to human immunodeficiency virus/acquired immunodeficiency syndrome (HIV/AIDS).

      (2) Personal history risk factors include intravenous (IV) substance abuse, sexual activity, and exposure to allergens.

      (3) Family history risk factors include immunosuppression or autoimmune disease.

2. Physical examination

  a. **Vital signs.** Assess temperature for hyperthermia.

  b. **Inspection**

    (1) Inspect the skin and mucous membranes for edema and lesions, including urticaria.

    (2) Observe the face for signs of "allergic facies."

      (a) Allergic shiners are dark circles under the eyes.

      (b) An allergic crease is a line on the nose caused by constant repetition of the allergic salute (ie, the child wipes her nose in an upward motion with her hand).

    (3) Inspect the eyes for periorbital edema and conjunctival redness.

  c. **Palpation**

    (1) Palpate the abdomen for splenomegaly.

    (2) Assess the joints for swelling, redness, tenderness, and decreased mobility.

    (3) Palpate the lymph nodes for adenopathy.

  d. **Auscultation**

    (1) Auscultate the lungs for abnormal breath sounds and adventitious sounds.

    (2) Auscultate the heart for tachycardia.

3. Laboratory studies and diagnostic tests

  a. A **complete blood count (CBC)** may show abnormal white blood cell (WBC) count and differential or an elevated eosinophil count.

  b. **Erythrocyte sedimentation rate (ESR)** and **C-reactive protein (CRP)** may be elevated.

B. Nursing diagnoses

  1. Risk of infection

  2. Altered nutrition: less than body requirements

  3. Pain

  4. Impaired physical mobility

  5. Impaired social interaction

  6. Altered sexuality patterns

  7. Altered family processes

  8. Anticipatory grieving

C. Planning and outcome identification

  1. The child will experience a minimized risk of infection.

  2. The child will participate in family and peer interactions and activities.

  3. The family will be able to meet the child's needs.

D. Implementation

  1. Prevent infection.

    a. Use proper handwashing techniques and observe medical asepsis.

    b. Keep the child away from people with infectious diseases.

    c. Encourage adequate nutrition and rest.

    d. Administer appropriate immunizations.

    e. Administer antibiotics when appropriate.

  2. Encourage activities with family and peers.

    a. Assist the child in identifying personal strengths to build self-esteem.

b. Assist the child in developing coping skills.
c. Allow the child to verbalize fears and concerns.
d. Help the child cope with body image disturbance.
e. Encourage the family to treat the child normally.
f. Encourage the family to foster normal growth and development.

3. Assist the family in meeting the child's needs.

a. Ensure that the family and school personnel have a good understanding of the child's disorder and its therapies.
b. Address the family's fears and concerns either directly or through referrals to appropriate personnel.
c. Reinforce the family's attempts to support the child.
d. Encourage the family to use other family members to assist with the child's needs.
e. Assess and support the family's learning needs.
f. Include the family in planning and problem-solving.
g. Refer the family to appropriate community agencies.

E. Outcome evaluation

1. The child experiences minimal infection.
2. The child participates in family and peer interactions and activities as appropriate for age and within the limits of the disorder.
3. The family is able to meet the child's physical and emotional needs.

III. **Human immunodeficiency virus (HIV) and acquired immunodeficiency syndrome (AIDS)**

A. Description

1. HIV causes a broad spectrum of disease and varied clinical courses. AIDS is the most severe end of the spectrum.
2. AIDS in children and adolescents accounts for approximately 2% of all reported AIDS cases in the United States. However, the numbers are increasing. The majority of children with HIV infection are less than 7 years of age.

B. Etiology

1. The predominant modes of transmission in children and adolescents are:
a. **Mother-to-infant transmission**. The risk of contracting HIV for an infant of an HIV-positive mother is 15% to 30%. Transmission occurs through one of the following ways:
(1) Via placental spread perinatally
(2) Exposure to blood and mucous membranes during delivery
(3) Breast-feeding (possibly)
b. **Sexual contact** (both homosexual and heterosexual)
c. **Transfusion of blood, blood components, or clotting factor concentrates**. This is now a rare mode of transmission. However, 11% to 13% of HIV-infected children were infected by blood transfusions (especially hemophiliacs receiving clotting factor) before 1985.

2. Most infected children are born to families where one or both parents are infected with HIV. The remainder of infected children includes children who received contaminated blood and blood products, children who have been sexually abused, or adolescents with adult risk factors (sexual transmission and IV drug abuse). The number of adolescents who are HIV positive is rapidly increasing.

C. Pathophysiology

1. AIDS is caused by infection with HIV, a retrovirus that produces lymphopenia and an inversion of the normal helper to suppressor lymphocytes.
2. Immunosuppression is the result of functional defects and a decrease in the number of CD4 T cells.
3. Helper T cells control B-cell function; therefore, young children with HIV are deficient in both cellular and humoral immunity. Abnormal B-cell function is apparent early in pediatric HIV infection.
4. Immunoglobulins are nonfunctional, leaving the body defenseless to recurrent bacterial infections.
5. Children are also unable to form antibodies after immunizations.

D. Assessment findings

1. **Clinical manifestations.** The incubation period of symptomatic HIV infection is variable and ranges from months to years. Infants who were infected perinatally are usually symptomatic by 18 to 24 months of age. About 20% of prenatally infected children have an accelerated course of the disease and are symptomatic in the first year; most of these children die by 4 years of age.
   a. Failure to thrive and multiple nutritional deficiencies are common.
   b. Lymphadenopathy, hepatosplenomegaly, and recurrent bacterial infections occur in two thirds of HIV-infected children.
   c. Pulmonary diseases occur in two thirds of HIV-infected children and include:
      (1) *Pneumocystis carinii* pneumonia (PCP)
      (2) Lymphocytic interstitial pneumonitis (LIP)
      (3) Pulmonary lymphoid hyperplasia (PLH)
   d. Chronic diarrhea may be primary or secondary to opportunistic gastrointestinal (GI) infections.
   e. Neurologic problems occur in 75% to 90% of HIV children and include:
      (1) Developmental delays
      (2) Loss of milestones and reflexes
      (3) Lack of coordination
      (4) Memory loss
      (5) Ataxia
      (6) Irritability
      (7) Visual disturbances
      (8) Decreased brain growth evidenced by microcephaly
2. **Laboratory and diagnostic study findings**. Diagnosis of infants is complicated by the presence of maternal IgG, which may result in false-positive readings.
   a. Viral assays will detect HIV in virtually all infected infants by 6 months of age. A positive virologic test (such as HIV detection by culture or DNA or RNA polymerase chain reaction [PCR]) indicates possible HIV infection and should be confirmed by a second virologic test as soon as possible.
   b. Enzyme-linked immunosorbent assay (ELISA) and Western blot tests are used in children over 18 months of age because the maternal stores of IgG will be depleted.
   c. Early peripheral smear may be normal; lymphopenia is noted later.
   d. Immune function tests will reveal decreased CD4 counts, increased CD8 counts, and a decreased CD4/CD8 ratio.

E. Nursing management

1. **Prevent opportunistic infections.**
   a. Assess for signs of opportunistic infections. The recommended zidovudine (AZT) chemoprophylaxis should begin as soon as possible after birth, and PCP pro-

phylaxis should be initiated at 4 to 6 weeks of age in all infants of HIV-infected women.

b. Assist in the identification of neonates at risk. The HIV-exposure status of neonates should be established rapidly to improve the chance of longer survival.

c. Administer prescribed medications, including:

    (1) Antiretrovirals, such as nucleoside reverse transcriptase inhibitors (zidovudine [AZT], didanosine [DDI], stavudine, lamivudine [3TC]); nonnucleoside reverse transcriptase inhibitors (neverapine, delavirdine); and protease inhibitors (indinavir, saquinavir, ritonavir, nelfinavir).

    (2) Other medications used to treat or prevent infection. Trimethoprim/sulfamethoxazole (Bactrim/Septra) is used to treat *P. carinii*; gamma globulin administration is helpful to compensate for B-cell deficiency.

d. Administer immunizations against childhood infections. All are recommended except varicella. IPV is used instead of OPV. MMR is given unless the child is severely immunocompromised. Pneumococcal and influenza vaccines are also recommended. Children may still need prophylaxis against childhood infections because antibody production is poor.

e. Promote pulmonary hygiene (eg, chest physiotherapy and deep breathing) to prevent secretions from pooling and causing infection.

2. Provide adequate nourishment.

a. Offer high-calorie, high-protein foods that the child likes. Nutrition supplements may be given. Child should only eat peeled or cooked fruits and vegetables to avoid infectious organisms. Children may also be placed on enteral feedings or hyperalimentation, which will require monitoring.

b. Provide mouth care because of candidal infections.

c. Monitor weight and height.

3. Foster healthy growth and development.

a. Assist the child in maintaining self-esteem, and enhance growth and development by encouraging the child to perform at an optimal level.

b. Allow the child and family to verbalize. Provide support and assist them in developing coping mechanisms.

c. Assist the child and family with the grieving process.

4. Assist the family in meeting the child's needs.

5. Provide child and family teaching (Child and Family Teaching 9-1).

CHILD AND FAMILY TEACHING 9-1

Minimizing the Risk of HIV Transmission

- Clarify misconceptions on modes of transmission.
- Avoid mixing the ill child's secretions with the rest of the family's (eg, separate linens, use a separate toothbrush and separate razor for the adolescent, and do not share eating utensils).
- Use blood and excretion precautions (eg, use gloves to change dressings; clean spills with a 1:10 bleach solution; keep trash in a closed container; flush feces, urine, and other body fluids down the toilet; and use proper container for needles).
- Use proper handwashing.
- Place restrictions on the behaviors and contacts of affected children who bite or who do not have control of their bodily secretions.
- Teach adolescents about safe sex.

IV. Juvenile rheumatoid arthritis (JRA)

A. Definition

1. JRA is an autoimmune inflammatory disorder.
2. It is one of the more common chronic diseases in children.
3. The outcome is variable and unpredictable in individual children. Even in its most severe form, JRA is rarely life-threatening.
4. There are three major forms of JRA:
   a. **Systemic**
   b. **Pauciarticular**. This form involves a few joints, usually less than five, and has three variations—type I, type II, and type III.
   c. **Polyarticular**. This form involves four or more joints and has two variations—type I and type II.

B. Etiology. The cause is unknown, but infectious and genetic origins have been implicated.

C. Pathophysiology

1. The synovial joints are primarily involved.
2. Immune complexes initiate the inflammatory response by activating plasma protein complement.
3. Kinin and prostaglandin are released, increasing blood vessel permeability and attracting leukocytes and lymphocytes to the synovial membrane.
4. Neutrophils and macrophages ingest immune complexes, releasing enzymes and damaging joints.
5. The synovial becomes inflamed, excessive fluid is produced, and thickened villi and nodules are produced into the joint cavity.

D. Assessment findings

1. **Clinical manifestations**
   a. **Systemic**
      (1) Any joint can be involved.
      (2) Extra-articular manifestations include fever, malaise, myalgia, rash, pleuritis, pericarditis, adenomegaly, and hepatosplenomegaly.
   b. **Pauciarticular**
      (1) Joint involvement is usually confined to the lower extremities.
      (2) Extra-articular manifestations include iridocyclitis, sacroiliitis, and eventual ankylosing spondylitis.
   c. **Polyarticular**
      (1) Any joint can be involved; smaller joints are usually affected.
      (2) Systemic symptoms are mild and may include low-grade fever, fatigue, and slowed growth.
2. **Laboratory and diagnostic study findings**
   a. **Systemic**
      (1) CBC will reveal leukocytosis and anemia.
      (2) ESR will be elevated.
      (3) CRP will be elevated.
      (4) RF (rheumatoid factor) is negative.
      (5) ANA (antinuclear antibody) is negative.
   b. **Pauciarticular**
      (1) CBC will reveal mild leukocytosis.
      (2) ESR will be elevated.
      (3) ANA may be positive.

       (4) *Type I*—**HLA** (human leukocyte antigen) **DRW5** is positive.

       (5) *Type II*—**HLA-B27** is positive.

       (6) *Type III*—**HLA-TMo** is positive.

   c. Pauciarticular

       (1) ESR will be elevated.

       (2) RF is positive.

E. Nursing management

   1. Assess joint function and extra-articular manifestations.

   2. Administer prescribed medications, which include those found in Drug Chart 9-1.

      a. Corticosteroids neither cure nor prevent long-term complications and they have numerous side effects. Their use is limited to rare, life-threatening complications (eg, profound anemia and vasculitis).

      b. Immunosuppressive agents are reserved for children who do not respond to conventional therapy.

   3. Relieve pain.

      a. Provide heat (eg, warm soaks, tub baths, whirlpool, or paraffin baths) to painful joints.

      b. Avoid overexercising painful joints.

DRUG CHART 9-1. Medications for Juvenile Rheumatoid Arthritis

Classifications	Used for	Selected Interventions

NSAIDs (nonsteroidal anti-inflammatory drugs)
  acetylsalicylic acid
    (aspirin, ASA)
  ibuprofen (Motrin, Advil)
  naproxen sodium (Naprosyn)
	Inflammation	Administer with food

		Monitor the drug level and assess for signs of viral syndrome (Reye syndrome prevention) for ASA.
		Monitor coagulation studies.
		Monitor and instruct the family on side effects, which include gastric upset, nausea and vomiting, bleeding, and tinnitus (ASA).

SAARDs (slow-acting antirheumatic drugs)
  penicillamine (Cuprimine)
  gold salts (Aurolate)
  hydroxychloroquine
    (Plaquenil Sulfate)
	Inflammation	Promote oral hygiene

		Encourage monthly eye exams.

		Monitor and instruct the family on side effects:
		  D-penicillamine—GI (gastrointestinal) upset, rash, leukopenia, thrombocytopenia, hematuria, and oral ulcers
		  Gold salts—same as above, but no GI upset
		  Hydroxychloroquine—nausea and vomiting, anorexia, diarrhea, and retinal deposits

c. Use nonpharmacologic pain relief measures.

d. Use a preventive schedule of medication administration.

4. Promote adequate joint function.

a. Assist with the physical therapy regimen.

b. Use splints if needed.

c. Use a firm mattress and maintain joint extension to reduce flexion deformity.

d. Use the prone position without a pillow to maintain spinal alignment.

e. Encourage physical activity without excess stress to affected joints.

5. Promote self-care.

a. Encourage maximum independence.

b. Use assistive devices (eg, utensils, modified toys, handrails, and so on).

c. Teach splint application.

d. Include school personnel in the child's plan.

 6. Encourage activities with family and peers.

7. Assist the family in meeting the child's needs.

V.   Allergy (atopy, type I hypersensitivity reaction)

A. Description

1. Allergic disorders occur as a result of abnormal antigen–antibody response.

2. Allergic disorders include, but are not limited to, allergic rhinitis, eczema, and allergic asthma.

B. Etiology

1. Allergies tend to have a familial predisposition.

2. Allergen exposure is necessary to trigger an allergic response.

C. Pathophysiology

1. The immune response is activated when IgE antibodies attached to the surface of mast cells bind with an antigen.

2. Histamine, a slow-reacting substance of anaphylaxis (SRS-A), and chemotactic substances are released.

3. Histamine causes permeability of blood vessels and peripheral vasodilation resulting in vascular congestion and edema.

4. SRS-A causes bronchial constriction.

D. Assessment findings

1. Clinical manifestations

a. **Allergic rhinitis** (symptoms may be acute or chronic)

(1) Watery rhinorrhea

(2) Nasal obstruction

(3) Sneezing

(4) Nasal pruritus

(5) Allergic facies and salute

b. **Eczema** (atopic dermatitis)

(1) Distribution of lesions

(a) Infantile eczema is generalized, especially on the scalp, cheeks, trunk, and extensor surfaces of the extremities.

(b) Childhood eczema is commonly seen on the flexor areas, wrists, and ankles and feet.

(c) Adolescent eczema is commonly seen on the face, sides of neck, hands, feet, and antecubital and popliteal fossa.

        (2) Appearance of lesions

           (a) Infantile eczema is characterized by erythema, vesicles, papules, weeping, oozing, crusting, and scaling. The lesions are often symmetrical.

           (b) Childhood eczema is characterized by symmetrical involvement, clusters of papules or minimally scaly patches, dry and hyperpigmented areas, lichenification (thickened skin with accentuation of creases), and keratosispilaris (follicular hyperkeratosis).

           (c) Adolescent eczema is characterized by the same signs seen during childhood with the addition of lichenified plaques (dry, thick lesions) and confluent papules.

        (3) Other manifestations

           (a) Intense itching

           (b) Dry unaffected skin

           (c) Lymphadenopathy, increased palmar creases, atopic pleats (extra groove of lower eyelid), pityriasis alba (patches of hypopigmentation), facial pallor, allergic shiners, and increased susceptibility to skin infections.

    c. **Asthma** (see Chap. 11)

2. Laboratory and diagnostic study findings

    a. CBC will reveal an increased eosinophil count (in most atopic children).

    b. A radioallergosorbent test (RAST) may be positive for the child's particular allergies. The RAST allows the child's serum IgE to react with specific allergens impregnated in laboratory disks.

    c. Skin testing detects the presence of IgE in the skin or isolates antigens to which the child is sensitive. An allergen is introduced into the child's skin via either a scratch or an intracutaneous injection. If the child is sensitive, a wheal develops, indicating a positive reaction and thus an allergy. The wheal size is graded as 1+ to 4+, or as slight, moderate, or marked.

E. Nursing management

1. Prevent severe allergic reaction or anaphylaxis from skin testing.

    a. Keep a syringe with epinephrine ready.

    b. Monitor the child's respiratory status during and after skin testing.

    c. Keep the child in the health care setting for 30 minutes after testing so that he is there during the time in which a reaction is likely to occur.

2. Minimize itching.

    a. Use distraction.

    b. Administer antihistamines, antipruritics, or topical steroids.

    c. Use wet dressings for children with eczema to keep skin moist. Emollients also may be used.

    d. Dress the child in soft clothing; wash clothes in mild detergents. Avoid rough fabrics and wool.

    e. Bathe the child in an oatmeal solution.

    f. Use a room humidifier to relieve dry skin and irritated respiratory mucous membranes.

3. Prevent infection.

    a. Keep nails trimmed to prevent scratching and secondary infection.

    b. Use elbow restraints if scratching is difficult to prevent.

    c. Maintain good skin hygiene.

4. Assist with hyposensitization therapy (immunotherapy).

    a. Administer subcutaneous injections while the child is in a health care setting that contains emergency equipment.

CHILD AND FAMILY TEACHING 9-2

Allergy Proofing the Home

- Keep the humidity level between 30% and 50% to minimize mold.
- Encase pillows and mattresses with allergen-impermeable cases to minimize mite exposure.
- Do not keep "dust collectors" such as stuffed animals, heavy drapes, and carpets in the child's room.
- Do not have pets.
- Use vacuums and air cleaners with high efficiency particulate arrestance filters.
- Cover the walls with washable paint or wallpaper.
- Wet-mop and wet-dust regularly.
- Avoid odors or sprays such as perfumes.

   b. Have emergency equipment and medication readily accessible.
   c. Keep the child in the health care setting for at least 30 minutes after the injection.
5. **Teach the child and family how to avoid allergen exposure and how to "allergy-proof" the home** (Child and Family Teaching 9-2).

STUDY QUESTIONS

1. Which of the following immune responses is a nonspecific response to invasion?
   (1) Inflammatory response
   (2) Antibody response
   (3) Humoral response
   (4) Cell-mediated response

2. Which of the following identifies the risk of transmission of HIV from an HIV-positive mother to her unborn child?
   (1) No risk
   (2) <13%
   (3) 15% to 30%
   (4) >39%

3. Which of the following interventions would be **inappropriate** when caring for a child with HIV?
   (1) Offering large amounts of fresh fruits and vegetables
   (2) Encouraging child to perform at optimal level
   (3) Teaching family about disease transmission
   (4) Using good handwashing before handling child

4. Which of the following would the nurse include in the plan of care for a child with juvenile rheumatoid arthritis?
   (1) Administration of corticosteroids to decrease joint damage
   (2) Prevention of contractures by keeping extremities in a flexed position
   (3) Vigorous range of motion (ROM) exercises with affected joints
   (4) Application of heat to minimize pain and stiffness

5. When assessing an infant with atopic dermatitis, the nurse notes that the child is scratching herself with her fingernails. To prevent infection, the nurse would avoid doing which of the following?
   (1) Covering the child's hands
   (2) Administering antipruritics
   (3) Using elbow restraints
   (4) Keeping the skin as dry as possible

6. A 16-year-old girl cannot understand why she cannot administer her own immunotherapy injections at home. The nurse's response is based on the knowledge of which of the following?
   (1) There is always a chance of her having a severe allergic reaction to the injection.
   (2) Intracutaneous injections are far too difficult for a 16-year-old to administer.
   (3) Only hyposensitization therapy may be administered outside the health care setting.
   (4) Injections must be administered by persons over 18 years of age.

7. Which of the following tests would be used to diagnose HIV in a 4-month-old child whose mother is HIV positive?
   (1) ELISA
   (2) Western blot
   (3) Virus assay
   (4) Complete blood count

8. When addressing a PTA group, a nurse is asked about the need to disallow children who are HIV positive to attend school. Which of the following statements by the nurse would be **most** appropriate?
   (1) "Since HIV is highly contagious, the children should be withheld from school."
   (2) "The child can attend school, but the child must be isolated from others."
   (3) "There is absolutely no risk of transmission between children at school."
   (4) "The risk of HIV transmission in schools is minimal."

9. Which of the following immunizations would the nurse expect to administer to a child who is HIV positive and severely immunocompromised?
   (1) Varicella
   (2) Rotavirus
   (3) MMR
   (4) IPV

ANSWER KEY

1. The answer is (1). The inflammatory response is a nonspecific response to injury or infection. This response is activated in a manner similar to any foreign substance. A humoral response, also called an antibody response occurs in response to specific antigens. With this response, B lymphocytes synthesize antibodies to specific proteins. Cell-mediated responses are varied but involve specific actions of the T lymphocytes.

2. The answer is (3). Current statistics report that the risk of contracting HIV for an infant of an HIV-positive mother is 15% to 30%. Transmission occurs through one of the following ways: placental spread perinatally, exposure to blood and mucous membranes during delivery, and possibly breast-feeding. The risk of transmission is always present.

3. The answer is (1). The child with HIV is immunosuppressed. Fresh fruits and vegetables, which may be contaminated with organisms and pesticides, can be harmful, if not fatal to the child. Therefore, these items should be avoided. Children with HIV infection should be encouraged to perform at their optimal level to increase their self-esteem. Families need to learn about transmission modes to prevent the spread of infection and to dispel possible myths. Good handwashing, always a means of infection control, plays an even greater role when caring for the child with HIV. Because the child is immunosuppressed, good handwashing decreases the chance of transmitting an infection to the child.

4. The answer is (4). Applications of heat are used to minimize joint pain in JRA. The use of corticosteroids is limited to rare, life-threatening complications (eg, profound anemia and vasculitis). These agents neither cure nor prevent long-term joint damage. Extending extremities, not keeping them in a flexed position prevents contractures. Vigorous ROM exercises with affected joints increases pain and should be avoided.

5. The answer is (4). Keeping the skin as dry as possible increases itching, which, in turn, increases the risk of the child scratching and breaking the skin leading to possible infection. The skin needs to be kept moist. Covering the child's hands, keeping nails short, administering antipruritics, and using elbow restraints if necessary, help to minimize the child's scratching and thereby lessen the chance of infection.

6. The answer is (1). With immunotherapy, there is always a chance of the child having a severe allergic reaction to the injection. Therefore, the injections must be administered in a setting where emergency equipment is readily available should a severe reaction occur. Immunotherapy, also known as hyposensitization therapy, involves injections that are given subcutaneously. Children are capable of administering their own injections once taught how to do so, as demonstrated by children with diabetes mellitus.

7. The answer is (3). The presence of maternal IgG antibodies in infants may result in false-positive readings. Therefore, viral assays are used to detect HIV in virtually all infected infants by 6 months of age. A positive virologic test (such as HIV detection by culture or DNA or RNA polymerase chain reaction) indicates possible HIV infection and should be confirmed by a second virologic test as soon as possible. ELISA and Western blot tests are used in children over 18 months of age because the maternal stores of IgG will be depleted. These two tests do, however, detect maternal antibodies to the virus. CBC results may suggest immunodeficiency, but it does not confirm a diagnosis.

8. The answer is (4). When talking with parents about the possible risk of HIV transmission in schools, they need to be informed that the risk of HIV transmission in schools is minimal. HIV is not highly contagious and there is no need to isolate children with HIV disease. There can be a risk of transmission, especially if child is a "biter."

9. The answer is (4). For the child with HIV, IPV rather than OPV, is administered. Children with HIV may still need prophylaxis against childhood infections because antibody production is poor. However, MMR vaccine is not administered to a child who is HIV positive and severely immunocompromised. Varicella and rotavirus vaccines are not recommended for any child who is HIV positive.

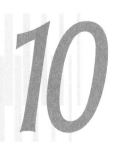

Infectious Diseases

 Infectious process and immunizations

A. Infectious process and the chain of infection

1. A **causative organism** can be any microorganism (eg, bacteria, virus, fungi, and so on).
2. **Reservoir** is the term used for any human, animal, plant, or substance that provides the causative organism with both nourishment and a mode for dispersal.
3. The causative organism requires a **means of exit** from the reservoir. Thus, the host must shed the organism through the respiratory, gastrointestinal, or genitourinary tracts.
4. A **route of transmission** is needed to connect the organism to its new host. Transmission routes include direct skin-to-skin, close contact, or exposure; sexual or parenteral fluids; or infected particles in the air. Different organisms require different routes.
5. The **host must be susceptible** for infection to occur. Young age, organism virulence, and impaired body defenses increase susceptibility to infection. Vaccines and previous infection can render a potential host immune (ie, not susceptible).
6. The organism must gain entry to the susceptible host through a **portal of entry**, such as the respiratory tract.

B. Stages of infectious diseases

1. The **communicability period** is the stage when the disease is transmissible to others (ie, contagious).
2. The **incubation period** is the time between the invasion of the organism and the onset of infection. The organisms grow and multiply during this period.
3. The **prodromal period** is the time between the beginning of nonspecific symptoms, such as lethargy and fever, and disease-specific symptoms. Prodromal stages usually last only a few days, and they are not found in all infectious diseases.
4. The **illness stage** is the period when disease-specific symptoms are manifested. Rashes on the skin are called **exanthems**, whereas rashes on mucous membranes are termed **enanthems**.
5. The **convalescent period** is the interval between the time when the symptoms begin to disappear and the complete return to wellness.

C. Immunizations

1. **Types of immunity**
   a. **Naturally acquired active.** The immune system makes antibodies after exposure to disease.

      b. **Naturally acquired passive.** Antibodies to disease are received passively and naturally (eg, via the placenta and colostrum).

      c. **Artificially acquired active.** Ingested or injected medically engineered substances stimulate the immune response against specific diseases.

      d. **Artificially acquired passive.** Injected antibodies provide immunity without stimulating an immune response.

2. Types of immunizations

    a. **Live attenuated**

        (1) Pathogen is treated with chemicals or heat to reduce the virulence, but not kill, the organism.

        (2) Examples of live attenuated immunizations include the measles, mumps, rubella (MMR) vaccine and the oral polio virus (OPV; Sabin) vaccine.

    b. **Inactivated**

        (1) A toxoid (eg, tetanus, diphtheria) is a bacterial exotoxin that has been treated with formalin or heat, which yields a nontoxic (inactivated), but still antigenic, agent.

        (2) Inactivated viral vaccines (eg, inactivated poliovirus [IPV; Salk], pertussis, Hib, HB) use killed viral organisms, or parts of organisms, to produce immunity.

    c. **Immunoglobulins**

        (1) Immune globulin (IG) or intravenous immune globulin (IVIG) is a solution that contains antibodies from large pools of human blood plasma. It is primarily used for maintenance of immunity of certain immunodeficient persons and for passive immunization against measles and hepatitis A.

        (2) Specific immune globulins are special preparations obtained from preselected donor pools that contain a high antibody content against a specific antigen. Examples include varicella-zoster immune globulin, hepatitis B immune globulin, tetanus immune globulin, and respiratory syncytial virus (RSV) immune globulin (Respigram).

        (3) Contraindications to use include hypersensitivity; safety in pregnancy has not been established.

        (4) Side effects include pain, tenderness, muscle stiffness at site, and possible systemic reactions such as light-headedness, headache, chest pain, nausea, urticaria, and arthralgia.

3. Recommended routine immunizations (Table 10-1). Immunization recommendations and scheduling change regularly. It is recommended that readers refer to the American Academy of Pediatric's Web site for up-to-date information on this topic (www.aap.org).

    a. **Diphtheria**

        (1) Commonly administered with tetanus (in children <7 years as dT) or with tetanus and pertussis (in children >7 years as DaPT).

        (2) Contraindications are previous immediate anaphylaxis or encephalopathy within 7 days. It is not contraindicated during pregnancy, but women should wait until the second trimester.

        (3) There are relatively no side effects.

    b. **Pertussis**

        (1) An acellular form is used that contains one or more immunogens derived from *Bordetella pertussis*. This form is associated with fewer local and systemic side effects. Current licensed forms include Acel-Immune, Tripedia, and Infantrix (diphtheria, acellular pertussis conjugate, and tetanus toxoid; DaPT).

TABLE 10-1
Recommended Childhood Immunization Schedule

RECOMMENDED AGE	IMMUNIZATION	ROUTE
Birth–2 months	HB (1st)	IM
2–4 months	HB (2nd)	IM
2 months	DaPT, Hib, IPV	IM, IM, IM
4 months	DaPT, Hib, IPV	IM, IM, IM
6 months	DaPT, Hib	IM, IM, IM
6–18 months	HB (3rd), IPV	IM, PO
12–15 months	Hib, MMR, Var	IM, SQ, SQ
12–18 months	DaPT or dtaP (at 15 months)	IM, IM
4–6 years	DaPT or dtaP, MMR, IPV	IM, SQ, PO
11–12 years	MMR, Var (if not received at 4–6 years)	SQ, SQ
11–16 years	Td	IM

From the American Academy of Pediatrics (2000) www.aap.org. Approved by the Advisory Committee on Immunization Practices (ACIP), the American Academy of Pediatrics (AAP), and the American Academy of Family Physicians (AAFP).

    (2) Contraindications are previous severe reactions and neurologic problems, such as uncontrolled or poorly managed seizure disorders.

    (3) Side effects can be local, mild, or severe.

        (a) Local side effects include redness, tenderness, and swelling at the site.

        (b) Mild side effects include fever (temperature >105°F), crying, and irritability.

        (c) Severe side effects include a high-pitched cry, fever (temperature 105°F), convulsions, hypotonia, and encephalopathy with brain damage and death.

  c. **Tetanus**

    (1) The toxoid is used for routine immunization. Tetanus immunoglobulin provides passive immunity and is used for wound management.

    (2) Contraindications are previous anaphylaxis or severe reaction.

    (3) Side effects are pain at the injection site and anaphylaxis (rare).

  d. **Polio**. Both the injected and oral vaccine forms are trivalent (ie, containing all three forms of the poliovirus).

    (1) **Inactivated polio vaccine (IPV)** (eg, Salk)

        (a) IPV is currently used for the primary immunization of healthy infants at 2, 4, and 6 months of age, and for children with immunodeficient disorders and their close contacts. Presently OPV is used for the boosters at 12 to 18 months, and 4 to 6 years, of age.

        (b) Contraindications include anaphylactic reaction to streptomycin (IPV is prepared in streptomycin).

    (2) **Oral polio vaccine (OPV)** (eg, Sabin)

        (a) The live, attenuated vaccine is more effective than IPV.

        (b) Contraindications include congenital immunodeficiency diseases, acquired immunodeficiency diseases, altered immune response (steroids, leukemia, or chemotherapy), family members with any of these (OPV may shed in stools and be transmitted to others), and pregnancy.

    (c) Side effects are few if any. However, children vaccinated with OPV risk developing the rare condition called vaccine-associated polio paralysis (VAPP).

        (i) **In an effort to eliminate VAPP, a decision was made to discontinue use of the Sabin vaccine in favor of the inactivated form (Salk).**

        (ii) If this decision is followed through on, the Salk vaccine will be the polio vaccine of choice starting in January 2000.

e. **MMR** (measles, mumps, rubella). The MMR vaccine should be administered after 12 months of age when the effectiveness of maternal antibodies subsides.

    (1) Contraindications include immunosuppression (except human immunodeficiency virus [HIV]), pregnancy, and allergy to eggs and neomycin.

    (2) Side effects include transient rash, pruritus, low-grade fever, and arthralgia and transient arthritis from rubella (especially in adults). The measles vaccine can cause a false-negative tine test (tuberculosis test) result.

f. **Haemophilus influenzae type B (Hib)**

    (1) This immunization protects against a number of serious diseases caused by Hib, including meningitis, epiglottitis, pneumonia, sepsis, and septic arthritis.

    (2) Types of licensed Hib vaccines include:

        (a) Oligosaccharide conjugate Hib vaccine (HbOC; HibTITER) is administered on a four-dose schedule of three primary injections plus a booster at 15 months of age.

        (b) Haemophilus b conjugate vaccine meningococcal protein conjugate (PRP-OMP, PedvaxHIB) is administered on a three-dose schedule of two primary injections plus a booster at 12 months of age.

        (c) Polyribosylribitol phosphate-tetanus toxoid conjugate (PRP-T, ActHib, OmniHib) is not licensed for children under age 12 months.

        (d) ComVax, a combination of Hib and hepatitis vaccines is available to decrease the number of injections that infants receive.

    (3) There are no contraindications and the associated side effects are minor (eg, possible discomfort and low-grade fever)

g. **Hepatitis B (HB)**

    (1) Recommended for universal immunization starting at birth and thereafter as follows:

        (a) Infants born to hepatitis B surface antigen (HbsAg)-negative mothers receive a second dose of HB vaccine at least 1 month after the first. The third dose is administered at least 4 months after the first dose, 2 months after the second, and not before 6 months of age.

        (b) Infants born to HbsAg-positive mothers receive hepatitis vaccine and 0.5 mL of hepatitis B immune globulin (HBIG) within 12 hours of birth at separate sites. The second dose is recommended at 1 to 2 months; the third dose is recommended at 6 months of age.

        (c) Infants born to mothers whose HbsAg status is unknown should receive hepatitis B vaccine within 12 hours of birth. Maternal blood is drawn at the time of delivery to determine status. If the mother is positive, the infant receives HBIG as soon as possible (no later than 1 week of age).

    (2) Children and adolescents who have not been immunized against hepatitis B may begin the series at any time. Three doses are recommended at 0-, 1-, and 6-month intervals.

    (3) Side effects include redness and tenderness at the site (rare).

    j. **Varicella**
- (1) Varicella-zoster vaccine (VZV) is a live vaccine given after 12 months of age. Nonimmunized children over 13 years of age who have not had the disease require two doses, 4 to 8 weeks apart.
- (2) Precautions are the same as those for MMR.

    k. **Rotavirus**
- (1) The rotavirus vaccine is a live vaccine administered at 2, 4, and 6 months of age for the prevention of rotavirus gastroenteritis.
- (2) Contraindications include altered immunity, allergy to vaccine components, acute gastroenteritis, and moderate to severe febrile illness. The rotavirus vaccine should not be given to children of mothers with HIV infection unless the child is confirmed HIV negative.
- (3) The rotavirus vaccine was removed from the market in late 1999. It is presently not in use.

4. Immunization schedule. Children should have most of their scheduled immunizations by the time they enter elementary school (see Table 10-1 for the recommended order of immunizations).

5. General contraindications, precautions, and recommendations
- a. Do not administer immunizations during severe febrile illness.
- b. Avoid giving live-virus immunizations to children with an impaired immune system (the exception is MMR for children with HIV disease) and to children who live with an immunosuppressed person.
- c. Postpone live-virus immunizations for 3 to 7 months in children who have just received passive immunity through blood transfusions, immunoglobulin, or maternal antibodies.
- d. Avoid administering live-virus immunizations during pregnancy and in women likely to become pregnant within 3 months.
- e. Do not give the vaccine if the child is allergic to the vaccine or to any of its components.
- f. Doses of live vaccines must be separated by a minimum of 30 days, but more than one live vaccine may be given on the same day. Shorter intervals limit the antibody response and render the second dose ineffective.
- g. Preterm infants are immunized at appropriate chronological ages regardless of weight.

6. Nonmandatory immunizations
- a. **Influenza virus vaccine**
  - (1) The vaccine provides protection against strains of influenza.
  - (2) It is recommended for children older than 6 months old who have chronic illnesses (such as cardiac or respiratory disorders, renal disease, and diabetes mellitus), HIV disease, and children who are receiving long-term aspirin therapy (risk for Reye syndrome).
  - (3) The vaccine should be administered in the fall and repeated yearly; two doses 4 weeks apart for children under 12 years of age; one dose for those over 12 years of age.
  - (4) It is contraindicated in children allergic to eggs.
  - (5) The vaccine may be given with other childhood immunizations.
- b. **Pneumococcal vaccine**
  - (1) The vaccine provides protection against several strains of *Streptococcus pneumoniae*.
  - (2) The vaccine is recommended for children 2 years and older who have sickle cell anemia, asplenia, HIV, and Hodgkin lymphoma.

(3) The vaccine can be administered via the subcutaneous (SQ) or intramuscular (IM) route; revaccination is not recommended.

(4) The vaccine should be deferred in pregnancy.

c. **Meningococcal vaccine**

(1) The vaccine provides protection against *Neisseria meningitides*.

(2) It is recommended for children 2 years old and older with terminal complement deficiencies and anatomic or functional asplenia.

(3) The duration of protection is unknown; safety during pregnancy has not been established.

II. NURSING PROCESS OVERVIEW FOR Infectious diseases

A. Assessment

1. Health history

a. Elicit a description of symptoms including onset, duration, location, and precipitation. **Cardinal signs and symptoms** may include:

(1) Fever

(2) General malaise

(3) Vomiting and diarrhea

b. Explore prenatal, personal, and family history for **risk factors** for respiratory disorders.

(1) Prenatal history risk factors include a maternal infectious disease history.

(2) Personal history risk factors include an immunization history, history of recurrent or chronic illness, previous communicable diseases and exposure to communicable disease, malnutrition, and eating raw or undercooked meats or seafood.

(3) Family history risk factors include early infant mortality, immunodeficiency, autoimmune disease, or malignancy.

2. Physical examination

a. **Vital signs**. Monitor temperature for hyperthermia.

b. **Inspection**

(1) Inspect the skin and mucous membranes for jaundice and rashes. If a rash is present, note its appearance, location, and distribution.

(2) Observe the eyes for conjunctival redness and discharge.

(3) Inspect tympanic membranes for redness, bulging, distorted landmarks, and immobility.

(4) Assess the tongue, tonsils, buccal mucosa, and pharynx for redness, lesions, and exudate.

c. **Palpation**

(1) Palpate the lymph nodes for adenopathy.

(2) Assess the abdomen for hepatosplenomegaly.

d. **Auscultation**

(1) Auscultate the heart for tachycardia and assess if rate is above the expected level for fever.

(2) Auscultate the lungs for abnormal breath sounds and adventitious sounds. Listen for cough, and note characteristics.

3. Laboratory studies and diagnostic tests

a. **Culture and sensitivity tests** are performed on bodily fluids and exudates to identify organisms and the antibiotics to which they are most susceptible.

b. **Enzyme-linked immunosorbent assay (ELISA)** and **enzyme immunosorbent assay (EIA)** detect viral antigens in body fluids.

c. **Direct fluorescent antibody (DFA) tests** detect specific enzyme-labeled antibodies.

d. A **complete blood count (CBC) with differential** provides a detailed evaluation of the white blood cell count and morphology.

e. The **erythrocyte sedimentation rate (ESR) and C-reactive protein (CRP)** may be elevated during infectious processes.

f. A **lumbar puncture** (spinal tap) is performed to identify organisms in the cerebrospinal fluid.

B. Nursing diagnoses

1. Hyperthermia
2. Altered nutrition: less than body requirements
3. Risk for infection

C. Planning and outcome identification

1. The child will maintain a stable body temperature.
2. The child will have an adequate nutritional intake.
3. The infection will not spread to other family members, and the family will be aware of the necessity of childhood immunizations.

D. Implementation

1. **Maintain a stable body temperature**.
   a. Assess and monitor temperature.
   b. Administer antipyretic medications.
   c. Encourage fluids.
   d. Dress the child lightly unless she has chills.
   e. Give tepid sponge baths (85°–90°F), as needed. Do not use ice water or alcohol.

2. **Promote an adequate nutritional intake**.
   a. Encourage small, frequent, nutritional meals.
   b. Allow the child to eat what he likes and provide nutritional supplementation when needed.

3. **Prevent the spread of infection to others**.
   a. Encourage the family to have children immunized according to the recommendations above.
   b. Administer antibiotics as prescribed (Drug Chart 10-1).
   c. Teach proper handwashing.
   d. Follow appropriate infection control precautions.

E. Outcome evaluation

1. The child maintains a stable body temperature, experiences no discomfort related to fever, and experiences no febrile convulsions.
2. The child maintains an adequate nutritional intake to meet growth needs.
3. Siblings do not develop infection, the family understands the importance of immunizations, and the child is adequately immunized.

DRUG CHART 10-1. Medications Used to Treat Infections

Classifications	Used for	Selected Interventions
Antibiotics	Inflammation	Assess for medication allergies.
		Obtain cultures before administering antibiotics.
		Encourage family to complete entire course of medication.

Cephalosporins
First-Generation
  cefadroxil (Duricef)
  cefazolin (Ancef)
  cephalexin (Biocef)
  cephapirin (Cefadyl)
  cephradine (Velosef)
	Sepsis and meningitis; pharyngitis; tonsillitis; UTI; skin infections; respiratory infections	Assess for penicillin and cephalosporin allergies.
		
		Administer oral medication with food to minimize GI upset.

Second-Generation
  cefaclor (Ceclor)
  cefmetazole (Zefazone)
  cefonicid (Monocid)
  cefoxitin (Mefoxin)
  cefpodoxime (Vantin)
  cefproxil (Cefzil)
  cefuroxime (Kefurox)
  loracarbef (Lorabid)
		Do not crush tablets.
		
		Monitor for side effects: GI upset, hypersensitivity, superinfections, disulfran-like reaction with alcohol.
		
		Assess for superinfection.
		
		Instruct adolescents to avoid alcohol during, and 3 days after, completing medication.

Third-Generation
  cefdinir (Omnicef)
  cefepime (Maxipime)
  cefixime (Suprax)
  cefoperazone (Cefobid)
  cefotaxime (Claforan)
  ceftazidime (Ceptaz)
  ceftizoxime (Cefizox)
  ceftriaxone (Rocephin)		

Macrolides
  azithromycin (Zithromax)
  clarithromycin (Biaxin)
  dirithromycin (Dynabac)
  erythromycin (EryPed)
	Respiratory infections; skin infections; chlamydia infections	Administer on an empty stomach (except erythromycin estolate, ethylsuccinate, and certain enteric-coated tablets
		
		Monitor for side effects: GI upset, uncontrollable emotions, abnormal thinking

(continued)

DRUG CHART 10-1. Medications Used to Treat Infections *(Continued)*

Classifications	Used for	Selected Interventions

Penicillins
  amoxicillin (Amoxil)
  ampicillin (Principen)
  bacampicillin (Spectrobid)
  carbenicillin (Geocillin)
  cloxacillin (Cloxapen)
  dicloxacillin (Dynapen)
  mezlocillin (Mezlin)
  nafcillin (Nallpen)
  oxacillin (Bactocill)
  penicillin G (Bicillin L-A)
  penicillin V (Pen-Vee-K)
  piperacillin (Pipracil)
  ticaracillin (Ticar)
	Respiratory infections
	Streptococcal infections
		Monitor electrolytes and cardiac status if penicillin G is administered IV
		
		Monitor for penicillin side effects: GI irritation, hypersensitivity, and superinfection.

Sulfonamides
  sulfadiazine
  sulfamethizole
    (Thiosulfil Forte)
  sulfamethoxazole (Gantanol)
  sulfasalazine (Azulfidine)
  sulfisoxazole
	Meningitis, UTI, ulcerative colitis, Crohn's disease	Monitor for sulfadiazine side effects: GI irritation, headache, crystalluria, photosensitivity, and agranulocytosis.
		
		Encourage use of sunscreens and protective clothing.
		
		Encourage fluids

Anti-inflammatories Aspirin	Anti-inflammatory effects	Monitor for side effects such as GI disturbance, decreased platelet count, tinnitus, and headache. Warn parents not to use aspirin for pain or fever, and to notify the physician if the child has signs of influenza or varicella due to the association with Reye syndrome when taking aspirin during these illnesses.

Corticosteroids
  methylprednisolone
    (Solu-Medrol)
  hydrocortisone (Solu-Cortef)
  prednisolone (Pediapred)
  dexamethasone (Decadron)
	Anti-inflammatory effects	Monitor for side effects, including fluid retention, edema, hypokalemia, GI irritation, hyperglycemia, altered growth patterns, and Cushing syndrome

(continued)

DRUG CHART 10-1 Medications Used to Treat Infections *(Continued)*

Classifications	Used for	Selected Interventions
Analgesics and antipyretics acetaminophen (Tylenol, Tempra)	Analgesic and antipyretic effects	Avoid using multiple preparations containing acetaminophen.
		Give with food if GI upset occurs.
		Avoid exceeding the recommended dosage.
ibuprofen (Motrin, Advil)	Analgesic and antipyretic effects	Monitor for side effects, which include headache, GI upset, rash, and renal impairment.
	May be used as an anti-inflammatory for certain disorders	Monitor for hypersensitivity.
		Administer with food if GI upset occurs.
		Avoid using multiple preparations containing ibuprofen.

GI; gastrointestinal; UTI, urinary tract infection

 Fever

A. Definition

1. Fever is an abnormally elevated rectal body temperature of at least 100.4°F (38°C). It is a sign of an underlying problem and is not a disease in and of itself.
2. Associated clinical findings provide clues regarding the seriousness of the fever (eg, an active, alert child with a temperature of 104°F [40.0°C] generally is of less concern than a listless, lethargic infant with a temperature of 102.2°F [39.0°C]).

B. Etiology.
Fever most commonly results from disruption of the hypothalamic set point, which can, in turn, be caused by any of the following disorders.

1. Common causes of fever in infants include upper and lower respiratory tract infections, pharyngitis, otitis media, and generalized and enteric viral infections. Vaccination reactions and overdressing are also common causes of fever in the infant.
2. More serious causes of fever include urinary tract infections, pneumonia, bacteremia, meningitis, osteomyelitis, septic arthritis, cancer, immunologic disorders, poisoning or drug overdose, and dehydration.

C. Pathophysiology.
Disrupted thermoregulation leads to increased heat production and decreased heat loss.

D. Assessment findings

1. **Clinical manifestations**
   a. Temperature over 100.4°F, typically 102°F to 105°F (38.9°–40.6°C) measured by the axillary route.
   b. Skin flushing, diaphoresis, and chills
   c. Restlessness or lethargy

2. **Laboratory and diagnostic study findings.** Tests and results will vary depending on the underlying cause of fever.

E. **Nursing management**

1. **Maintain a stable body temperature**.
2. **Administer prescribed medications,** including antipyretics, acetaminophen, or ibuprofen. Aspirin is contraindicated because of the association between aspirin and Reye syndrome (see Drug Chart 10-1).
3. **Teach parents how to take the child's temperature and implement fever control measures.**

IV. Febrile seizures

A. **Definition**

1. Febrile seizures are seizures that are associated with an illness characterized by a high fever (temperature of 102°–104°F [38.9°–40.0°C]). They last less than 15 minutes, are generalized, and occur in children without neurologic disability.
2. This type of seizure affects 3% to 5% of children and usually occurs after 6 months of age and before 3 years of age. Febrile convulsions are unusual after the child is 5 years old.

B. **Etiology**. The cause is unknown. Febrile convulsions are usually associated with upper respiratory tract infections, urinary tract infections, and roseola.

C. **Pathophysiology**

1. Typically, the seizure is characterized by an active tonic-clonic pattern. It usually lasts less than 1 minute and is associated with an acute, benign febrile illness.
2. The convulsion usually results from the rapid rise in temperature, with the initial fever.
3. Febrile convulsions are considered benign if underlying neurologic and physical problems are ruled out.

D. **Assessment findings**

1. **Clinical manifestations**
   a. Most seizure activity ceases by the time the child is brought in for medical attention, but the child may be unconscious.
   b. Parents or caregivers will describe tonic-clonic seizure manifestations (ie, tonic—contraction of muscles, extension of extremities, loss of bowel and bladder control, cyanosis, and loss of consciousness; clonic—rhythmic contraction and relaxation of the extremities; postictal phase is characterized by persistent unconsciousness).
   c. There is often a family history of febrile convulsions.
2. **Laboratory and diagnostic study findings**
   a. Electroencephalography (EEG) is usually normal, ruling out the likelihood of a seizure disorder.
   b. Lumbar puncture may be done to rule out meningitis.
   c. Computed tomography (CT) and magnetic resonance imaging (MRI) may be performed to rule out abnormalities.

E. **Nursing management**

1. **Maintain a stable body temperature.**
2. **Prevent injury and the recurrence of seizures** by providing child and family teaching (Child and Family Teaching 10-1)
3. **Administer anticonvulsant therapy if prescribed.** Keep in mind that prophylactic therapy does not reduce the risk of future seizures. Anticonvulsant therapy may be

> **Protection During Febrile Seizures and Prevention of Recurring Febrile Seizures**
>
> - Protect your child from injury during a seizure.
>   - Provide a safe environment by removing potentially harmful objects.
> - Prevent the recurrence of febrile seizures.
>   - Observe for signs and symptoms of febrile illness.
>   - Implement temperature control methods.

prescribed for children who meet certain criteria, which include a focal or prolonged seizure, neurologic abnormalities, afebrile seizures in a first-degree relative, age under 1 year, and multiple seizures in less than 24 hours.

 V.   Sepsis

A. Description

1. Sepsis is a generalized bacterial infection that usually occurs in the first month of life.
2. Neonates are highly susceptible due to their immature immune response.
3. Mortality rates have diminished, but incidences have not.
4. Risk factors include prematurity, invasive procedures, steroid use for chronic lung problems, and nosocomial exposure to pathogens.
5. The antibodies found in colostrum are effective against gram-negative organisms; thus, breast-feeding has a protective benefit against infection.

B. Etiology

1. All neonatal infections are considered opportunistic and any bacteria are capable of causing sepsis.
2. Group B streptococcus is the most common cause of sepsis, followed by *Escherichia coli*, group A streptococcus, and *Streptococcus viridans*. Other pathogens include gonococci, *Candida albicans*, herpes simplex virus (type II), and *Listeria* organisms.

C. Pathophysiology

1. Immune defense mechanisms in neonates are immature, posing the potential for rapid invasion, spread, and multiplication of infecting organisms.
2. The newborn is unable to localize infections.

D. Assessment findings

1. Clinical manifestations

  a. Subtle, vague signs and symptoms characterize infant systemic infections. The only presenting complaint may be that the infant does not look or act right. There is rarely a sign of localized infection.

  b. Initial signs and symptoms may include:
  (1) Poor sucking and feeding
  (2) Weak cry
  (3) Lethargy
  (4) Irritability

  c. Subsequent signs and symptoms may include:
  (1) Pallor, cyanosis, or mottling
  (2) Decreased pain response
  (3) Hypotension
  (4) Abnormal heartbeat (tachycardia)

(5) Irregular respirations

(6) Jaundice

(7) Dehydration

(8) Temperature instability (may be hypothermic or hyperthermic)

(9) Gastrointestinal disturbances

(10) Seizures

(11) Hypotonia

(12) Tremors

(13) Full fontanelle

(14) Cardiac arrest

b. The most common presentation for late onset sepsis (up to 4 months of age) is meningitis.

2. Laboratory and diagnostic study findings

a. Blood culture may disclose the offending organism.

b. Urine culture and cerebrospinal fluid (CSF) analysis (by lumbar puncture) will detect organisms.

c. CBC will reveal elevated a white blood cell (WBC) count with increased immature neutrophils, which suggests infection.

d. Erythrocyte sedimentation rate (ESR) and C-reactive protein (CRP) will be increased, signifying inflammation.

E. Nursing management

1. Promote normal physiologic functioning by providing care similar to that given to a high-risk newborn.

a. Maintain a patent airway.

b. Provide a neutral thermal environment.

c. Protect the infant from increased infection. Administer antibiotic therapy for 7 to 10 days if culture results are positive and discontinue therapy as prescribed if culture results are negative (usually in 3 days).

d. Provide adequate nutrition.

2. Administer prescribed medications (see Drug Chart 10-1).

3. Monitor for signs of impending shock.

 4. Anticipate sepsis in risk populations. Immediate recognition of the onset of sepsis is crucial.

VI. Meningitis

A. Description

1. Meningitis is an infection of the meninges that is usually caused by bacterial invasion and less commonly by viruses.

2. Prognosis depends on the child's age, the organism, and the child's response to therapy. Bacterial meningitis is fatal if it is not treated immediately.

3. Most cases occur between 1 month and 5 years of age. Infants younger than 12 months of age are the most susceptible to bacterial meningitis.

B. Etiology

1. *E. coli*, group B *Streptococcus*, and *Listeria monocytogenes* are the most common organisms that cause meningitis in the neonate.

2. *Haemophilus influenzae*, *Neisseria meningitidis*, and *Diplococcus pneumoniae* are the most common organisms that cause meningitis in infants and children. However, the Hib vaccine has dramatically decreased the incidence of *H. influenzae* meningitis.

Other causative organisms include β-hemolytic *Streptococcus*, and *Staphylococcus aureus*.

3. Viral meningitis (due to coxsackievirus, echovirus, or mumps) is a self-limiting disease lasting 7 to 10 days.

C. Pathophysiology

1. In bacterial meningitis, the bacteria enter the meninges through the bloodstream and spread through the CSF; the infection may also infect the meninges directly through trauma or neurosurgery.

2. The pathogen acts as a toxin, creating a meningeal inflammatory response and a resultant release of purulent exudate. The infection spreads quickly through the exudate. Exudate can cover the choroid plexus and obstruct the arachnoid villi, causing hydrocephalus.

3. Vascular congestion and inflammation lead to cerebral edema, which may produce increased intracranial pressure (ICP). Necrosis of brain cells can cause permanent damage and death.

4. Complications can include obstructive hydrocephalus, thrombi in meningeal veins or venous sinuses, brain abscesses, deafness, blindness, and paralysis.

5. Meningococcal meningitis can result in meningococcal sepsis. If severe, sudden, and fulminate, it is called Waterhouse-Friderichsen syndrome characterized by disseminated intravascular coagulation (DIC), massive bilateral adrenal hemorrhages, and purpura. Mortality is as high as 90%.

D. Assessment findings

1. Clinical manifestations

a. Children younger than 2 years old do not display the characteristic signs of meningitis. Instead, they may exhibit:

(1) Poor feeding

(2) Irritability and lethargy

(3) High-pitched cry

(4) Bulging fontanelle

(5) Fever or low temperature

(6) Resistance to being held

(7) Opisthotonos (hyperextension of the neck and spine; may be apparent later in the course of disease)

b. Older children may exhibit:

(1) Respiratory or gastrointestinal problems (initially)

(2) Nuchal rigidity (stiff neck)

(3) Headache

(4) Tripod posturing

(5) Kernig sign (pain and resistance to knee extension when the child is in the supine position with knees and hips flexed)

(6) Brudzinski sign (flexion of the knees and hips when the neck is flexed with the child in the supine position)

(7) Petechial rash

2. Laboratory and diagnostic study findings

a. **CSF analysis (by lumbar puncture) establishes both the diagnosis (CSF may be cloudy, WBC count is elevated, protein level is elevated, and glucose level is decreased) and the causative agent. Lumbar puncture is not performed if the child has increased ICP. This is a measure to prevent brain herniation.**

b. CBC reveals an increased WBC count.

c. Blood culture may also identify the causative agent.

E. Nursing management

1. **Perform careful assessments to note clinical characteristics in their early stages.**
2. **Monitor temperature and vital signs frequently.**
3. **Monitor intake and output (I&O) and fluid and electrolyte balance.**
   a. Children with diminished consciousness should receive nothing by mouth; others are allowed liquids and diet progression as tolerated.
   b. Fluid intake may be limited to two thirds of normal maintenance to prevent cerebral edema.
   c. Overhydration is avoided to prevent the occurrence of syndrome of inappropriate diuretic hormone (SIADH).
4. **Check for neurologic signs and monitor the level of consciousness.**
   a. Measure head circumference to monitor for subdural effusions and obstructive hydrocephalus, which may develop as complications.
   b. Assess for signs of ICP (see Chap. 17).
5. **Administer prescribed medications,** such as antibiotics (type depends on the organism), steroids (to relieve cerebral edema), and anticonvulsants (see Drug Chart 10-1).
6. **Provide supportive interventions,** including measures to maintain a stable body temperature.
7. **Prevent the spread of infection to others.** Implement isolation with respiratory precautions for 24 to 48 hours after antibiotic administration begins.
8. **Keep the room as quiet as possible to decrease environmental stimuli**.

VII. Communicable diseases with rashes

A. Rubeola (measles)

1. The **infectious agent** is a virus.
2. The **mode of transmission** is usually through direct contact with droplets.
3. The **incubation period** is 10 to 20 days.
4. The **period of communicability** is from 4 days before to 5 days after the rash appears.
5. **Clinical manifestations**
   a. The **prodromal stage** consists of fever and malaise, followed by coryza, cough and conjunctivitis, and photophobia in 24 hours. Koplik spots first appear as red spots on the inside of the cheek. They evolve into pinpoint white papules with an erythematous base.
   b. The **rash** appears 3 to 4 days after the onset of the prodromal stage. It begins as an erythematous (reddened) maculopapular rash on the face and gradually spreads downward. The rash is more severe in earlier sites and less severe in later sites. It then turns brownish after 3 to 4 days when fine desquamation occurs over severe areas.
6. **Complications**
   a. Otitis media
   b. Pneumonia and laryngotracheitis
   c. Encephalitis
7. **Nursing implications**
   a. Show parents how to provide supportive management for fever and discomfort.
   b. Use a dimly lit room or sunglasses for photophobia.
8. **Prevention** is through vaccine (MMR).

B. Rubella (German measles)

1. The **infectious agent** is the rubella virus.
2. The **mode of transmission** is through direct and indirect contact.
3. The **incubation period** is from 14 to 21 days.
4. The **period of communicability** is from 7 days before to about 5 days after the rash appears.
5. **Clinical manifestations**
   a. There is no **prodromal stage** in children.
   b. The **rash** starts on face and rapidly spreads downward. It is a discrete, pinkish red maculopapular rash, and it disappears in the same order as it appeared.
   c. **General symptoms** include low-grade fever, headache, malaise, and lymphadenopathy.
6. **Complications** include possible teratogenic effects on a **fetus**.
7. **Nursing implications.** Provide supportive care.
8. **Prevention** is through vaccine (MMR).

C. Varicella (chickenpox)

1. The **infectious agent** is the varicella-zoster virus.
2. **Modes of transmission** are through direct contact and contact with contaminated objects.
3. The **incubation period** is from 2 to 3 weeks.
4. The **period of communicability** is from 1 to 2 days before the rash develops until all lesions are crusted.
5. **Clinical manifestations**
   a. Low-grade fever, malaise, and anorexia characterize the **prodromal stage**.
   b. A multilesion **rash** includes maculas, papules, vesicles, pustules, and crusts. It is centripetal, spreading to face and proximal extremities, and sparsely covering distal extremities. The rash may affect mucous membranes, and the pruritus is severe.
   c. **General symptoms** include fever, lymphadenopathy, and irritability from pruritus.
6. **Complications**
   a. Secondary infections, encephalitis, and pneumonia
   b. Hemorrhagic varicella (in high-risk children)
7. **Nursing implications**
   a. Maintain strict isolation in the hospital setting; isolate children at home until all vesicles dry.
   b. Provide skin care; provide cool or Aveeno baths and loose clothing.
   c. Administer antipyretics (do not use aspirin) and antihistamines. Administer acyclovir (for high-risk child) as well as zoster immune globulin (ZIG).
8. **Prevention** is through vaccine (VZV).

D. Erythema infectiosum (fifth disease)

1. The **infectious agent** is the human parvovirus B19 (HPV).
2. **Modes of transmission** are unknown; probably via the respiratory tract and blood.
3. The **incubation period** is 4 to 14 days, may be as long as 20 days.
4. The **period of communicability** is uncertain, but usually before the onset of symptoms and for approximately 1 week after the onset of symptoms in children with aplastic crisis.
5. **Clinical manifestations**
   a. **Three-stage rash**
      (1) The first stage begins with erythema on the face that gives the cheeks a "slapped face" appearance. Facial rash disappears in 1 to 4 days.

(2) The second stage begins approximately 1 day after the facial rash appears. It is a symmetrical, red maculopapular rash that appears on upper and lower extremities. The rash has proximal to distal progression and may last a week.

(3) During the third stage, the rash subsides but it can resurface if skin is irritated or traumatized.

b. The rash may be absent in children with aplastic crisis. These children may also experience prodromal symptoms, which include lethargy, fever, myalgia, nausea, vomiting, and abdominal pain.

6. Complications
a. Self-limited arthritis and arthralgia
b. Aplastic crisis (in children with hemolytic disease or immune deficiency)
c. Myocarditis (rare)
d. Encephalitis (rare)
e. Fetal death (if the mother is infected during pregnancy; however, there is no evidence of congenital anomalies.)

7. Nursing implications
a. Administer antipyretic and analgesic medications.
b. Isolation is not necessary, and pregnant women need not be excluded from the workplace where HPV infection is present; however, they should understand the risks.
c. Hospitalized children with HIV infection or aplastic crisis who are suspected of HPV infection are placed on precautions.

8. Prevention. There is no vaccine at present.

E. Exanthema subitum (roseola)

1. The **infectious agent** is human herpes simplex virus type 6 (HHV-6).
2. **Modes of transmission** are unknown.
3. The **incubation period** is usually 5 to 15 days.
4. The **period of communicability** is unknown.
5. **Clinical manifestations**
   a. A **general symptom** is a high fever (temperature 102°F) that persists for 3 to 4 days in a child who appears well. A precipitous drop in the fever is followed by the appearance of a rash.
   b. The **rash** is a discrete, nonpruritic pink macular or maculopapular rash, first appearing on trunk, then face, neck, and extremities. The rash fades on pressure and lasts 1 to 2 days.
   c. **Associated symptoms** include cervical adenopathy, injected pharynx, coryza, and cough.
6. **Complications**
   a. Recurrent febrile seizures
   b. Mononucleosis-like illness
   c. Encephalitis (rare)
7. **Nursing implications**
   a. Teach parents temperature regulation measures.
   b. Discuss seizure precautions if the child is seizure-prone (see Child and Family Teaching 10-1).
8. **Prevention**. There is no vaccine at present.

E. Scarlet fever

1. The **infectious agent** is group A β-hemolytic streptococci.
2. **Modes of transmission** are direct contact, droplet spread, and indirect contact.

3. The **incubation period** is from 2 to 4 days, but can range from 1 to 7 days.
4. The **period of communicability** is during the incubation phase and clinical illness, and during first 2 weeks of the carrier phase.
5. **Clinical manifestations**
   a. The **prodromal stage** consists of a sudden high fever, pulse increased out of proportion to fever, headache, vomiting, general malaise, abdominal pain, and chills.
   b. The **rash** appears within 12 hours after the prodromal stage. Red pinpoint punctuate lesions rapidly become generalized except for face. The rash is more intense in joint folds, and the face is usually flushed with significant circumoral pallor. By end of the first week, the skin desquamates ("sandpaper" feel with "sheetlike' sloughing). Desquamation may last 3 weeks.
   c. **General symptoms**. The tonsils are enlarged, red, and covered with exudate. In severe cases, exudate may resemble the membrane of diphtheria. The pharynx is beefy red and the palate is covered with erythematous punctate lesions. The tongue is coated, and papilla are red and swollen (white strawberry tongue). By the fourth day, the coat sloughs off, leaving prominent papilla (red strawberry tongue).
6. **Complications**
   a. Otitis media
   b. Peritonsillar abscess
   c. Sinusitis
   d. Glomerular nephritis
   e. Carditis and polyarthritis (rare)
7. **Nursing implications**
   a. Administer the full course of antibiotics (usually penicillin, or erythromycin if child allergic to penicillin), analgesics, and antipyretics.
   b. Initiate respiratory precautions until the child has taken antibiotics for 24 hours.
   c. Encourage fluids.
8. **Prevention**. There is no vaccine at present.

VIII. Communicable diseases without rashes

A. Diphtheria
1. The **infectious agent** is *Corynebacterium diphtheriae*.
2. **Modes of transmission** include direct contact, air, and personal articles.
3. The **incubation period** is 2 to 5 days or longer.
4. The **period of communicability** exists until bacilli are no longer present (2–4 weeks without treatment or 1–2 days after the start of treatment).
5. **Clinical manifestations** (depend on the site of membrane)
   a. **Nasal**. Manifestations resemble the common cold; drainage becomes serosanguineous then mucopurulent with a foul odor.
   b. **Tonsillar-pharyngeal**. There is malaise, anorexia, sore throat, low-grade fever, pulse higher than expected for fever, and lymphadenitis ("bull neck"). When severe, there is toxemia, septic shock, and death.
   c. **Laryngeal.** There is fever, hoarseness, cough, and potential airway obstruction.
6. **Complications**
   a. Myocarditis
   b. Neuritis
7. **Nursing implications**
   a. Maintain strict isolation.

b. Maintain a patent airway and observe for signs of obstruction. Administer oxygen if needed. Tracheostomy may be needed for obstruction.

c. Promote hydration, administer antibiotics as prescribed, and maintain bed rest.

d. Institute orders for antitoxin and antibiotics.

8. **Prevention** is through vaccine, and is maintained by boosters (DaPT, DT, dT).

B. Whooping cough (pertussis)

1. The **infectious agent** is *Bordetella pertussis.*
2. **Modes of transmission** are through direct contact, air, and personal objects.
3. The **incubation period** is 5 to 21 days (average 10).
4. The **period of communicability** is from the catarrhal stage through the fourth week (greatest during the catarrhal stage).
5. **Clinical manifestations**
   a. **Catarrhal stage**. This stage consists of symptoms of upper respiratory tract infection. It continues for 1 to 2 weeks at which point the hacking cough becomes more severe.
   b. **Paroxysmal stage** (generally 4–6 weeks). The characteristic paroxysmal "whooping" cough (usually at night) develops, and is accompanied by flushed or cyanotic cheeks, bulging eyes, and a protruding tongue. The cough continues until a thick mucous plug is dislodged. There is usually vomiting after an attack.
   c. **Convalescent stage**. During this stage the cough gradually decreases, the vomiting stops, and strength generally returns.
6. **Complications**
   a. Pneumonia, atelectasis, otitis media, convulsions, hemorrhage, weight loss, dehydration, and rectal prolapse
   b. Respiratory arrest caused by mucous plug or apnea in young infants
7. **Nursing implications**
   a. Institute isolation and respiratory precautions and bed rest when febrile.
   b. Provide reassurance during coughing; provide a quiet environment to decrease paroxysmal spells.
   c. Encourage fluids, provide humidity, observe for signs of obstruction, and administer antibiotics and pertussis immune globulin.
8. **Prevention** is through vaccine (DaPT).

C. Poliomyelitis

1. The **infectious agents** are three types of enteroviruses.
2. **Modes of transmission** are through direct contact and the fecal-oral route.
3. The **incubation period** is from 7 to 14 days.
4. The **period of communicability** is not known. However, the virus is in the throat for 1 week after onset and in the feces intermittently for 3 to 4 weeks.
5. **Clinical manifestations** (three forms)
   a. **Abortive or apparent**. Brief fever, malaise, anorexia, nausea, vomiting, constipation, headache, and abdominal pain manifest this form.
   b. **Nonparalytic**. This is the same as abortive or apparent but there is more severe pain. It progresses to nuchal and spinal rigidity with changes in reflexes.
   c. **Paralytic.** This is the same as nonparalytic but there is muscular weakness progressing to paralysis, including paralysis of bowel and bladder muscles and paresis of respiratory muscles.
6. **Complications**
   a. Permanent paralysis
   b. Respiratory arrest
   c. Hypertension

    d. Kidney stones

    e. Pulmonary edema and pulmonary emboli

  7. Nursing implications

    a. Promote anxiety relief, participate in physiotherapy techniques, and maintain body alignment.

    b. Observe for respiratory paralysis.

    c. Supply supportive treatment with airway maintenance and bowel and bladder programs when needed.

    d. Position the child to maintain body alignment and prevent contractures and decubiti.

  8. Prevention is through vaccine (TIPV, TOPV).

D. Parotitis (mumps)

  1. The **infectious agent** is the paramyxovirus.

  2. The **modes of transmission** are through direct contact and droplet.

  3. The **incubation period** is from 14 to 21 days.

  4. The **period of communicability** is immediately before to immediately after swelling appears.

  5. Clinical manifestations

    a. **Prodromal stage**. Fever, headache, and anorexia, followed by earache aggravated by chewing manifest this stage.

    b. **Acute stage.** By the third day, glandular (parotid) swelling reaches maximal size and is accompanied by pain and tenderness.

    c. **Other symptoms** include malaise, anorexia, and general lymphadenopathy.

  6. Complications

    a. Meningoencephalitis

    b. Orchitis, epididymitis, and sterility in males (rare)

    c. Arthritis

    d. Obstructive laryngitis

    e. Otitis media and pneumonia

  7. Nursing implications

    a. Institute isolation, respiratory precautions, and bed rest.

    b. Administer analgesics and fluids; administer intravenous fluids if prescribed and if the child refuses to drink.

    c. Provide warmth and support for orchitis.

    d. Dim the lights if the child has photophobia.

  8. Prevention is through vaccine (MMR).

STUDY QUESTIONS

1. Which of the following types of immunity does an infant receive when given a DaPT injection?
   (1) Natural, active
   (2) Natural, passive
   (3) Artificial, active
   (4) Artificial, passive

2. The nurse would administer the varicella vaccine to a 15-month-old who had which of the following?
   (1) Acquired immunodeficiency syndrome (AIDS)
   (2) Upper respiratory tract infection
   (3) Leukemia
   (4) Long-term steroid therapy

3. After administering DaPT to a child, the nurse should instruct the mother about which of the following?
   (1) Monitoring the child for a rash in 7 to 10 days
   (2) Decreasing milk intake to prevent diarrhea
   (3) Giving acetaminophen for fever and discomfort
   (4) Warning that the virus may be shed in the child's stool

4. According to the routine immunization schedule, which of the following immunizations should a child 15 to 18 months of age receive?
   (1) DaPT, IPV, Var
   (2) Hib, MMR, Var
   (3) HB, MMR,
   (4) Hib, HB

5. When administering an antipyretic to a child, the nurse knows that aspirin is contraindicated for children with viral syndromes because of the possibility for development of which of the following?
   (1) Reye syndrome
   (2) Reflux syndrome
   (3) Raynaud syndrome
   (4) Reiter syndrome

6. Which of the following would the nurse expect to be performed for a child with possible febrile convulsions to rule out a seizure disorder?
   (1) Brain scan
   (2) Electroencephalogram (EEG)
   (3) Serum chemistry
   (4) Lead level analysis

7. Which of the following organisms is the **most** common cause of neonatal sepsis?
   (1) *Staphylococcus aureus*
   (2) *Streptococcus viridans*
   (3) Group B streptococcus
   (4) *Haemophilus influenzae*

8. When evaluating the laboratory test results of an infant with sepsis, which of the following would the nurse expect to find?
   (1) Leukopenia
   (2) Decreased erythrocyte sedimentation rate (ESR)
   (3) Increased C-reactive protein (CRP)
   (4) Hyperglycemia

9. Which of the following would the nurse expect to assess as common early manifestations of meningitis in a 2-month-old infant?
   (1) Opisthotonos
   (2) Nuchal rigidity
   (3) Kerning sign
   (4) Hypothermia

10. A child, whose parents seek attention for the child's generalized confluent red-pink maculopapular rash, appears ill and exhibits conjunctivitis and photophobia. Which of the following would the nurse suspect?
    (1) Rubella
    (2) Roseola
    (3) Rubeola
    (4) Varicella

11. A thick whitish gray pseudomembrane and a "bull neck" are characteristic of which of the following?
    (1) Pertussis
    (2) Diphtheria
    (3) Mumps
    (4) Tetanus

12. A mother brings her infant into the clinic for evaluation of a discrete rash on the trunk and spreading to the face that appeared shortly after the child's fever suddenly subsided. Which of the following would the nurses suspect?
    (1) Roseola
    (2) Fifth disease
    (3) Scarlet fever
    (4) Pertussis

ANSWER KEY

1. The answer is (3). Artificially acquired, active immunity results from the use of ingested or injected vaccines, medically altered substances, which stimulate the immune system to produce antibodies. Naturally acquired, active immunity occurs when antibodies develop naturally (through nature), for example, when an infectious disease develops in an individual. In response, the body's immune system makes antibodies. Naturally acquired, passive immunity occurs when antibodies are directly received naturally, such as through the placenta or breast milk. Artificially acquired immunity results when antibodies are artificially delivered to the body, such as with the administration of tetanus immunoglobulin. In this case, there is no immune response by the body.

2. The answer is (2). The varicella vaccine is a live virus vaccine and may be administered to children with mild episodic illnesses, such as upper respiratory tract infections. However, the vaccine is contraindicated in children who are immunosuppressed, such as those with AIDS, leukemia, or receiving long-term steroid therapy because of the increased risk for developing the disease.

3. The answer is (3). Following administration of DaPT, fever and discomfort are possible. Therefore, the nurse should instruct the mother to give acetaminophen. Acetaminophen assists in decreasing the fever that may accompany the pertussis vaccine and the pain that may accompany the tetanus vaccine. A rash may be seen 7 to 10 days after the measles, mumps, and rubella (MMR) vaccine. Diarrhea is not associated with the DaPT vaccine. The live polio vaccine may be shed into the stools.

4. The answer is (2). Hib (HibTITER), MMR, and Var are scheduled to be given at 15 to 18 months of age. DaPT and IPV booster are scheduled at 18 months. HB is given at 0, 2, and 6 months or at 2, 4, and 6 months.

5. The answer is (1). In children with viral illnesses, the use of aspirin is linked with the development of Reye syndrome, an acute encephalitis with fatty infiltrates of the internal organs. The use of aspirin in children with viral illness is not associated with any type of reflux syndrome. Raynaud disease is a condition involving ischemia of the extremities. Reiter syndrome is an arthritic disorder of adult men.

6. The answer is (2). For the child with possible febrile convulsions, evaluation focuses on ruling out other disease processes. An EEG is used to determine if a child has a seizure disorder. A brain scan may be used to rule out a mass or lesion. Serum chemistry findings may rule out electrolyte imbalance. Lead level determination will rule out lead poisoning.

7. The answer is (3). Group B β-hemolytic streptococcus is the most common cause of bacterial meningitis and sepsis in the neonate. Staphylococcus can cause sepsis in the neonate, but it is not the most common causative organism. *S. viridans* is not a common cause of sepsis. *H. influenzae* can cause sepsis and meningitis, but it is less common in the neonate and now is less frequent in the older child as a result of the Hib vaccine.

8. The answer is (3). For the infant with sepsis, laboratory results typically reveal leukocytosis (increased WBC count) with an increase in immature neutrophils suggesting infection, and an increased ESR and CRP indicating inflammation. Hyperglycemia is not usually associated with sepsis.

9. The answer is (4). Hypothermia and hyperthermia are early signs of meningitis in the young infant. Opisthotonos is a late and ominous sign. Nuchal rigidity and Kerning sign are seen in older children and adults with meningitis. Infants do not localize infections.

10. The answer is (3). A confluent red-pink maculopapular rash along with an ill appearance is a classic presentation of rubeola or measles. Rubella, or German measles, presents with a similar rash but the child does not appear ill. Roseola presents with a mild rash after the child's fever subsides. Varicella, or chickenpox, is a multilesion rash.

11. The answer is (2). The pseudomembrane and the characteristic lymphadenitis ("bull neck") are seen in diphtheria. Pertussis is whooping cough characterized by a severe "whooping" cough usually at night. Mumps begins with enlarged parotid glands and neck swelling, but there is no pseudomembrane. Tetanus is lockjaw characterized by trismus.

12. The answer is (1). The development of a discrete rash first on the trunk and then spreading to the face, neck, and extremities following a precipitous or sudden drop in fever is characteristic of roseola. Fifth disease is characterized by erythema on the face that gives the cheeks a "slapped face" appearance. Scarlet fever is associated with a rash that appears within 12 hours after prodromal stage, beginning as red pinpoint punctuate lesions that rapidly become generalized except for the face. The rash is more intense in joint folds, and the face is usually flushed with significant circumoral pallor. Pertussis does not involve a rash.

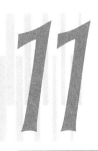

Respiratory Dysfunction

Structure and function of the respiratory system

A. Structures

1. The **upper respiratory tract** consists of the nose, sinuses, pharynx, larynx, trachea, and epiglottis.

2. The **lower respiratory tract** consists of the bronchi, bronchioles, and lungs. Table 11-1 presents information on development of the respiratory system.

B. Function. The major function of the respiratory system is to deliver oxygen (O_2) to arterial blood and remove carbon dioxide (CO_2) from venous blood, a process known as **gas exchange**.

1. **Normal gas exchange depends on three processes**.

   a. **Ventilation** is movement of gases from the atmosphere into and out of the lungs. This is accomplished through the mechanical acts of **inspiration** and **expiration**.

   b. **Diffusion** is movement of inhaled gases in the alveoli and across the alveolar capillary membrane.

   c. **Perfusion** is movement of oxygenated blood from the lungs to the tissues.

2. **Control of gas exchange** involves neural and chemical processes.

   a. The **neural system**, composed of three parts located in the pons, medulla, and spinal cord, coordinates respiratory rhythm and regulates the depth of respirations.

   b. **Chemical processes** perform several vital functions, such as:

      (1) Regulating alveolar ventilation by maintaining normal blood gas tension

      (2) Guarding against hypercapnia (excessive CO_2 in the blood) as well as hypoxia (reduced tissue oxygenation caused by decreased arterial oxygen [Pao_2]). An increase in arterial CO_2 ($Paco_2$) stimulates ventilation; conversely, a decrease in $Paco_2$ inhibits ventilation.

      (3) Helping to maintain respirations (through peripheral chemoreceptors) when hypoxia occurs

3. **Differences in respiratory response**. The normal functions of respiration, O_2 and CO_2 tension, and chemoreceptors are similar in children and adults. However, children respond differently than adults to respiratory disturbances; major areas of difference include:

   a. **Poor tolerance of nasal congestion**, especially in infants who are obligatory nose breathers up to 4 months of age

   b. **Increased susceptibility to ear infection** due to shorter, broader, and more horizontally positioned eustachian tubes

   c. **Increased severity of respiratory symptoms** due to smaller airway diameters

   d. **A total body response to respiratory infection**, with such symptoms as fever, vomiting, and diarrhea

TABLE 11-1
Development of the Respiratory System

AGE	RESPIRATORY RATE	STRUCTURE AND FUNCTION
Fetal development	NA	Appearance of the laryngotracheal groove around the fourth week of gestation is closely followed by development of the larynx and trachea.
		Development of the bronchial tree occurs predominantly between weeks 5 and 16 of gestation.
		In weeks 6 through 12 of gestation, luminal and blood vessel growth occurs in the bronchi and bronchioles.
		Production of surfactant (a phospholipid protein complex that reduces alveolar surface tension, thereby decreasing the tendency of the alveoli to collapse during expiration) occurs at about 24 weeks of gestation.
		Two surface tension-reducing substances, lecithin and sphingomyelin, can be detected in amniotic fluid and are useful predictors of lung maturity; a lecithin/sphingomyelin ratio of 2:1 or greater indicates fetal lung maturity.
		The detection of phosphatidylglycerol in amniotic fluid also indicates fetal lung maturity.
Infant (0–1 year)	30–35	At birth, the lungs contain fluid; this is replaced by air as the infant begins respiration.
		The respiratory tract is small and relatively delicate, and it provides inadequate protection against infection. The close proximity of one structure to another eases the spread of infection. There is limited alveolar surface for gas exchange.
Toddler/Preschooler (1–6 years)	20–30	Lung volume increases and susceptibility to infection decreases.
Schoolager (6–12 years)	18–21	Respiratory system achieves adult maturity. The respiratory rate slows as the amount of air exchanged increases with each breath. Lung capacity becomes proportionate to body size.
Adolescent (12–21 years)	16–20	Inadequate oxygenation occurs as the respiratory system grows slowly in proportion to the rest of the body. Males have greater vital capacity due to greater chest size, and their lung capacity matures later than females who reach adult capacity at 17 or 18.

II.   **NURSING PROCESS OVERVIEW FOR**
The respiratory system

A. Assessment

1. Health history

a. Elicit a description of symptoms including onset, duration, location, and precipitation. **Cardinal symptoms** may include:
   - (1) Shortness of breath
   - (2) Difficulty breathing
   - (3) Chest pain
   - (4) Feeding and sucking difficulty in an infant
   - (5) Nasal congestion, runny nose, and sneezing
   - (6) Cough

b. Explore prenatal, personal, and family history for **risk factors** for respiratory disorders.
   - (1) Prenatal risk factors include maternal infections, maternal smoking, or maternal use of marijuana, cocaine, or heroin.
   - (2) Personal risk factors include perinatal history of meconium staining or mechanical ventilation at birth, or prematurity; history of respiratory illnesses; number of colds per year; history of chronic illnesses, such as cardiac disorder, asthma, cystic fibrosis, or human immunodeficiency virus (HIV) and acquired immunodeficiency syndrome (AIDS); or exposure to passive tobacco smoke or other environmental irritants.
   - (3) Family risk factors include family history of allergies, asthma, tuberculosis, or cystic fibrosis.

2. Physical examination

a. **Vital signs**
   - (1) Monitor temperature for hyperthermia and hypothermia, which may indicate infection.
   - (2) Monitor respirations for rate, depth, and quality. Prolonged inspiration may indicate upper airway obstruction; prolonged expiration may indicate an obstructive disorder, such as asthma.

b. **Inspection**
   - (1) Observe for alertness, changes in mental status, activity level, and signs of fatigue. Anxiety and restlessness are early signs of respiratory distress. Observe body position that the child maintains. Note any signs of dehydration.
   - (2) Note presence and characteristics of cough (ie, productive versus nonproductive and type [harsh, croupy, paroxysmal, tight, or moist]).
   - (3) Observe skin color changes, especially cyanosis.
   - (4) Observe respiratory effort, noting dyspnea, stridor, grunting, nasal flaring, and presence and severity of intracostal, suprasternal, sternal, and substernal retractions.
   - (5) Observe for an elongated, anteroposterior chest diameter, which may indicate air trapped in the alveoli.

c. **Percussion**. Percuss for signs of dullness. Dullness indicates that fluid or solid tissue has replaced air.

d. **Auscultation**
   - (1) Note quality of breath sounds.
   - (2) Note presence of adventitious lung sounds (eg, crackles [rales], rhonchi, and wheezes).

3. Laboratory and diagnostic studies
   a. **Chest x-ray films** remain the best initial imaging technique to detect abnormalities of the pulmonary, mediastinal, and musculoskeletal structures of the thorax.
   b. **Pulse oximetry** measures arterial hemoglobin saturation (SaO_2).
   c. **Pulmonary function tests** (ie, spirometry, gas dilution, and body plethysmography) measure airway function, lung volumes, and gas exchange. They are used to determine the presence, nature, and extent of pulmonary disease; however, they do not indicate the cause of the dysfunction.
   d. **Peak flow measurement** is used to measure the greatest flow velocity during a forced expiration. The child is instructed to exhale quickly and forcefully into the meter after deep inspiration (total lung capacity).
   e. **Electrocardiograms (ECGs) and echocardiograms** are obtained to assess secondary cardiac changes.
   f. **Sputum, throat, or nasal cultures** identify infectious organisms.
   g. **Nasal washings** are also used to identify pathogens.
   h. **Blood gas analysis** involves the drawing of blood to determine information about the oxygenation of the blood and its acid–base status. (Normal values are provided in Appendix A.)
   i. **Bronchography** involves x-ray films of the lung after instillation of an opaque medium into a bronchus.
   j. **Computed tomography (CT) scan** is a sequence of x-ray films that show a cross-sectional view of the thorax. It is used to indicate tumors and may indicate infections such as tuberculosis.
   k. **Magnetic resonance imaging (MRI)** uses magnetic waves to detect thoracic soft tissue abnormalities.

B. Nursing diagnoses
   1. Ineffective breathing pattern
   2. Ineffective airway clearance
   3. Pain
   4. Risk for infection
   5. Risk for altered body temperature
   6. Risk for fluid volume deficit
   7. Altered nutrition: less than body requirements
   8. Fear
   9. Anxiety
   10. Knowledge deficit
   11. Risk for altered growth
   12. Risk for altered development
   13. Activity intolerance

C. Planning and outcome identification
   1. The child will resume an optimal breathing pattern.
   2. The child will exhibit no signs of secondary infection.
   3. The child will consume adequate fluids and nutrition.
   4. The child and family will experience minimal fear and anxiety.
   5. The child will not deviate from developmental norms due to illness.

D. Implementation
   1. **Promote adequate oxygenation and a normal breathing pattern.**
      a. Administer bronchodilators, anti-inflammatories, mucolytics, and expectorants (Drug Chart 11-1).
      b. Elevate the head of the bed or allow the child to maintain a position of comfort.

DRUG CHART 11-1. Medications Used in Respiratory Disorders

Classifications	Used for	Selected interventions

Bronchodilators
Beta-adrenergic agonists
  albuterol (Proventil)
  epinephrine (Sus-Phrine)
  metaproterenol sulfate
    (Alupent)
  terbutaline sulfate (Brethaire)
  theophylline (Bronkydl)
	Used to promote pulmonary smooth muscle relaxation and improve respiratory function.	Correct inhaler technique is important.
		
		If used to prevent exercise-induced asthma, it must be given at least 15 minutes before exercise.
		
		IV aminophylline must be administered slowly. Monitor for toxicity, which may be exhibited by vomiting, thirst, tinnitus, palpitations, and elevated serum theophylline levels.
		
		Instruct regarding side effects, which include nervousness, tremors, tachycardia, hypertension, cramps, dizziness, headache, and insomnia.

Anti-inflammatory Medications
  Antiallergics
    cromolyn sodium
      (Intal)
    nedrocromil sodium (Tilade)
  Corticosteroids
    prednisolone (Prelone)
    prednisone (Deltasone)
	Used to reduce airway reactivity and inflammation.	Anti-inflammatory agents have no bronchodilating effect and thus the inhalant forms are used after the bronchodilator inhalers.
		
		Instruct child and family on side effects:
		
		Steroidal and nonsteroidal inhalers: Oral candidiasis (rinsing mouth after use minimizes this)
		
		Nonsteroidals: Virtually no side effects but may have unpleasant taste, headache, cough, and throat irritation.

	Steroids are sometimes used to treat recurrent otitis media	*Steroids:* (Depends on dose and duration) mood changes, increased appetite, fluid retention, infection, GI distress, and impaired growth. Instruct family to not abruptly stop oral preparations of steroids and to have child take them with food or milk to minimize gastric irritation.

Mucolytic agents
  acetylsysteine (Mucomyst)
  dornase alfa (recombinant
    human deoxyribonuclease,
    DNase; Pulmozyme)
	Used to reduce the viscosity of sputum, chiefly in patients with cystic fibrosis.	Administer via nebulizer.
		
		Refrigerate medication and protect it from light.
		
		Ensure proper use of inhalation device.
		
		Instruct family on side effects, which include stomatitis, nausea, vomiting, chest pain, pharyngitis, and increased cough.

(continued)

DRUG CHART 11-1. Medications Used in Respiratory Disorders *(Continued)*

Classifications	Used for	Selected interventions

Antibiotics
  Penicillins
  Macrolides
    azithromycin (Zithromax)
    erythromycin (EryPed)
  Cephalosporins (sometimes the treatment of choice because of their broad-spectrum activity and bactericidal effect on β-lactamase-producing pathogens)
  Aminoglycosides
  Combination antibacterials
    sulfamethoxazol-trimethoprim (Bactrim-Septra)
    erythromycin-sulfisoxazole (Pediazole)
	Antibiotics are used for respiratory infections such as pneumonia and epiglottitis.
	
	Long-term antibiotic therapy is often used for recurrent otitis media
		General nursing implications:
		1. Obtain all culture and sensitivity specimens before giving antibiotics.
		2. Check for allergies.
		3. Check storage of medications.
		4. Monitor child's temperature.
		5. Provide instruction for the child and family, as follows: Advise child to take the antibiotic exactly as prescribed for the entire time period prescribed; antibiotics are not used to treat viral infections; most antibiotics work best on an empty stomach; antibiotics may decrease the effects of oral contraceptives; fungal superinfections are possible, especially thrush and monilial diaper rash.
		
		Specific nursing implications:
		1. Penicillin: give amoxicillin with food; child may break out in nonallergic rash between days 7 and 10 of amoxicillin therapy.
		2. *Macrolides:* do not give with fruit juice; do not give intramuscularly (IM); erythromycin increases theophylline levels.
		3. *Cephalosporins:* 15% of all clients who are allergic to penicillin are allergic to cephalosporins.
		4. *Aminoglycosides:* assess for ototoxicity and nephrotoxicity; increase fluid intake; monitor intake and output, keep urine alkaline.

(continued)

DRUG CHART 11-1. Medications Used in Respiratory Disorders *(Continued)*

Classifications	Used for	Selected interventions
Antivirals ribavirin (Virazole)	Used for the treatment of respiratory syncytial virus (RSV) in a specific population of infants and young children: 1. Use for children at high risk for complications caused by other conditions (premature infants, immunosuppressed children, and children with severe RSV infection) 2. Consider using for infants at increased risk for progressing from mild to severe disease (ie, infants < 6 weeks of age or infants with underlying conditions)	This drug is administered via small particle aerosol generator. Monitor apical pulse and respirations every 1–2 hours. Pregnant nurses should not care for these children. Observe precautions for health care workers and visitors; provide information about potential but unknown risks of drug; advise pregnant women to avoid giving direct care to infants receiving ribavirin; minimize environmental exposure to ribavirin (temporarily stop medication when tent is open, administer drug in well-ventilated rooms).
Expectorants guaifenesin (Robitussin)	Used to enhance the output of respiratory tract excretions	Water is still the best expectorant. Instruct parents not to administer for more than 1 week. *Monitor for side effects:* nausea, vomiting, headache, and dizziness.

   c. Administer oxygen as needed.

   d. Perform chest physiotherapy consistent with the child's tolerance level, which can be monitored by pulse oximetry. Chest physiotherapy consists of three techniques—postural drainage, percussion, and vibration—that are used to loosen mucus for expectoration.

   e. Periodically change the child's position from side to side and front to back to improve bronchial drainage and promote expansion and ventilation of all lung fields.

   f. Use incentive spirometry and suction airway secretions as needed.

   g. Administer appropriate pain management techniques when pain interferes with coughing mechanisms.

   h. Encourage the child to expectorate.

   i. Promote rest by scheduling nursing activities so that they do not coincide with rest periods, and encourage activities appropriate to tolerance level.

2. Prevent secondary infection.

   a. Maintain an aseptic technique and use appropriate isolation precautions when warranted.

   b. Administer antibiotics (see Drug Chart 11-1).

   c. Minimize the child's contact with infected persons.

3. Promote desired fluid and nutritional intake.
   a. Monitor the fluid intake and output.
   b. Ensure adequate hydration by encouraging or administering fluids, or monitoring intravenous (IV) infusion.
   c. Allow the child to eat a diet as tolerated and desired; provide nutritional supplements when necessary. Serve desirable foods in a pleasant atmosphere.

4. Minimize fear and anxiety.
   a. Provide a quiet environment. Use a calm, reassuring manner.
   b. Explain procedures and equipment, and encourage parents to participate in the child's care.
   c. Provide diversional activities and encourage verbalization.
   d. Provide child and family teaching to minimize episodes of respiratory distress, which, in turn, will minimize fear and anxiety (Child and Family Teaching 11-1).

5. Promote growth and development.
   a. Acute respiratory illness is frightening to both the child and the parents and calls for effective crisis intervention by the nurse.
   b. Chronic respiratory illness in children is commonly accompanied by a history of acute crisis episodes and chronic stress.
   c. The respiratory-impaired child's developmental needs can best be met by maintaining optimal exercise and activity levels.

E. Outcome evaluation

   1. The child maintains adequate oxygenation and exhibits a normal breathing pattern.
   2. The child does not develop a secondary infection.
   3. The child's fluid and nutritional status is optimal.
   4. The child verbalizes fears and anxieties, and deals with them in a healthy manner.
   5. The child continues to grow and develop despite the crisis and stress associated with a respiratory illness.

III. Bronchopulmonary dysplasia (BPD)

A. Description

   1. BPD is a chronic pulmonary disease of infancy marked by the need for oxygen therapy beyond 28 days after birth.
   2. BPD most commonly affects very low-birth-weight (VLBW [under 2500 g]) and extremely low-birth-weight (ELBW [under 1000 g]) infants with lung disorders (eg, res-

CHILD AND FAMILY TEACHING 11-1

Minimizing Episodes of Respiratory Distress

- Detail measures to prevent respiratory infection by avoiding exposure to persons with known infections and by maintaining good hygiene and sound health patterns.
- Explain the diagnosis.
- Express ways to identify and prevent known attack precipitants, including passive tobacco smoke.
- Define the need for hydration to keep mucous secretions thin.
- Discuss ways to perform physical activities commensurate with tolerance level.
- Demonstrate and explain rationale for breathing exercises, inhalation therapy, and chest physiotherapy.
- Outline dosage, administration, and possible side effects of medications.

piratory distress syndrome ([RDS]), also called hyaline membrane disease, and meconium aspiration).

3. A premature infant who is mechanically ventilated and receives high concentrations of oxygen is at greatest risk.

B. Etiology

1. The exact cause of BPD is unknown, but it is thought that it is the response of a premature lung to early injury.

2. Mechanical ventilation and a high inspired oxygen concentration are thought to be two major causes of BPD. BPD may occur after mechanical ventilation therapy for conditions such as RDS, meconium aspiration, persistent pulmonary hypertension, and cyanotic heart disease.

C. Pathophysiology

1. Positive inspiratory pressures and high concentrations of oxygen can injure the alveolar saccules and small airway epithelium and lead to fibrosis of these structures.

2. Areas of cystic foci and atelectasis appear in the lung parenchyma. In addition, airway smooth muscle hypertrophy results in bronchospasm and endothelial cell damage, causing interstitial edema.

3. These changes further aggravate airway obstruction and necessitate long-term oxygen therapy.

D. Assessment findings

1. Clinical manifestations

a. BPD is characterized by cyanosis when breathing room air, tachypnea, retractions, grunting, nasal flaring, increased anteroposterior diameter of the chest, wheezing, rales, and copious secretions.

b. Manifestations of right-sided heart failure may be present, including periorbital edema, hepatomegaly, and jugular vein distention. Pulmonary edema may occur. Clubbing of the fingers is seen with severe disease.

c. The child with BPD is usually thin with height and weight measurements in the bottom 50th percentile. Growth and development usually are delayed secondary to poor nutrition and prolonged hospitalization.

2. Laboratory and diagnostic study findings

a. Pulmonary function tests (PFTs) will reveal increased airway resistance, decreased compliance (increased lung stiffness), and increased functional residual capacity (FRC).

b. Chest x-ray films show characteristic streakiness with areas of hyperinflation and atelectasis.

c. ECG and echocardiogram may show evidence of right-sided cardiac hypertrophy.

E. Nursing management

1. Assess all at-risk neonates for signs of BPD. Assess for signs of increased distress and heart failure in infants who have BPD.

2. Administer prescribed medications, such as bronchodilators, anti-inflammatories, and antibiotics. Diuretics may be prescribed to treat congestive heart failure and cor pulmonale (see Drug Chart 11-1).

3. Administer respiratory syncytial virus (RSV) immune globulin (Respigam) to diminish the effects of RSV should infant be exposed to the organism.

4. Provide respiratory support through continuous mechanical ventilation and administration of oxygen via oxygen hood, nasal catheter, or cannula.

5. Support safe weaning from oxygen, which will be indicated by clinical manifestations of readiness:

     a. Maintenance of normal arterial blood gas, Pao_2, and $Paco_2$ levels

     b. No increase in the work of breathing

     c. Normal growth and development

6. Promote adequate oxygenation and a normal breathing pattern.

7. Promote desired fluid and nutritional intake.

  8. Provide family teaching, which includes instruction on cardiopulmonary resuscitation because of the high mortality rate associated with BPD during the first year of life (see Child and Family Teaching 11-1).

IV. Sudden infant death syndrome (SIDS)

A. Description

  1. SIDS is the term used to describe sudden, unexpected death of any infant for whom a postmortem examination fails to determine the cause of death. Death usually occurs during sleep.

  2. Infants at greatest risk for SIDS include premature infants, infants with apneic episodes, infants with prenatal drug exposure, siblings of infants who have died of SIDS, infants exposed to prenatal and postnatal maternal smoking, infants of adolescent mothers, infants of closely spaced pregnancies, underweight infants, infants with BPD, twins, Native American infants, Alaskan native infants, and economically disadvantaged black infants. Home monitoring is suggested for infants at risk.

  3. SIDS is the most common cause of death in children 1 month to 1 year of age.

B. Etiology

  1. Numerous theories have been proposed, but the etiology of SIDS remains unknown.

  2. It has been related to hypoxemia, apnea, an immature nervous system, and brain stem abnormality in neuroregulation of cardiorespiratory control.

  3. Recent findings suggest an increased incidence of SIDS in infants who sleep in the prone position. There has been a dramatic decrease in the incidence of SIDS since parents and caregivers started putting infants to sleep on their backs.

C. Pathophysiology. Autopsies reveal consistent findings, such as pulmonary edema and intrathoracic hemorrhages that are used to make a diagnosis of SIDS.

D. Assessment findings. Clinical manifestations may include:

  1. There are no characteristic findings before death. Parents or caregivers usually discover that the child has died in her sleep.

  2. Typically, the infant is huddled in a corner of a disheveled bed, with blankets over the head and hands clutching the sheets. Frothy, blood-tinged fluid fills the infant's mouth and nostrils, the infant may be lying in secretions, and the diaper is filled with urine and stool. The suddenness of the death and the appearance of the infant add to the horror that parents face.

E. Nursing management

  1. Evaluate family coping and grieving patterns.

  2. Provide anticipatory guidance for typical feelings.

  3. Allow the parents to verbalize; listen and validate feelings.

  4. Refer family for counseling, if needed.

  5. Refer to appropriate community self-help groups.

  6. Monitor infants at risk for apnea.

  7. Teach parents how to minimize the risk of SIDS:

     a. Avoid smoking during and after pregnancy.

b. Encourage putting infants to sleep in the prone position unless contraindicated; the side-lying position also may be used,

c. Avoid soft, moldable mattresses.

d. Avoid use of pillows.

e. Avoid overheating during sleep.

V. Upper respiratory tract infections

A. Definition

1. Upper respiratory tract infections include **nasopharyngitis**, **pharyngitis**, and **tonsillitis**.

a. Also called the common cold, nasopharyngitis is a viral infection of the nose and throat.

b. Pharyngitis is an infection (viral or bacterial) and inflammation of the pharynx.

c. Tonsillitis is an infection (viral or bacterial) and inflammation of the tonsils.

2. Of the upper respiratory tract inflammations, nasopharyngitis is the most common illness in infancy and childhood. Uncommon in infants younger than 1 year of age, incidence of pharyngitis peaks between 4 and 7 years of age. Incidence of tonsillitis peaks in school-age children.

B. Etiology

1. Nasopharyngitis is caused by a virus. Viruses most likely to cause the infection include rhinovirus, coxsackievirus, RSV, adeno-associated virus, and parainfluenza and influenza viruses.

2. Pharyngitis and tonsillitis can be either viral or bacterial in origin. The organism most commonly associated with bacterial infection is group A β-hemolytic *Streptococcus*, which has the potential to lead to complications such as rheumatic fever or acute glomerulonephritis.

C. Pathophysiology. Invading organisms initiate an inflammatory process in the epithelial cells of the mucous membrane layers of the nasopharynx and oropharynx.

D. Assessment findings

1. **Clinical manifestations**

a. **Nasopharyngitis**

(1) Nasal congestion

(2) Watery rhinitis

(3) Low-grade fever

(4) Difficulty breathing secondary to edema and congestion

(5) Enlarged cervical lymph nodes

(6) Respiratory distress (in young infants because they are obligatory nose breathers)

(7) Secondary symptoms, such as vomiting and diarrhea

b. **Pharyngitis**

(1) **Viral pharyngitis** manifestations are generally mild.

(a) Symptoms include sore throat, fever, and general malaise.

(b) Physical examination reveals erythema of the pharynx and palatine arch, and regional adenopathy.

(2) **Bacterial pharyngitis** manifestations include:

(a) Symptoms include severe sore throat, high fever, and lethargy.

(b) On examination, the pharynx is red. Palatine tonsils are enlarged and markedly erythematous, and may have white exudate. Petechiae may be noted on the palate.

(c) The child usually looks sick and may have difficulty swallowing.

(d) Other manifestations may include headache and abdominal pain.

 c. **Tonsillitis**

  (1) **Viral tonsillitis** is a mild disorder characterized by a gradual onset, low-grade fever, mild headache, sore throat, hoarseness, and a cough.

  (2) Bacterial tonsillitis is a more dramatic disorder marked by rapid onset of high fever, headache, generalized muscle aches, and vomiting.

 d. **Bacterial and viral pharyngitis and tonsillitis can not be differentiated by physical assessment alone. A throat culture is needed to confirm a diagnosis of streptococcal pharyngitis.**

2. Laboratory and diagnostic study findings. Throat culture may be positive for streptococcal organisms.

E. Nursing management

1. Assess respiratory status.

2. Minimize symptoms.

 a. Keep nasal passages clear in nasopharyngitis, especially in infants younger than 4 months, who are obligatory nose breathers, by using normal saline nose drops and a nasal aspirator.

 b. Provide liquids and soft foods.

 c. Use a cool mist vaporizer to keep mucous membranes moist.

3. Administer prescribed medications. A 10-day course of antibiotics (usually penicillin, but may be erythromycin if child is allergic to penicillin) is prescribed for bacterial infections to prevent the complication of rheumatic fever (see Drug Chart 11-1).

4. Provide child and family teaching (see Child and Family Teaching 11-1).

5. Provide preoperative and postoperative nursing care if surgery is performed (eg, to remove the tonsils). Tonsillectomy or adenoidectomy, or both, may be indicated for chronic enlargement of the tonsils that interferes with swallowing or breathing, or for recurrent streptococcal infections, peritonsillar abscess, or retropharyngeal abscess.

 a. Preoperative nursing care

  (1) Prepare the child for hospitalization and surgery according to his developmental level.

  (2) Explain that the child will have a sore throat after surgery, but he will be able to talk and swallow.

  (3) Explain the postoperative care measures (eg, proper positioning, ingesting cool liquids, and using an ice collar).

 b. Postoperative nursing care.

  (1) Observe for, and report, unusual bleeding.

  (2) Intervene for bleeding as appropriate.

  (3) Monitor vital signs.

  (4) Assess the child's color.

  (5) Help prevent bleeding by discouraging the child from coughing and clearing throat.

  (6) Position the child on the side or the abdomen to facilitate drainage from the throat.

  (7) Provide appropriate teaching. Instruct the child and parents to:

   (a) Observe activity restrictions, including when the child can return to school.

   (b) Avoid persons with known infections.

   (c) Provide a soft diet with an adequate fluid intake.

   (d) Avoid acidic or other irritating foods.

   (e) Monitor the child for bleeding, especially immediately postoperatively and 5 to 10 days postoperatively when tissues sloughing occurs.

VI.   Acute otitis media (AOM)

A. Description

1. AOM is inflammation of the middle ear.
2. It is one of the most prevalent diseases of early childhood, with peak incidence occurring between 6 months and 2 years of age. Approximately 70% of all children will experience at least one episode of otitis media.

B. Etiology

1. AOM is usually caused by *Haemophilus influenzae* or *Streptococcus pneumoniae.*
2. Contributing factors predisposing infants and children to otitis media include:
   a. Short, horizontally positioned eustachian tubes
   b. Poorly developed cartilage lining, which makes eustachian tubes more likely to open prematurely
   c. Enlarged lymphoid tissue, which obstructs eustachian tube openings
   d. Immature humoral defense mechanism, which increases the risk of infection
   e. Bottle-feeding an infant in the supine position, which allows formula to pool in the pharyngeal cavity; breast-fed infants have a lower incidence of AOM compared with formula-fed infants.
   f. Passive smoking, which is recognized as a significant contributing factor in acute otitis media

C. Pathophysiology

1. Eustachian tube dysfunction enables bacterial invasion of the middle ear and obstructs drainage of secretions.
2. Possible complications include hearing loss, tympanosclerosis (scarring), tympanic perforation, adhesive otitis ("glue-ear"), chronic suppurative otitis media, mastoiditis, meningitis, and cholesteatoma.

D. Assessment findings

1. Clinical manifestations

a. Infants characteristically do not localize infections.
b. Otitis media typically follows an upper respiratory infection and is characterized by the following:
   (1) Pain
   (2) Fever
   (3) Irritability
   (4) Loss of appetite
   (5) Nasal congestion
   (6) Cough
   (7) Vomiting and diarrhea
c. The infant will exhibit pain by crying and rubbing or pulling at the affected ear. Older children will verbally express complaints of ear pain.
d. Otoscopic findings disclose:
   (1) Injected or erythematous tympanic membrane; bulging tympanic membrane with no visible landmarks, including no light reflex; and diminished tympanic membrane mobility
   (2) Purulent discharge

2. Laboratory and diagnostic study findings

a. Culture and sensitivity tests may be done to identify the organism in aural discharge.
b. Audiometric testing establishes a baseline or detects any hearing loss secondary to recurring infection.

E. Nursing management

1. **Assess the child for fever and pain level**, and assess for possible complications.
2. **Administer prescribed medications.** Antibiotic therapy, usually amoxicillin, remains the standard pharmacologic treatment for acute AOM (see Drug Chart 11-1).
3. **Reduce fever** by administering antipyretics as prescribed and by having the child remove extra clothing. Be careful to avoid chilling.
4. **Relieve pain** by administering prescribed analgesics, offering soft foods to help the child limit chewing, and applying local heat or warm compresses to the affected ear.
5. **Facilitate drainage** by having the child lie with affected ear in a dependent position.
6. **Prevent skin breakdown** by keeping the external ear clean and dry.
7. **Provide preoperative and postoperative care,** if needed. Occasionally, a myringotomy (incision in the posterior inferior aspect of the tympanic membrane) may be necessary for draining exudate and releasing pressure. Tympanoplasty ventilating tubes or pressure-equalizing tubes may be inserted into the middle ear to create an artificial auditory canal that equalizes pressure on both sides of the tympanic membrane.
8. **Provide patient and family teaching.**
   a. Explain dosage, administration techniques, and possible side effects of medications.
   b. Emphasize the importance of completing the entire course of antibiotics.
   c. Identify signs of hearing loss and stress the importance of audiologic testing, if needed.
   d. Discuss preventive measures, such as holding the child upright for feedings, gentle nose blowing, blowing games, and chewing sugarless gum.
   e. Point out the need for follow-up care after completing antibiotic therapy to check for persistent infection.

VII. Acute laryngotracheobronchitis (LTB) and spasmodic croup

A. Description

1. **Acute LTB** is characterized by inflammation and narrowing of the laryngeal and tracheal areas. It is the most common form of croup and usually affects children younger than *8* years old.
2. **Spasmodic croup** is similar to acute LTB, but it tends to occur at night and recurs with respiratory tract infections. *usually affects children from age 6 mos. to 3 yrs. old.*

B. Etiology — *self-limiting*

1. **Acute LTB** is usually caused by a virus. Common organisms include parainfluenza viruses, adeno-associated viruses, RSV, and influenza viruses.
2. **Spasmodic croup** is ~~not~~ caused by a virus, but may *be caused by viruses and* have associated genetic, allergic, or emotional predisposing factors.

C. Pathophysiology

1. **Acute LTB** is usually preceded by an upper respiratory infection, which progresses to laryngitis and then descends into the trachea and, sometimes, the bronchi.
   a. The flexible larynx of a young child is particularly susceptible to spasm, which may cause complete airway obstruction.
   b. Profound airway edema may lead to obstruction and seriously compromised ventilation.
2. **Spasmotic croup.** The pathophysiology is similar to acute LTB except that there is no infectious cause. *, but may be caused by viruses c̄ allergic component. — self-limiting*

D. **Assessment findings. Clinical manifestations** will differ slightly for acute LTB and spasmodic croup.

1. **Acute LTB** is characterized by:
   a. Gradual onset from upper respiratory tract infection, which progresses to signs of distress
   b. Hoarseness (dysphonia) ↓ barking cough/brassy croupy cough (croaking frog)
   c. Inspiratory stridor
   d. Retractions
   e. Severe respiratory distress
   f. Low-grade fever (possible)
   g. Restlessness and irritability
   h. Pallor or cyanosis
   i. Wheezing, rales, rhonchi, and localized areas of diminished breath sounds

2. **Spasmodic croup** is characterized by signs and symptoms similar to acute LTB, but the child is afebrile, the onset is sudden, and the child is awakened at night with a barklike cough./croupy cough.

E. **Nursing management**

1. **Assess for airway obstruction** by evaluating respiratory status. Note color, respiratory effort, evidence of fatigue, and vital signs. (↑temp for LTB)

2. **Keep emergency equipment (tracheotomy and intubation tray) near the bedside**.

3. **Administer oxygen and increase atmospheric humidity** to alleviate hypoxia, as prescribed. This is usually done with a mist tent.

4. **Promote desired fluid intake.**

5. **Administer prescribed medications**, which may include aerosol (racemic) bronchodilators, such as epinephrine; anti-inflammatory medications, such as corticosteroids; or both (see Drug Chart 11-1).

6. **Minimize fear and anxiety.**

7. **Provide child and family teaching.**
   a. When the child awakens with a barklike cough, tell the parents to place the child in the bathroom and to run hot water to produce steam. to soothe inflammed membranes
   b. Instruct the parents to stay in the bathroom with the child to prevent accidental injury.
   c. See Child and Family Teaching 11-1 for general child and family teaching points.

VIII. Epiglottitis

A. **Description**

1. Epiglottitis is an acute, severe inflammation of the epiglottis.

2. This emergency situation occurs most commonly in children between 3 and 6 years of age.

B. **Etiology.** Epiglottitis is primarily caused by the bacterium *H. influenzae*, type B.

C. **Pathophysiology**

1. The soft tissue of the epiglottis becomes inflamed, which causes life-threatening marked obstruction.

2. Progressive obstruction results in hypoxia, hypercapnia, and acidosis, closely followed by decreased muscle tone, altered level of consciousness, and, if obstruction becomes complete, sudden death.

D. Assessment findings

1. **Clinical manifestations**
   a. Sudden onset of fever, lethargy, and dyspnea
   b. Restlessness and anxiety
   c. Hyperextension of the neck, drooling, and severe sore throat with refusal to drink
   d. Stridor and hoarseness
   e. Rapid thready pulse
   f. Characteristic "tripod" position, which consists of child sitting upright, leaning forward, with chin thrust out, mouth open, and tongue protruding (Fig. 11-1)
   g. Late signs of hypoxia, which include listlessness, cyanosis, bradycardia, and decreased respiratory rate with decreased aeration
   h. Red and inflamed throat with a large, cherry red, edematous epiglottis

2. **Laboratory and diagnostic study findings**
   a. X-ray films of the lateral neck show epiglottal enlargement, which confirms the diagnosis.
   b. Complete blood count (CBC) with differential (DIFF) reveals elevated white blood cell (WBC) count and increased bands and neutrophils.
   c. Blood culture may identify the causative bacteria.

E. Nursing management

1. **Closely monitor respiratory status to ensure airway patency.** If the child presents with symptoms of epiglottitis, ensure that appropriate personnel perform a throat examination and that emergency equipment is at hand.

2. **Prepare for emergency hospitalization.** After diagnosis is confirmed, an endotracheal intubation or tracheostomy typically is performed to maintain a patent airway. Swelling usually decreases after 24 hours and the child is generally extubated by the third day.

3. After the child is intubated, **monitor closely and maintain a patent airway** by suctioning as needed and providing oxygen therapy as prescribed.

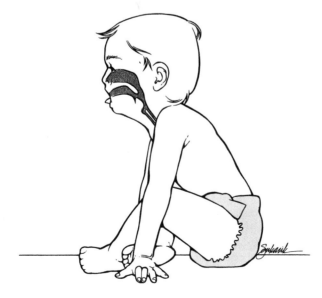

FIGURE 11-1
Classic tripod position of a child with epiglottitis: forward sitting, balanced on hands, mouth open, tongue protruding, and head tilted in sniffing position to relieve airway obstruction.

4. **Administer prescribed medications,** which may include antibiotics and anti-inflammatories, such as steroids (see Drug Chart 11-1).

5. **Minimize fear and anxiety.** Assist the child in finding a comfortable position for breathing before intubation, and administering a sedative, as prescribed, during intubation.

6. Recommend that all children receive *H. influenzae* type B (Hib) conjugate vaccine, beginning at 2 months of age, because *H. influenzae* is the most common cause of epiglottitis (see Chap. 10).

IX. Foreign body aspiration

A. Description

1. Aspiration occurs when a foreign body lodges somewhere in the upper respiratory tract. It can occur at any age but is most common in children between 1 and 3 years of age.

2. The severity of foreign body aspiration is determined by the location and extent of obstruction and the type of object aspirated. Objects such as peanuts and popcorn not only swell when wet, increasing obstruction, but are coated with oil, which adds to the risk of development of lipid pneumonia.

3. Common aspirates, besides peanuts and popcorn, include hot dogs, candy, grapes, cookies, carrots, peanut butter, latex balloons, coins, bullets, nails, and small toy parts.

4. The right bronchus is usually the site of bronchial obstruction because it is shorter and straighter than the left bronchus.

B. Etiology

1. Infants and children younger than 4 years of age are more likely to put small objects in their mouths.

2. Older children may aspirate when laughing while eating, or when engaging in risk-taking activities. This is especially true of adolescents who may be intoxicated.

C. Pathophysiology

1. Most foreign bodies lodge in a mainstem or lobar bronchus; the trachea is the next common site of obstruction. The site of obstruction is determined by the size, weight, and configuration of the object.

2. Three mechanisms of obstruction exist.
   a. **First-degree obstruction** occurs when the foreign body allows for passage of air in both directions.
   b. **Second-degree obstruction** occurs when air is able to move past the foreign body in one direction only. Air passages enlarge during inspiration, then diminish during expiration. This produces obstructive emphysema.
   c. **Complete obstruction** occurs when air is unable to move in either direction because the foreign body and edema obliterate passage. Air distal to the obstruction is absorbed, creating an area of obstruction atelectasis.

D. Assessment findings

1. **Clinical manifestations**
   a. Initially, foreign body aspiration causes choking and coughing.
   b. Additional signs and symptoms depend on the site and degree of obstruction.
      (1) Laryngotracheal obstruction causes dyspnea, hoarseness, cough, and stridor. Cyanosis occurs if it worsens.
      (2) Bronchial obstruction causes dyspnea, paroxysmal cough, wheezing, and asymmetric breath sounds.

    c. Secondary symptoms, which occur as a result of persistent obstruction, include signs of infection (eg, lipid pneumonia).

    d. If the object is not removed, the child may lose consciousness and die of asphyxiation.

  2. Laboratory and diagnostic study findings

    a. Chest x-ray films will reveal radiopaque objects.

    b. Bronchoscopy will reveal objects that are lodged in the trachea and larynx; fluoroscopy will reveal objects that are lodged in the bronchi.

E. Nursing management

  1. Assess signs and symptoms to determine location and degree of obstruction.

  2. Perform emergency measures for children who are choking.

    a. Abdominal thrusts for children older than 1 year of age

    b. Back blows and chest thrusts for children younger than 1 year of age

  3. Provide preprocedure and postprocedure care for the child undergoing bronchoscopy, which is used not only to visualize the foreign body, but to remove it as well. (See Appendix B)

  4. Encourage prevention of aspiration by teaching parents the following:

    a. Do not allow small children access to small objects.

    b. Use Mylar instead of latex balloons.

    c. Do not use adhesive bandages on small children.

    d. Spread peanut butter on bread; do not allow the child to eat it from a spoon because it can obstruct the airways and stick to the mucous membranes.

    e. Act as a positive role model and do not engage in behaviors such as holding pins, nails, or toothpicks in the mouth.

X. Bronchiolitis

A. Description

  1. Bronchiolitis is a viral infection of the lower respiratory tract characterized by inflammation of the bronchioles and production of mucus. It usually follows an upper respiratory tract infection.

  2. It is rare in children older than 2 years of age, and usually occurs between 2 months and 12 months of age, peaking at 6 months of age during the winter.

B. Etiology. RSV is responsible for more than half of all cases of bronchiolitis. RSV is a paramyxovirus that contains a single strand of ribonucleic acid (RNA). Two major subgroups exist—A, which is the most virulent and the more common, and B. Other viral causes include adeno-associated viruses and parainfluenza viruses.

C. Pathophysiology

  1. Inflammation of the bronchiole mucosa and presence of mucus cause varying degrees of obstruction of the bronchiolar lumen. This leads to air trapping and hyperinflation. If enough alveoli collapse, hypercapnia, hypoxemia, and respiratory acidosis may follow.

  2. The walls of the bronchi and bronchioles become infiltrated with inflammatory cells.

  3. Peribronchial interstitial pneumonitis is usually present.

D. Assessment findings

  1. Clinical manifestations

    a. Early signs and symptoms include irritability, rhinorrhea, pharyngitis, coughing, sneezing, wheezing, diffuse rhonchi and rales, and intermittent fever.

    b. As illness progresses, increased coughing and sneezing, air hunger, tachypnea and retractions, and cyanosis occur.

    c. Severe illness is characterized by tachypnea greater than 70 breaths per minute, list-lessness, apneic spells, poor air exchange, and markedly diminished breath sounds.

  2. Laboratory and diagnostic study findings

    a. Nasal washing may identify RSV by enzyme-linked immunosorbent assay (ELISA).

    b. Chest x-ray films show hyperaeration and areas of consolidation.

E. Nursing management

  1. Assess for respiratory distress. Note respiratory rate and rhythm, breath sounds, and adventitious sounds (especially wheezing). Check skin coloration.

  2. Institute contact isolation to prevent the spread of infection.

  3. Administer prescribed medications, such as bronchodilators and antivirals (see Drug Chart 11-1).

 4. Promote adequate oxygenation and a normal breathing pattern. Ensure high humidity with oxygen, as prescribed.

5. Promote desired fluid intake. The child may need IV fluids if tachypnea imposes risk of aspiration.

  6. Provide child and family teaching (see Child and Family Teaching 11-1).

XI. Pneumonia

A. Description

  1. Pneumonia is an acute inflammation of the lung parenchyma (ie, bronchioles, alveolar ducts and sacs, and alveoli) that impairs gas exchange.

  2. Pneumonia is classified according to etiologic agent (see below), but also according to location and extent of pulmonary involvement.

    a. Lobar pneumonia involves a large segment of one or more lobes.

    b. Bronchopneumonia begins in the terminal bronchioles and involves the nearby lobules.

    c. Interstitial pneumonia is confined to the alveolar walls and peribronchial and interlobular tissues.

  3. Pneumonia occurs at a rate of two to four children in 100 and is most commonly seen during the late winter and early spring.

B. Etiology

  1. Pneumonia most commonly results from infection with bacteria, viruses, or mycoplasmas, or from aspiration of foreign substances.

  2. The major organisms that cause bacterial pneumonia in infants younger than 3 months of age are *Streptococcus pneumoniae*, group A *Streptococcus*, *Staphylococcus*, gram-negative bacilli, enteric bacilli, and *Chlamydia*. In children between 3 months and 5 years of age, *S. pneumoniae*, *H. influenzae* (decreased since vaccine), and *Staphylococcus* are the typical causative organisms of bacterial pneumonia.

  3. Viral pneumonia occurs more frequently than bacterial pneumonia. The most common cause of viral pneumonia in infants is RSV. In older children, adeno-associated viruses, influenza, and parainfluenza viruses are typical causative organisms.

  4. Mycoplasma pneumonia is similar to viral pneumonia, except that the *Mycoplasma* organisms are somewhat larger than viral organisms. Mycoplasma pneumonia occurs more often in children older than 5 years of age.

C. Pathophysiology

1. Pneumonia typically begins with a mild upper respiratory tract infection. As the disorder progresses, parenchymal inflammation occurs.

2. Bacterial pneumonia most often causes lobular involvement and sometimes consolidation; viral pneumonia usually causes inflammation of interstitial tissue.

D. Assessment findings

1. Clinical manifestations

a. Common findings in **bacterial pneumonia** include:

(1) High fever

(2) Respiratory signs and symptoms, including cough (nonproductive to productive with whitish sputum), tachypnea, rhonchi, rales, dullness on percussion, chest pain, retractions, nasal flaring, and pallor or cyanosis (depending on severity)

(3) Irritability, restlessness, and lethargy

(4) Nausea, vomiting, anorexia, diarrhea, and abdominal pain

(5) Meningeal signs (meningism)

b. Common findings in **viral pneumonia** include:

(1) Variations ranging from mild fever, slight cough, and malaise to high fever, severe cough, and prostration

(2) Nonproductive or productive cough with whitish sputum

(3) Rhonchi or fine rales

c. Common findings in **mycoplasma pneumonia** include:

(1) Sudden or insidious onset

(2) Fever, chills, malaise, headache, anorexia, and myalgia

(3) Hacking cough, rhinitis, and sore throat

(4) Cough progresses from nonproductive to productive with seromucoid sputum that later becomes mucopurulent or blood-streaked

2. Laboratory and diagnostic study findings

a. Chest x-ray films may reveal diffuse or patchy infiltrates, consolidation, disseminated infiltration or patchy clouding, depending on the type of pneumonia.

b. CBC may reveal elevated a WBC count.

c. Blood culture, Gram stain, and sputum culture may reveal the causative organisms.

d. Positive antistreptolysin-O (ASO) titer is diagnostic of streptococcal pneumonia.

E. Nursing management

1. Assess for respiratory distress by monitoring vital signs and respiratory status.

2. Administer prescribed medications (see Drug Chart 11-1).

a. Antibiotics are indicated for the treatment of bacterial pneumonia. Penicillin G usually is used for pneumococcal and streptococcal pneumonia; a penicillinase-resistant penicillin (methicillin) usually is used for staphylococcal pneumonia.

b. Antibiotics are not used to treat viral pneumonia, but they may be recommended to reduce the risk of a secondary bacterial infection.

3. Promote adequate oxygenation and a normal breathing pattern.

4. Recommend the pneumococcal vaccine for children 2 years of age and older who are at risk (see Chap. 10).

5. Provide child and family teaching (see Child and Family Teaching 11-1).

XII.   Asthma

A. Description

1. Asthma is a chronic, reversible, obstructive airway disease, characterized by wheezing. It is caused by a spasm of the bronchial tubes, or the swelling of the bronchial mucosa, after exposure to various stimuli.
2. Asthma is the most common chronic disease in childhood. Most children experience their first symptoms by 5 years of age.

B. Etiology

1. Asthma commonly results from hyperresponsiveness of the trachea and bronchi to irritants. Allergy influences both the persistence and the severity of asthma, and atopy or the genetic predisposition for the development of an IgE-mediated response to common airborne allergens is the strongest predisposing factor for the development of asthma.
2. Common irritants include:
   a. Allergen exposure (in sensitized persons). Common allergens include:
      (1) Dust mites
      (2) Molds
      (3) Animal danders
   b. Viral infections
   c. Irritants, which include:
      (1) Air pollution
      (2) Smoke
      (3) Perfumes
      (4) Laundry detergents
   d. Certain foods (especially food additives)
   e. Rapid changes in environmental temperatures
   f. Exercise
   g. Psychological stress

C. Pathophysiology

1. An asthma attack may occur spontaneously or in response to a trigger. Either way, the attack progresses in the following manner.
   a. There is an initial release of inflammatory mediators from bronchial mast cells, epithelial cells, and macrophages, followed by activation of other inflammatory cells.
   b. Alterations of autonomic neural control of airway tone and epithelial integrity occur and the increased responsiveness in airway smooth muscle results in clinical manifestations (eg, wheezing and dyspnea).
2. Three events contribute to clinical manifestations.
   a. Bronchial spasm
   b. Inflammation and edema of the mucosa
   c. Production of thick mucus, which results in increased airway resistance, premature closure of airways, hyperinflation, increased work of breathing, and impaired gas exchange
3. If not treated promptly, status asthmaticus—an acute, severe, prolonged asthma attack that is unresponsive to the usual treatment—may occur, requiring hospitalization.

D. Assessment findings

1. Clinical manifestations (Box 11-1)
   a. Increased respiratory rate
   b. Wheezing (intensifies as attack progresses)
   c. Cough (productive)
   d. Use of accessory muscles
   e. Distant breath sounds
   f. Fatigue
   g. Moist skin
   h. Anxiety and apprehension
   g. Dyspnea

BOX 11-1. **Steps of Clinical and Diagnostic as per National Asthma Education and Prevention Program**

Mild Intermittent Asthma
- Symptoms $\leq$ 2 times per week
- Brief exacerbations
- Nighttime symptoms $\leq$ 2 times a month
- Asymptomatic and normal PEF (peak expiratory flow) between exacerbations
- PEF or FEV_1 (forced expiratory volume in 1 second) $\geq$ 80% of predicted value
- PEF variability $<$ 20%

Mild Persistent Asthma
- Symptoms $>$ 2 times/week, but less than once a day
- Exacerbations may affect activity
- Nighttimes symptoms $>$ 2 times a month
- PEF/FEV_1 $\geq$ 80% of predicted value
- PEF variability 20%–30%

Moderate Persistent Asthma
- Daily symptoms
- Daily use of inhaled short-acting β_2-agonists
- Exacerbations affect activity
- Exacerbations $\geq$ 2 times a week
- Exacerbations may last days
- Nighttime symptoms $>$ once a week
- PEF/FEV_1 $>$60%–$<$80% of predicted value
- PEF variability $>$ 30%

Severe Persistent Asthma
- Continual symptoms
- Frequent exacerbations
- Frequent nighttime symptoms
- Limited physical activity
- PEF or FEV_1 $\leq$ 60% of predicted value
- PEF variability $>$ 30%

2. **Laboratory and diagnostic study findings.** Spirometry will detect:
   a. Decreased forced expiratory volume (FEV)
   b. Decreased peak expiratory flow rate (PEFR)
   c. Diminished forced vital capacity (FVC)
   d. Diminished inspiratory capacity (IC)

E. **Nursing management**

1. **Assess respiratory status** by closely evaluating breathing patterns and monitoring vital signs.
2. **Administer prescribed medications**, such as bronchodilators, anti-inflammatories, and antibiotics (see Drug Chart 11-1).
3. **Promote adequate oxygenation and a normal breathing pattern.**
4. **Explain the possible use of hyposensitization therapy** (see Chap. 9).
5. **Help the child cope with poor self-esteem** by encouraging him to ventilate feelings and concerns. Listen actively as the child speaks, focus on the child's strengths, and help him to identify the positive and negative aspects of his situation.
6. **Discuss the need for periodic PFTs** to evaluate and guide therapy and to monitor the course of the illness.
7. **Provide child and family teaching.** Assist the child and family to name signs and symptoms of an acute attack and appropriate treatment measures (see Child and Family Teaching 11-1 for general child and family teaching information).
8. **Refer the family to appropriate community agencies for assistance.**

XIII. Cystic fibrosis (CF)

A. **Description**

1. CF is a chronic, multisystem disorder of the exocrine glands characterized by abnormally thick pulmonary secretions. CF affects the pancreas, respiratory system, gastrointestinal tract, salivary glands, and reproductive tract.
2. CF is considered the most common cause of chronic lung disease in children. It is the most common fatal inherited disease affecting whites; incidence is approximately 1/2500 live births, and about 5% of persons are asymptomatic carriers. CF occurs rarely in blacks and Asians.

B. **Etiology**

1. CF is an autosomal recessive hereditary disorder caused by a defective gene.
2. The gene responsible for CF is located on chromosome 7 with its protein product, cystic fibrosis transmembrane regulator (CFTR). Numerous alterations that diverge from the original sequence of the gene have been reported.

C. **Pathophysiology**

1. The underlying defect is thought to be related to a protein or enzyme alteration.
2. Several mechanisms result in the CF process.
   a. Exocrine glands become obstructed by thick mucus; electrolyte concentrations in the exocrine secretions are abnormal.
   b. The ciliary lining in the respiratory tract moves 5 to 10 times slower than normal.
   c. Secretions accumulate in respiratory passages, causing obstruction, air trapping, and increasing the incidence of respiratory infections (which are most commonly caused by *Pseudomonas aeruginosa, Pseudomonas cepacia* [*Burkholderia cepacia*], *Staphylococcus aureus, H. influenza, Escherichia coli,* and *Klebsiella pneumoniae*).
   d. Recurrent respiratory infections lead to bronchiectasis and fibrosis.

e. The small intestine, bile ducts, salivary glands, and the reproductive system also are affected negatively by thickened secretions.

D. Assessment findings

1. **Clinical manifestations.** Manifestations vary with severity and time of emergence; they may appear at birth or take years to develop.

a. **Respiratory signs and symptoms** include:

(1) Wheezing, dyspnea, cough, and cyanosis

(2) Atelectasis and generalized obstructive emphysema, which occur as the disease progresses and result from mucoid obstruction in small airways; these conditions produce the characteristic features of barrel chest and finger clubbing.

(3) Chronic sinusitis, bronchitis, bronchopneumonia, and ear, nose, and throat problems

b. **Gastrointestinal signs** include:

(1) Meconium ileus at birth

(2) Rectal prolapse (most common gastrointestinal sign)

(3) Loose, bulky, frothy, fatty stools; voracious appetite; weight loss; marked tissue wasting; failure to thrive; distended abdomen; thin extremities; and evidence of vitamin A, D, E, and K deficiencies

(4) Partial or complete intestinal obstruction (known in CF as distal intestinal obstruction syndrome [DIOS])

c. **Reproductive signs** include:

(1) Females will have delayed puberty and decreased fertility (apparently from increased viscosity of cervical mucus, which blocks the entry of sperm).

(2) Males, with few exceptions, are infertile; sterility is caused by blockage of the vas deferens with abnormal secretions, which prevents sperm from forming.

d. **Cardiovascular signs** include:

(1) Cor pulmonale, right-sided heart enlargement, and congestive heart failure resulting from obstruction of pulmonary blood flow

(2) Signs and symptoms of hyponatremia, necessitating rapid IV electrolyte replacement to prevent circulatory collapse

e. **Integumentary signs** include:

(1) Increased concentrations of sodium and chloride in sweat; parents report a "salty" taste when they kiss their babies.

(2) Failure to thrive may result in hypoalbuminemia, which causes edema.

2. **Laboratory and diagnostic study findings**

a. Sweat test (iontophoresis with pilocarpine) reveals elevated chloride levels above 60 mEq/L.

b. Stool analysis will detect steatorrhea.

c. Chest x-ray films will show evidence of characteristic patchy atelectasis and generalized obstructive emphysema.

E. Nursing management

1. **Perform a multisystem assessment,** observing for symptom worsening and complications.

2. **Promote adequate oxygenation and a normal breathing pattern (good pulmonary hygiene).**

a. Encourage aerosol treatments with bronchodilators and breathing exercises.

b. Assist the child in the proper use of the Flutter Mucus Clearance Device (Scandipharm, Inc.), which is a small hand-held device that facilitates the removal of mucus. This is contraindicated in young children because it may pose a choking hazard if the device separates.

3. **Assess nutritional status** by maintaining calorie counts, monitoring intake and output, and recording daily weights.

4. **Promote desired nutritional intake.** The prescribed diet typically is high in calories and protein, with fats as tolerated and increased salt intake during hot weather or febrile periods.

5. **Administer prescribed medications,** including pancreatic enzymes, bronchodilators, antibiotics, and fat-soluble vitamins (A, D, E, K) (see Drug Chart 11-1).

6. **Allow the family and child to verbalize about the chronic nature of the disorder and its long-term implications,** including death and dying.

7. **Prepare the child and family for lung transplantation,** if necessary.

8. **Provide child and family teaching** (see Child and Family Teaching 11-1).
   a. Review the diagnosis, disease process, long-term implications, and chronic nature of the condition.
   b. Highlight the importance of good pulmonary hygiene, infection prevention, and general well-being.
   c. Outline special dietary instructions.

STUDY QUESTIONS

1. When caring for a very low-birth-weight newborn, the nurse carefully monitors inspiratory pressure and oxygen (O_2) concentration to prevent which of the following?
   (1) Respiratory distress syndrome (RDS)
   (2) Respiratory syncytial virus (RSV)
   (3) Bronchopulmonary dysplasia (BPD)
   (4) Meconium aspiration syndrome

2. Which of the following infants is **least** likely to develop sudden infant death syndrome (SIDS)?
   (1) An infant who was premature
   (2) A sibling of an infant who died of SIDS
   (3) An infant with prenatal drug exposure
   (4) An infant who sleeps on his back

3. Which of the following instructions should be included in the teaching plan for parents of an young child with otitis media?
   (1) Cleaning the inside of the ear canals with cotton swabs
   (2) Placing the child in the supine position to bottle feed
   (3) Avoiding contact with people who have upper respiratory infections
   (4) Giving prescribed amoxicillin (Amoxcil) on an empty stomach

4. Ribavirin (Virazole) is used to treat which of the following?
   (1) Bronchiolitis
   (2) Respiratory syncytial virus (RSV)
   (3) Otitis media
   (4) Cystic fibrosis

5. Which of the following respiratory conditions is always considered a medical emergency?
   (1) Laryngotracheobronchitis (LTB)
   (2) Epiglottitis
   (3) Asthma
   (4) Cystic fibrosis (CF)

6. Immunization of children with the *H. influenzae* type B (Hib) vaccine decreases the incidence of which of the following conditions?
   (1) Laryngotracheobronchitis (LTB)
   (2) Epiglottitis
   (3) Pneumonia
   (4) Bronchiolitis

7. In a child with asthma, β-adrenergic agonist agents, such as albuterol, are administered primarily to do which of the following?
   (1) Decrease postnasal drip
   (2) Dilate the bronchioles
   (3) Reduce airway inflammation
   (4) Reduce secondary infections

8. Which of the following would the nurse expect to assess in an older child with pneumococcal pneumonia?
   (1) Bulging fontanelle
   (2) Mild cough
   (3) Slight fever
   (4) Chest pain

9. An acute, severe prolonged asthmatic attack that is unresponsive to usual treatment is referred to as which of the following?
   (1) Intrinsic asthma
   (2) Status asthmaticus
   (3) Reactive airway disease
   (4) Extrinsic asthma

10. Which of the following statements by the family of a child with asthma indicates a need for additional home care teaching?
   (1) "We need to identify what things trigger his attacks."
   (2) "He is to use his bronchodilator inhaler before the steroid inhaler."
   (3) "We'll make sure that he avoids exercise to prevent attacks."
   (4) "He should increase his fluid intake regularly to thin secretions."

11. When developing a plan of care for the child diagnosed with cystic fibrosis (CF), which of the following must the nurse keep in mind?

(1) CF is an autosomal dominant hereditary disorder.

(2) Pulmonary secretions are abnormally thick.

(3) Obstruction of the endocrine glands occurs.

(4) Elevated levels of potassium are found in the sweat.

ANSWER KEY

1. The answer is (3). Close monitoring of inspiratory pressure and oxygen concentration is necessary to prevent BPD, which is related to the use of high inspiratory pressures and oxygen concentrations especially in very low-birth-weight and extremely low-birth-weight infants with lung disorders. RDS, a disorder caused by lack of surfactant, usually is found in premature infants. RSV is a group of viruses that cause respiratory infections such as bronchiolitis and pneumonia. Meconium aspiration syndrome is a respiratory disorder created by the aspiration of meconium in the perinatal period.

2. The answer is (4). Infants who sleep on their back are least likely to develop SIDS. However, SIDS has been associated with infants who sleep on their abdomens. Prematurity, siblings of an infant who has died of SIDS, and those prenatally exposed to drugs are all considered to be at high risk for the development of SIDS.

3. The answer is (3). Otitis media is commonly precipitated by an upper respiratory tract infection. Therefore children prone to otitis should avoid persons known to have an upper respiratory tract infection. Cotton swabs can cause injuries, such as tympanic perforation. They may be used to clean the outer ear, but they should never be inserted into the ear canal. A bottle-fed child should be fed in an upright position because feeding the child in the supine position may actually precipitate otitis by allowing formula to pool in the pharyngeal cavity. Amoxicillin, when prescribed, should be given with food to prevent stomach upset.

4. The answer is (2). Ribavirin is an antiviral medication used for treating severe RSV infection and for children with RSV who are compromised (such as children with BPD or heart disease). The drug is not used to treat bronchiolitis, otitis media, or cystic fibrosis.

5. The answer is (2). Epiglottitis, acute and severe inflammation of the epiglottis, is always considered an acute medical emergency because it can lead to acute, life-threatening airway obstruction. Acute LTB requires close observation for airway obstruction, but this condition is not always an emergency. Asthma is a chronic disease; however, status asthmaticus and acute attacks require prompt treatment. CF is a chronic disease and is not considered an emergency.

6. The answer is (2). Epiglottitis is a bacterial infection of the epiglottis primarily caused by *H. influenzae* type B. Administration of the vaccine has decreased the incidence of epiglottitis. Acute LTB is of viral origin. The most common bacterial organisms causing pneumonia in children are pneumococci, streptococci, and staphylococci. Bronchiolitis is usually caused by RSV.

7. The answer is (2). β-Adrenergic agonists, such as albuterol, are highly effective bronchodilators and are used to dilate the narrow airways associated with asthma. Decongestants may be given to decrease postnasal drip. Corticosteroids may be used for their anti-inflammatory effect; antibiotics are used to prevent secondary infection.

8. The answer is (4). Older children with pneumococcal pneumonia may complain of chest pain. A bulging fontanelle may be seen in infants with meningitis or increased intracranial pressure. A mild cough and slight fever are more commonly assessed with viral pneumonia.

9. **The answer is (2).** Status asthmaticus is an acute, prolonged, severe asthmatic attack that is unresponsive to usual treatment. Often the child requires hospitalization. Intrinsic is a term used to denote internal precipitating factors, such as viruses. Reactive airway disease is another general term for asthma. Extrinsic is a term used to denote external precipitating factors, such as allergens.

10. **The answer is (3).** Additional teaching is needed if the family states that the child with asthma should avoid exercise to prevent attacks. Children with asthma should be encouraged to exercise as tolerated. Identifying triggers, using a bronchodilator inhaler before a steroid inhaler, and increasing fluid intake are appropriate measures to be included in a home care teaching program for the child with asthma and his family.

11. **The answer is (2).** CF is characterized by abnormally thick pulmonary secretions. It is a chronic inherited disorder, specifically an autosomal recessive hereditary disorder affecting the exocrine, not endocrine glands. The thick mucus obstructs the exocrine glands. Diagnosis of CF is based on elevated chloride levels found in sweat.

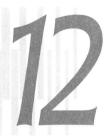

Gastrointestinal Dysfunction

Structure and function of the gastrointestinal (GI) system

A. Structures

1. The **upper GI system** includes the mouth, esophagus, and stomach.
2. The **lower GI system** includes the duodenum, liver, gallbladder, pancreas, jejunum, ileum, cecum, appendix, ascending colon, transverse colon, descending colon, sigmoid colon, rectum, and anus. Table 12-1 provides information on the development of the GI system.

B. Function. The primary functions of the digestive system are digestion and absorption.

1. **Digestion** involves physical and chemical breakdown of food into absorbable substances.
2. **Absorption** involves transfer of the end-products of digestion across the intestinal wall into the circulation for use by the cells.

 II. **NURSING PROCESS OVERVIEW FOR The Gastrointestinal System**

A. Assessment

1. **Health history**

   a. Elicit a description of symptoms including onset, duration, location, and precipitation. **Cardinal symptoms** may include:

   (1) Anorexia

   (2) Nausea and vomiting

   (3) Diarrhea or constipation

   (4) Abdominal pain

   (5) Recent weight gain or loss

   (6) Blood in stool

   b. Explore prenatal, personal, and family history for **risk factors** for GI disorders.

   (1) Prenatal history risk factors include maternal exposure to medications.

   (2) Personal history risk factors include low birth weight, prematurity, feeding difficulties, metabolic disorders, neuromuscular disorders, blood dyscrasias, immunosuppression, substance abuse, stress, or poisoning.

   (3) Family history risk factors include history of GI disorders, such as inflammatory bowel disease or malabsorption syndromes.

   c. Elicit a complete nutritional history, including a 24-hour dietary intake.

TABLE 12-1
Development of the Gastrointestinal System

AGE	STRUCTURE AND FUNCTION
Fetal development	Development of a primitive digestive system begins during the fourth week of gestation, with the most extensive development occurring in the last few weeks before birth. During intrauterine life, the GI tract can be divided into three parts: foregut (esophagus, stomach, and proximal duodenum), midgut (distal duodenum, jejunum, ileum, cecum, and proximal colon), and hind gut (distal colon and rectum). The salivary glands, liver, gallbladder, and pancreas grow from the foregut and midgut.
Infant (0–1 year)	The newborn GI system is immature with a stomach capacity of 90 mL that rapidly empties. The system matures slightly at about 3 months when the infant has more adult-like saliva composition and amount. Stomach capacity increases to reach 210–360 mL by age 1 year, and emptying time slows. Gastric acid secretion is low, and pepsinogen approximates adult levels by 3 months. The liver is proportionately larger than the adult's and is immature until age 1 year. Peristalsis matures by 8 months, causing stools to be more formed. Primary dentition starts about age 6 months.
Toddler/Preschooler (1–6 years)	Digestive glands reach maturity, and gastric acid secretion gradually increases. Stomach capacity is about 500 mL. Primary dentition is completed by age 2.5 years with full 20 teeth.
Schoolager (6–12 years)	The GI system becomes more efficient with better digestion, absorption, secretion, and excretion; thus, there is less stomach upset. Stomach capacity by age 10 years is 750–900 mL. Primary teeth shed, and secondary teeth erupt.
Adolescent (12–21 years)	Gastric acidity increases, and stomach capacity grows to 1000–1500 mL, correlating with increased appetite. The intestines increase in length and circumference, and abdominal musculatures become stronger and thicker. The liver reaches adult size and function. All 32 secondary teeth have erupted by age 21.

2. **Physical examination**
   a. **Vital signs**
      (1) Measure height and weight for signs of growth failure.
      (2) Temperature elevation may be indicative of infection or dehydration.
   b. **Inspection**
      (1) Inspect the skin for pallor, jaundice, and carotenemia.
      (2) Inspect the mouth for caries, periodontal disease, lesions, and clefts.
      (3) Inspect the abdomen for distention, depression, umbilical herniation, and visible peristaltic waves.
      (4) Inspect the anus for rectal bleeding and nonpatency.
   c. **Auscultation**
      (1) Auscultation of the abdomen must be performed before palpation or percussion to avoid altering bowel sounds.
      (2) Auscultate the abdomen to assess bowel sounds (note absence or hyperactivity).
   d. **Palpation**
      (1) Palpate the hard and soft palates for defects.

      (2) Palpate the abdomen to note for tenderness, rigidity, masses, and organomegaly.

    e. **Percussion.** Percuss the abdomen for presence of excessive gas, masses, fluid, and an enlarged liver span.

3. Laboratory studies and diagnostic tests (see Appendices A and B for normal findings and nursing considerations)

    a. **Stool analysis,** including tests for bacteria, ova and parasites, blood, mucus, fat, urobilogen, trypsin, leukocytes (Table 12-2), reducing substances, and pH, may be performed to determine the presence of infection, infestation, bleeding, or malabsorption disorders.

    b. **Erythrocyte sedimentation rate (ESR)** may be performed to determine the presence of inflammation.

    c. A **complete blood count (CBC)** may be ordered to evaluate presence of anemia in the case of bleeding.

    d. **Abdominal ultrasound** is used to visualize organ structure and to identify problems such as cysts, abscesses, tumors, gallstones, and appendicitis.

    e. **Gastric x-ray radiography**, **upper GI study**, **esophagus and stomach x-ray,** and a **small bowel study** may be performed to detect lesions, obstruction, and motility problems.

    f. **Barium enema** (large bowel study, colon x-ray) may be performed to detect lesions, obstruction, and motility problems of the lower GI system.

    g. **Computed tomography** identifies tumors, abscesses, and biliary duct obstruction.

TABLE 12-2
Stool Analysis

PARAMETER	NORMAL FINDINGS	IMPLICATIONS OF ABNORMAL FINDINGS
Color	Brown (shade varies with diet)	Black: GI bleeding
		Tan or clay: common bile duct blockage; pancreatic insufficiency
		Red streaked: lower GI bleeding
Blood	Negative	Positive: GI bleeding; ulcerative colitis
Mucus	Negative	Positive: ulcerative colitis; bacillary dysentery
Fat	*Fatty acids:* 0–6 years: <2 g/24 hours	Increase: malabsorption syndromes
	6 and over: 2–6 g/24 hours	
Urobilogen	30–200 mg/100 g feces	Increase: hemolytic anemia
		Decrease: biliary obstruction, severe liver disease, oral antibiotic therapy that alters intestinal flora, or disorders causing decreased hemoglobin turnover (eg, aplastic anemia)
Trypsin	Positive for a small amount in 95% of all children	Absence: pancreatic insufficiency
pH	7.0–7.5	Acid: carbohydrate fermentation
		Alkaline: protein breakdown
Nitrogen	1–2 g/24 hours	Increase (along with high fecal fat): chronic progressive pancreatitis

    h. **Esophagogastroduodenoscopy (EGD), endoscopy, and gastroscopy** are upper GI endoscopic procedures performed using a fiberoptic endoscope to examine the lumen and mucosal lining of the esophagus, stomach, and upper portion of the small intestine. These tests determine tissue abnormality, GI bleeding, and ulcers.

    i. **Colonoscopy, proctoscopy, anoscopy, sigmoidoscopy, and proctosigmoidoscopy** are lower GI endoscopic procedures performed to evaluate the colon and terminal cecum for the presence of inflammatory bowel disease, GI bleeding, and diarrhea. Biopsies may be performed during the procedure.

B. Nursing diagnoses

    1. Altered nutrition: less than body requirements

    2. Fluid volume deficit

    3. Pain

    4. Altered growth and development

C. Planning and outcome identification

    1. The child will receive adequate nutrition and gain weight.

    2. The child will achieve and maintain normal fluid and electrolyte status.

    3. The child will experience minimal or no pain.

    4. The child will experience no alterations in growth and development.

D. Implementation

    1. Provide adequate nutrition according to the child's age and nutritional requirements.

      a. Monitor feeding and eating patterns.

      b. Record daily food intake.

      c. Monitor daily weights.

      d. Encourage nutritious feedings appropriate for age and condition.

      e. Administer enteral or parenteral feedings as needed.

    2. Promote adequate hydration.

      a. Monitor hydration status by recording fluid intake and output (I&O), weighing the child daily, and evaluating urine specific gravity.

      b. Ensure adequate hydration by assessing for signs and symptoms of dehydration, monitoring fluid I&O, and administering intravenous (IV) fluids as prescribed.

    3. Relieve pain.

      a. Assess location, duration, frequency, and type of pain.

      b. Provide analgesics as needed.

      c. Use nonpharmacologic methods of pain relief, such as distraction and guided imagery.

    4. Promote healthy growth and development.

      a. **Infants.** Oral gratification may be compromised by an infant's inability to suck well owing to a cleft lip or palate, surgery, and alternate feeding methods.

      b. **Toddlers.** Locomotion is compromised in a child receiving long-term hyperalimentation or drug therapy.

      c. **Preschoolers.** Malnourishment may interfere with development of normal motor skills such as running.

      d. **School-age children and adolescents.** Body image and self-concept may be challenged by a child's altered body function and health maintenance needs.

E. Outcome evaluation

    1. The child receives adequate nutrition and gains weight.

    2. The child achieves and maintains normal fluid and electrolyte status.

    3. The child experiences minimal or no pain.

    4. The child experiences no alterations in growth and development.

III. Cleft lip and palate

A. **Description**

1. **Cleft lip (CL)** is a congenital anomaly that occurs at a rate of 1 in 800 births.
   a. It ranges in severity from a slight dimple to a large fissure that extends from the lip up into the nasal structures.
   b. Cleft lip can be unilateral or bilateral.
2. **Cleft palate (CP)** is a congenital anomaly that occurs in approximately 1 of every 2000 births, and it is more common in boys than girls.
   a. It ranges in severity from soft palate involvement alone to a defect including the hard palate and portions of the maxilla.
   b. Cleft palate may or may not be associated with cleft lip.
3. Children with these structural disorders may have associated dental malformations, speech problems, and frequent otitis media, the latter resulting from improper functioning of the eustachian tubes.

B. **Etiology**

1. Many factors are associated with the development of CL and CP, and CL with or without CP is developmentally and genetically different from isolated CP.
2. Most cases appear to be consistent with the concept of multifactorial inheritance as evidenced by an increased incidence in relatives and monozygotic twins.

C. **Pathophysiology**

1. During embryonic development the lateral and medial tissues forming the upper lip fuse between weeks 7 and 8 of gestation; the palatal tissues forming the hard and soft palates fuse between weeks 7 and 12 of gestation.
2. CL and CP result when these tissues fail to fuse.

D. **Assessment findings**

1. **Clinical manifestations**
   a. CL and CP are readily apparent at birth. Careful physical assessment should be performed to rule out other midline birth defects.
   b. CL and CP appear as incomplete or complete defects, and may be unilateral or bilateral.
2. **Laboratory and diagnostic study findings**. Obstetric ultrasound will reveal CL while the infant is in utero.

E. **Nursing management**

1. **Assess for problems with feeding, breathing, parental bonding, and speech**.
2. **Ensure adequate nutrition and prevent aspiration**.
   a. Provide special nipples or feeding devices (eg, soft pliable bottle with soft nipple with enlarged opening) for a child unable to suck adequately on standard nipples.
   b. Hold the child in a semiupright position; direct the formula away from the cleft and toward the side and back of the mouth to prevent aspiration.
   c. Feed the infant slowly and burp frequently to prevent excessive swallowing of air and regurgitation.
   d. Stimulate sucking by gently rubbing the nipple against the lower lip.
3. **Support the infant's and parents' emotional and social adjustment**.
   a. Help facilitate the family's acceptance of the infant by encouraging the parents to express their feelings and concerns and by conveying an attitude of acceptance toward the infant.
   b. Emphasize the infant's positive aspects and express optimism regarding surgical correction.

4. **Provide preoperative care**.
    a. Depending on the defect and the child's general condition, surgical correction of the CL usually occurs at 1 to 3 months of age; repair of the CP is usually performed between 6 and 18 months of age. Repair of the CP may require several stages of surgery as the child grows.
    b. Early correction of CL enables more normal sucking patterns and facilitates bonding. Early correction of CP enables development of more normal speech patterns.
    c. Delayed closure or large defects may require the use of orthodontic appliances.
    d. The responsibilities of the nurse are to:
        (1) Reinforce the physician's explanation of surgical procedures.
        (2) Provide mouth care to prevent infection.
5. **Provide postoperative care.**
    a. Assess airway patency and vital signs; observe for edema and respiratory distress.
    b. Use a mist tent, if prescribed, to minimize edema, liquefy secretions, and minimize distress.
    c. Position the child with CL on her back, in an infant seat, or propped on a side to avoid injury to the operative site; position the child with a CP on the abdomen to facilitate drainage.
    d. Clean the suture line and apply an antibacterial ointment as prescribed to prevent infection and scarring. Monitor the site for signs of infection.
    e. Use elbow restraints to maintain suture line integrity. Remove them every 2 hours for skin care and range-of-motion exercises.
    f. Feed the infant with a rubber-tipped medicine dropper, bulb syringe, Breck feeder, or soft bottle-nipple, as prescribed, to help preserve suture integrity. For older children, diet progresses from clear fluids; they should not use straws or sharp objects.
    g. Attempt to keep the child from putting tongue up to palate sutures.
    h. Manage pain by administering analgesics as prescribed.
6. **Provide child and family teaching** (Child and Family Teaching 12-1).

[handwritten margin note: side-lying position away from the corrected side is the best position for CL to prevent aspiration. as prescribed]

CHILD AND FAMILY TEACHING 12-1

Cleft Lip and Cleft Palate Care

- Demonstrate surgical wound care.
- Show proper feeding techniques and positions.
- Explain that temperature of feeding formulas should be monitored closely because new palate has no nerve endings; therefore, the child can suffer a burn to the palate easily and without knowing it.
- Explain handling of prosthesis if indicated.
- Stress the importance of long-term followup, including speech therapy, and preventing or correcting dental abnormalities.
- Discuss the need for, at least, annual hearing evaluations because of the increased susceptibility to recurrent otitis. The child may require myringotomy and surgical placement of drainage tubes.
- Teach infection control measures.

IV. Gastroesophageal reflux (GER)

A. Description

1. GER is the backflow of gastric contents into the esophagus resulting from relaxation or incompetence of the lower esophageal (cardiac) sphincter.

2. GER is the most common esophageal problem in infancy. Some reflux occurs normally in infants, children, and adults. GER is deemed pathologic when it is severe, persists into late infancy, or is associated with complications.

3. GER is not uncommon in children with tracheoesophageal or esophageal atresia repairs, prematurity, bronchopulmonary dysplasia, cerebral palsy, neurologic disorders, scoliosis, asthma, or cystic fibrosis.

B. Etiology. The cause is unknown, but GER may result from delayed maturation of lower esophageal neuromuscular function or impaired local hormonal, control mechanisms.

C. Pathophysiology

1. Inappropriate relaxation or failure of cardiac sphincter contraction leads to increased gastric or abdominal pressure and resultant reflux of gastric contents.

2. Delayed gastric emptying may be a contributing factor in GER.

3. Repeated reflux of acidic gastric contents can damage delicate esophageal mucosa.

D. Assessment findings

1. **Clinical manifestations**

    a. Forceful vomiting, possibly with hematemesis   *most common manifestation*
    b. Weight loss
    c. Aspiration and recurrent respiratory infections
    d. Cyanotic and apneic episodes that may be life-threatening
    e. Esophagitis and bleeding from repeated irritation of the esophageal lining with gastric acid
    f. Melena (dark stools)   *accumulated* *≈ (dff acid)*
    g. Heartburn, abdominal pain, and a bitter taste in the mouth *{ less common*

2. **Laboratory and diagnostic study findings**

    a. Upper GI study will reveal reflux following barium swallow and absence of gastric or duodenal obstruction, which is indicative of reflux.
    b. Esophageal manometry will reveal low resting lower esophageal sphincter pressure, which signifies reflux.
    c. CBC may reveal anemia, which may occur secondary to blood loss.
    d. Intraesophageal pH monitoring measures reflux acid from the stomach.
    e. Scintigraphy detects radiographic substances in the esophagus after feeding a compound to the child.

E. Nursing management

1. **Promote adequate hydration.**

2. **Assess the amount, frequency, and characteristics of emesis.**

3. **Assess the relationship between feeding and vomiting and the infant's activity level.**

4. **Improve nutritional status through feeding techniques.**

    a. Administer small frequent feedings.   *to prevent vomiting*
    b. Administer formula thickened with cereal using enlarged nipple holes. At this writing, thickened feedings are controversial; therefore, this intervention may change.
    c. Burp the infant frequently. *to prevent excessive swallowing of air and regurgitation.*

+ prone position c̄ head elevated is the most appropriate for child
c̄ GER

5. **Prevent reflux and respiratory complications.**
   a. Position the infant upright, *and (L) side* as prescribed, through feedings and afterward, in an infant seat. At this writing, upright positioning is controversial.
   b. Assess breath sounds before and after feedings.
   c. Keep suctioning equipment at bedside.
   d. Place the infant on a cardiac-apnea monitor, when needed.
6. **Administer prescribed medications**, including:
   a. Antacids and histamine receptor antagonists (H_2 blockers) such as cimetadine (Tagamet), rantidine (Zantac), or famotidine (Pepcid), which reduce acid and may prevent esophagitis
   b. Omerprazole (Prilosec), which blocks the proton pump in parietal cells of the gastric mucosa
   c. Prokinetic medications, such as metoclopramide (Reglan), which may decrease reflux   *↳ anti-emetic*
   d. Cisapride (Propulsid), which increases lower esophageal pressure, promotes gastric emptying, and has fewer side effects than metoclopramide.
7. **Provide child and family teaching** regarding feeding and positioning.
8. **Provide postoperative care**.
   a. GER commonly is self-limiting, usually resolving by age 1 year. In more severe cases, the child may require hospitalization and possibly surgery, such as a Nissen fundoplication, in which the gastric fundus is wrapped around the distal esophagus.
   b. Placement of a nonsurgical percutaneous gastrojejunostomy tube may be an alternative to surgery for children with neurologic impairment.
   ✳ c. Postoperative nursing responsibilities include:
      (1) Prevent gastric distention by monitoring the nasogastric tube or gastrostomy.
      (2) Vent the gastrostomy tube for several days if the child is to receive gastrostomy feedings.
      ✳ (3) Inform parents of problems that may follow surgery, which may include flatulence, inability to vomit, poor feeding habits, and choking on solid foods.

V. Pyloric stenosis

A. **Description**. Pyloric stenosis is the narrowing of the pyloric sphincter at the outlet of the stomach.

B. **Etiology.** The exact cause is unknown; however, heredity may play an important role.
   most affected are male (full term baby) than premature
C. **Pathophysiology**
   1. The pylorus narrows because of progressive hypertrophy and hyperplasia of the circular pyloric muscle. The muscle may grow to twice its size (Fig. 12-1).
   2. This leads to obstruction of the pyloric sphincter, with subsequent gastric distention, dilatation, and hypertrophy.

D. **Assessment findings**
   1. **Clinical manifestations**
      a. No abnormal signs in the first weeks after birth (usually)
      b. Regurgitation or nonprojectile vomiting beginning by 3 weeks of age; emesis is not bile stained and contains only gastric contents but may be blood tinged.
      c. Vomiting increases in frequency and force over the next 1 to 2 weeks until most of ingested food is expelled through projectile vomiting. *✳*
   ↑ d. No signs of anorexia; good appetite and feeding habits

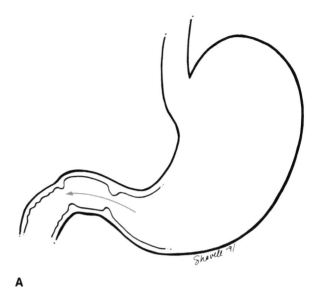

Shavell '91

A

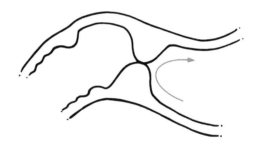

B

FIGURE 12-1
Pyloric stenosis. **(A)** *Arrow* represents normal passage through pyloric sphincter. **(B)** *Curved arrow* represents stoppage of flow because of stenotic sphincter.

e. No evidence of pain *because pt. always vomits*
f. Weight loss *d/t vomiting most of the ingested foods. and ↓ absorption of foods by the body because foods cannot pass through the intestines*
g. Upper abdominal distention
h. Palpable olive-shaped mass in the epigastrium just to the right of the umbilicus *the intestines*
i. Visible gastric peristaltic waves moving from left to right across the epigastrium
j. Decreased frequency and volume of stools *(pylorus is located slightly on the right side of the body.)*
k. Signs of malnutrition and dehydration

2. **Laboratory and diagnostic studies**
   a. Ultrasonography and an upper GI study may reveal delayed gastric emptying, an elongated and thin pylorus, or a pyloric mass.
   b. Arterial blood gases (ABGs) will reveal increased serum pH and bicarbonate levels, which indicate metabolic alkalosis. *as a result of vomiting (& prolonged ngt)*
   c. Electrolyte studies will reveal decreased serum chloride, sodium, and potassium levels if electrolyte depletion occurs. *d/t vomiting*
   d. CBC will reveal increased hematocrit and hemoglobin values, which reflect hemoconcentration. *compensatory mechanism for dehydration.*

E. Nursing management

1. **Monitor feeding pattern and the association between feedings and vomiting**.
2. **Assess the amount, character, and frequency of emesis**.
3. **Promote adequate hydration**. Administer parenteral fluids, as prescribed, to replenish potassium and correct alkalosis.
4. **Prevent aspiration**.
   a. Feed the infant slowly
   b. Burp the infant frequently
   c. Position the infant in the high Fowler position on the right side after feedings. *to promote movement of food from stomach (left) to the intestines (right) by the help of gravity*
5. **Provide postoperative care**.
   a. Pyloromyotomy, creation of an incision along the anterior pylorus to split the muscle, is commonly performed to relieve the obstruction.
   b. Nursing responsibilities include:
      (1) Provide nutrition as prescribed. Typically, small amounts of clear liquids are given every 4 to 6 hours, advancing to formula as tolerated.
      (2) Promote comfort.
         (a) Provide good oral care. *bec. pt. was NPO b4 surgery. Thus, pt. has dry mouth after.*
         (b) Offer a pacifier while the infant is receiving nothing by mouth (NPO).
         (c) Encourage parents to hold their infant.
         (d) Administer analgesics as prescribed.
6. **Provide family teaching**.
   a. Explain all procedures, scheduled surgical procedures, and preoperative and postoperative care measures.
   b. Demonstrate feeding and positioning techniques and surgical wound care.

VI. Celiac disease (gluten-sensitive enteropathy; celiac sprue)

A. Description

1. Celiac disease is a malabsorption syndrome that occurs when the mucosa of the proximal small intestine is sensitive to, or undergoes an immunologic response to, gluten.
2. Celiac disease occurs more frequently in Europe than in the United States, and it is rarely reported in African Americans or Asians.

B. Etiology

1. Celiac disease is believed to result from either an inborn error of metabolism or an abnormal immunologic response to the gluten factor of protein.
2. Most likely, there is an inherited predisposition influenced by environmental factors.
3. Episodes of celiac crises are precipitated by ingestion of gluten, infections, prolonged fasting, or exposure to anticholinergic drugs.

C. Pathophysiology

1. Intolerance for and inability to digest gluten (specifically the gliadin fraction of gluten found in wheat, barley, rye, and oats) results in the accumulation of the amino acid glutamine, which is toxic to intestinal mucosal cells.
2. As a result, intestinal villi eventually atrophy, which reduces the absorptive surface of the small intestine.
3. Celiac crisis may lead to electrolyte imbalance, rapid dehydration, and severe acidosis.

D. Assessment findings

1. **Clinical manifestations**
   a. Symptoms typically appear between 1 and 5 years of age, usually several months after the introduction of gluten to the diet.

b. Anorexia and abdominal pain are common.
c. Diarrhea can be either acute or insidious, and the stools are frequently watery, pale, and foul smelling. ~~and odoraive stree~~.
d. Vomiting, constipation, and anemia may occur.
e. Severe abdominal distention and muscle wasting may occur in some children.
f. Behavioral changes can include irritability and fretfulness.

2. Laboratory and diagnostic study findings

a. Biopsy of the jejunum reveals flat mucosal surface with hyperplastic villous atrophy. This is the definitive diagnosis of celiac disease. These characteristic lesions return to normal after dietary restriction of gluten, which helps confirm the diagnosis.
b. The diagnosis is aided by the presence of antigliadin, antireticulin, and antiendomysial IgG and IgA antibodies and their absence when gluten is removed from the diet.
c. A rapid detection test for serum IgG and IgA antigliadin antibodies permits screening for the disease and monitoring response to therapy.

E. Nursing management

1. Promote adequate hydration.

2. Promote adherence to dietary guidelines.

a. Explain the disease process to the child and family.
b. Explain that a lapse in dietary management may result in growth retardation, anemia, and osteomalacia.
c. Provide a gluten-free diet (Box 12-1).
d. Encourage the child and family to carefully read all food labels because gluten is a component of many foods, especially foods that children like (eg, cake, cookies, donuts, pies, hot dogs, and some types of ice creams).
e. Encourage the family to try new recipes, including Chinese and Mexican recipes that use rice and corn.
f. Consult a nutritionist to assist family with meal planning.

BOX 12-1. **Basics of a Gluten-Free Diet**

Foods Allowed

Meats: beef, pork, poultry, and fish

Eggs

Milk and dairy products: milk, cream, and cheese

Fruits and vegetables: all

Grains: rice, corn, gluten-free wheat flour, puffed rice, corn flakes, corn meal, and precooked gluten-free cereals

Foods Prohibited

Milk: commercially prepared ice cream, malted milk, and prepared puddings

Grains: anything made from wheat, rye, oats, or barley (eg, bread, rolls, cookies, cakes, crackers, cereal, spaghetti, macaroni, and noodles)

Beer and ale

    g. Enforce other dietary restrictions when necessary.

      (1) Provide a lactose-free diet (ie, no milk or milk products) for children with severe mucosal damage.

      (2) Encourage avoidance of high-fiber foods (eg, nuts, raisins, raw fruits, and raw vegetables) because the bowel is usually inflamed.

3. Support the parents and child by encouraging them to express their feelings and concerns. Refer them to the Celiac Sprue Association/United States of America for additional information and support.

4. Prevent complications from celiac crises.

    a. Monitor closely to prevent dehydration, electrolyte imbalance, and metabolic acidosis (eg, weakness, irritability, decreasing level of consciousness, irregular heartbeat, and poor muscle control).

    b. Administer steroids to decrease inflammation.

    c. Administer IV fluids.

    d. Administer hyperalimentation, if necessary.

VII. Hirschsprung disease (congenital aganglionic megacolon)

A. Description

  1. Hirschsprung disease is a congenital anomaly characterized by the absence of nerves to a section of the intestines. It results in mechanical intestinal obstruction due to inadequate motility in an intestinal segment.

  2. It is at least four times more common in boys than in girls and is seen more commonly in children with Down syndrome.

  3. It can be acute and life-threatening or chronic.

B. Etiology

  1. Hirschsprung disease is believed to be a familial, congenital defect.

  2. It results from failure of the craniocaudal migration of ganglion nerve cell precursors along the GI tract between the 5th and 12th weeks of gestation.

C. Pathophysiology

  1. Absence of autonomic parasympathetic ganglion cells in one segment of the colon causes lack of innervation in that segment.

  2. Lack of innervation leads to absence of propulsive movements, causing accumulation of intestinal contents and distention of the bowel proximal to the defect (Fig. 12-2).

  3. Enterocolitis, inflammation of the small bowel and colon, is the leading cause of death in children with Hirschsprung disease. It occurs as a result of intestinal distention and ischemia secondary to bowel wall distention.

D. Assessment findings

  1. Clinical manifestations

    a. Clinical findings vary with age at time of diagnosis, the length of affected bowel, and the occurrence of complications.

      (1) **Newborns.** Failure to pass meconium, reluctance to ingest fluids, abdominal distention, and bile-stained emesis

      (2) **Infants.** Failure to thrive, constipation, abdominal distention, vomiting, and episodic diarrhea

      (3) **Older children.** Anorexia, chronic constipation, foul-smelling and ribbon-like stools, abdominal distention, visible peristalsis, palpable fecal mass, malnourishment or poor growth, signs of anemia, and hypoproteinemia

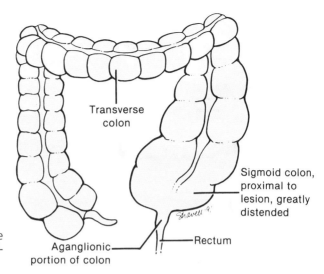

FIGURE 12-2
In Hirschsprung disease, the sigmoid colon is dilated proximal to bowel.

b. Rectal examination typically reveals a rectum empty of stool, a tight anal sphincter, and stool leakage.

c. Ominous signs signifying enterocolitis include explosive, bloody diarrhea, fever, and severe prostration.

2. Laboratory and diagnostic study findings

a. Barium enema reveals megacolon.

b. Rectal biopsy will reveal absence of ganglionic cells, which confirms the diagnosis.

c. Anorectal manometry, whereby a balloon catheter is inserted into the rectum, records the reflex pressure response of the internal anal sphincter. In Hirschsprung disease, the external sphincter contracts normally but fails to relax.

E. Nursing management

1. Assess for, and promptly report, any signs of enterocolitis.

2. Promote adequate hydration.

3. Assess bowel functioning.

a. Assess passage of meconium in neonates.

b. Note and record the frequency and characteristics of stools in infants and older children.

c. Periodically measure abdominal girth to assess for increasing distention.

4. Promote adequate nutrition according to the child's age and nutritional requirements. Provide smaller and more frequent feedings.

5. Administer enemas, as prescribed, **to relieve constipation.**

6. Avoid taking temperatures rectally because of the potential for damaging frail mucosa.

7. Administer prescribed medications, which may include:

a. Systemic antibiotics given with enemas to reduce intestinal flora

b. Stool softeners to relieve constipation

8. Decrease discomfort due to abdominal distention.

a. Elevate the head of the bed.

b. Change the child's position frequently.

c. Assess for any respiratory difficulty associated with distention.

9. **Support the child and parents.**
   a. Encourage the child and parents to express their feelings and concerns.
   b. Encourage parents to visit and participate in their child's care, as appropriate.
10. **Prepare the child and the parents for procedures and treatments**, which may include:
    a. Manual dilatation of the anus, dietary management, and cleansing enemas until the child can tolerate surgery
    b. Surgery to remove the aganglionic, nonfunctioning segment of the colon, followed by anastomosis in three stages:
       (1) A temporary colostomy before definitive surgery to allow the bowel to rest and the child to gain weight
       (2) Reanastomosis by means of an abdominoperineal pull-through about 9 to 12 months later
       (3) Closure of the colostomy about 3 months after the pull-through procedure.
    c. Nursing responsibilities for preoperative care include:
       (1) Assist with symptomatic treatment to improve the child's physical status to withstand surgery. Treatment may include enemas; low-fiber, high-calorie, high-protein diet; and, occasionally, the use of total parenteral nutrition (TPN).
       (2) Prepare the bowel for surgery with repeated saline enemas, systemic antibiotics, and colonic antibiotic irrigations to decrease bowel flora. Bowel prep is not necessary for the newborn whose bowel is sterile.
    d. Nursing responsibilities for postoperative care include:
       (1) Keep the child NPO during the initial postoperative period.
       (2) Monitor I&O, including nasogastric tube drainage.
       (3) Keep the infant's diaper away from the dressing to prevent contamination.
       (4) Initiate oral fluids once bowel functioning is established, usually after bowel sounds are identified.
       (5) Provide ostomy care if indicated. This includes preparation of the skin, application of the collecting appliance, care of the appliance, control of odor, and monitoring for problems such as ribbon-like stools, excessive diarrhea, bleeding, prolapse, and failure to pass stools or flatus.
       (6) Instruct the family regarding home care, including ostomy care and available resources.
11. **Educate the child and family**.
    a. Explain procedures and treatments, such as enemas, stool softeners, and a low-residue or low-fiber diet (eg, allowing tender meats, poultry, fish, white bread, and clear soups, and omitting highly seasoned foods, fruits and fruit juices, raw vegetables, and whole-grain cereals and breads).
    b. Discuss and answer questions about diagnosis, surgery, preoperative and postoperative care, and colostomy care, if applicable.
    c. Arrange for consultation with an ostomy nurse to assist with teaching, as indicated.

VIII. Intussusception

A. Description

1. Intussusception is an invagination or telescoping of one portion of the intestine into an adjacent portion, causing obstruction.
2. It is one of the most frequent causes of intestinal obstruction in children and typically affects children between 3 months and 5 years of age, most commonly between 3 and 12 months of age.

3. If treatment is delayed for longer than 24 hours, bowel strangulation may occur, leading to necrosis, hemorrhage, perforation, peritonitis, and shock. If untreated, intussusception is incompatible with life.

B. Etiology

   1. In most cases the cause of intussusception is unknown.

   2. It may be associated with viral infections, intestinal polyps, Meckel diverticulum, and lymphoma.

C. Pathophysiology

   1. Invagination typically begins with hyperperistalsis in an intestinal segment, most often at or near the ileocecal valve.

   2. Peristalsis continues to pull the invaginated segment along the bowel; intestinal edema and obstruction occur and blood supply to the area is cut off (Fig. 12-3).

D. Assessment findings

   1. Clinical manifestations

   a. **Severe paroxysmal abdominal pain, causing the child to scream and draw his knees to the abdomen**

   b. Vomiting of gastric contents

   c. **Tender, distended abdomen, possibly with a palpable mass**

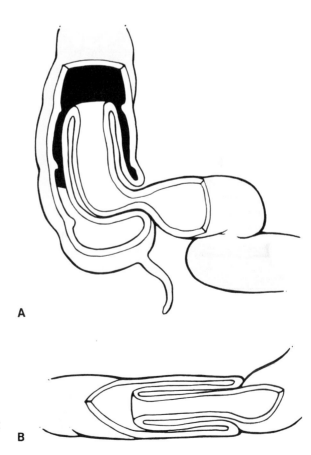

A

B

FIGURE 12-3
Intussusception. **(A)** Ileocolic variety. **(B)** Ileoileal variety.

     d. With continued obstruction, the following occur: lethargy, "currant jelly" stools (containing blood and mucus), bile-stained or fecal emesis, and shocklike syndrome, which may progress to death.

2. Laboratory and diagnostic study findings

     a. A contrast enema, using air, barium, or water-soluble contrast may be used for diagnosis or a therapeutic treatment tool. This test typically follows nasogastric decompression and the administration of IV fluids.

     b. Electrolyte studies will reveal electrolyte loss relative to symptoms.

E. Nursing management

1. Promote adequate hydration.

     a. Monitor nasogastric tube drainage, when appropriate.

     b. Encourage intake of clear liquids after surgery.

2. Promote adequate nutrition according to the child's age and nutritional requirements. Advance the diet as tolerated after surgery.

3. Monitor bowel elimination status for return to normal function.

     a. Assess stool amount and characteristics.

     b. Perform guaiac testing on all stools.

     c. Observe for abdominal distention.

     d. Auscultate for bowel sounds.

4. Monitor for infection.

     a. Assess the surgical wound for redness, swelling, and drainage.

     b. Monitor temperature.

5. Support the parents.

     a. Allow them to verbalize their anxieties and concerns.

     b. Encourage them to participate in their child's care as appropriate.

IX. Hernias and hydroceles

A. Description

1. A **hernia** is a protrusion of the bowel through an abnormal opening in the abdominal wall; in children, this occurs most commonly at the umbilicus and through the inguinal canal.

2. A **hydrocele** is the presence of abdominal fluid in the scrotal sac.

B. Etiology. These defects most commonly arise from congenital anomalies.

C. Pathophysiology *→ still covered by skin.*

1. In an **umbilical hernia**, incomplete closure of the umbilical ring results in protrusion of portions of the omentum and intestine through the opening. The defect usually closes spontaneously by the time the child is 3 to 4 years old. *→ outside the skin yet·*

2. Inguinal hernias result from incomplete closure of the tube (processus vaginalis) between the abdomen and the scrotum (or uterus in girls), leading to descent of an intestinal portion. Incarceration results when the descended portion becomes tightly caught in the hernia sac, which compromises blood supply.

3. Hydroceles may be communicating or noncommunicating.

     a. In a **noncommunicating hydrocele**, most commonly seen at birth, residual peritoneal fluid is trapped within the lower segment of the processus vaginalis (the tunica vaginalis). There is no communication with the peritoneal cavity. The fluid usually is absorbed during the first months after birth and requires no treatment.

     b. A **communicating hydrocele** is commonly associated with a hernia because the processus vaginalis remains open from the scrotum to the abdominal cavity.

D. Assessment findings. Clinical manifestations will vary depending on the disorder.

1. **Umbilical hernia.** Soft swelling or protrusion around the umbilicus, usually reducible with the finger
2. **Inguinal hernia.** Usually a painless swelling in the inguinal area; swelling reducible and possibly subsiding during periods of rest but visible when the infant is crying
3. **Incarcerated hernia.** Irritability, tenderness at the site, anorexia, abdominal distention, and difficulty defecating; may lead to complete intestinal obstruction and gangrene
4. **Noncommunicating hydrocele.** Painless swelling in scrotum that does not change in size or shape with the infant's activities; it is easily transilluminated.
5. **Communicating hydrocele.** Inguinal swelling that may vary in size with positioning and that is not reducible

E. Nursing management

1. **Assess for signs of incarceration and strangulation.**
2. **Perform postoperative care.**
   a. Surgical correction of an umbilical hernia is necessary if closure does not occur or if the herniated bowel becomes incarcerated.
   b. Inguinal hernias require surgical repair. An incarcerated inguinal hernia is considered a medical emergency requiring immediate surgical repair.
   c. In most cases of communicating hydroceles, a hydrocelectomy is performed if spontaneous resolution does not occur by 1 year of age.
   d. Nursing responsibilities for postoperative care include:
      (1) Assess for wound infection.
         (a) Observe the incision for redness or drainage.
         (b) Monitor temperature.
      (2) Maintain a good hydration status.
         (a) Administer IV fluids, if prescribed.
         (b) Monitor fluid I&O.
         (c) Advance the child's diet.
      (3) Promote comfort.
         (a) Administer analgesics as needed.
         (b) In a child who has undergone hydrocelectomy, apply ice bags and use a scrotal support to help relieve pain and swelling, if prescribed.
3. **Support the parents.**
   a. Allow them to verbalize their concerns.
   b. Encourage them to participate in their child's care, as appropriate.

STUDY QUESTIONS

1. While assessing a newborn with cleft lip, the nurse would be alert that which of the following will most likely be compromised?
   (1) Sucking ability
   (2) Respiratory status
   (3) Locomotion
   (4) GI function

2. When providing postoperative care for the child with a cleft palate, the nurse should position the child in which of the following positions?
   (1) Supine
   (2) Prone
   (3) In an infant seat
   (4) On the side

3. While assessing a child with pyloric stenosis, the nurse is likely to note which of the following?
   (1) Regurgitation
   (2) Steatorrhea
   (3) Projectile vomiting
   (4) "Currant jelly" stools

4. Which of the following nursing diagnoses would be **inappropriate** for the infant with gastroesophageal reflux (GER)?
   (1) Fluid volume deficit
   (2) Risk for aspiration
   (3) Altered nutrition: less than body requirements
   (4) Altered oral mucous membranes

5. Which of the following parameters would the nurse monitor to evaluate the effectiveness of thickened feedings for an infant with gastroesophageal reflux (GER)?
   (1) Vomiting
   (2) Stools
   (3) Urine
   (4) Weight

6. Discharge teaching for a child with celiac disease would include instructions about avoiding which of the following?

   (1) Rice
   (2) Milk
   (3) Wheat
   (4) Chicken

7. Which of the following would the nurse expect to assess in a child with celiac disease having a celiac crisis secondary to an upper respiratory infection?
   (1) Respiratory distress
   (2) Lethargy
   (3) Watery diarrhea
   (4) Weight gain

8. Which of the following should the nurse do **first** after noting that a child with Hirschsprung disease has a fever and watery explosive diarrhea?
   (1) Notify the physician immediately
   (2) Administer antidiarrheal medications
   (3) Monitor child every 30 minutes
   (4) Nothing, this is characteristic of Hirschsprung disease

9. A newborn's failure to pass meconium within the first 24 hours after birth may indicate which of the following?
   (1) Hirschsprung disease
   (2) Celiac disease
   (3) Intussusception
   (4) Abdominal wall defect

10. When assessing a child for possible intussusception, which of the following would be **least** likely to provide valuable information?
    (1) Stool inspection
    (2) Pain pattern
    (3) Family history
    (4) Abdominal palpation

11. Which of the following refers to the defect resulting from residual peritoneal fluid trapped within the lower segment of the processus vaginalis?
    (1) Noncommunicating hydrocele
    (2) Communicating hydrocele
    (3) Inguinal hernia
    (4) Incarcerated hernia

ANSWER KEY

1. The answer is (1). Because of the defect, the child will be unable to form the mouth adequately around nipple, thereby requiring special devices to allow for feeding and sucking gratification. Respiratory status may be compromised if the child is fed improperly or during postoperative period. Locomotion would be a problem for the older infant because of the use of restraints. GI functioning is not compromised in the child with a cleft lip.

2. The answer is (2). Postoperatively, children with cleft palate should be placed on their abdomens to facilitate drainage. If the child is placed in the supine position, he or she may aspirate. Using an infant seat does not facilitate drainage. Side-lying does not facilitate drainage as well as the prone position.

3. The answer is (3). Projectile vomiting is a key symptom of pyloric stenosis. Regurgitation is seen more commonly with GER. Steatorrhea occurs in malabsorption disorders such as celiac disease. "Currant jelly" stools are characteristic of intussusception.

4. The answer is (4). GER is the backflow of gastric contents into the esophagus resulting from relaxation or incompetence of the lower esophageal (cardiac) sphincter. No alteration in the oral mucous membranes occurs with this disorder. Fluid volume deficit, risk for aspiration, and altered nutrition are appropriate nursing diagnoses.

5. The answer is (1). Thickened feedings are used with GER to stop the vomiting. Therefore, the nurse would monitor the child's vomiting to evaluate the effectiveness of using the thickened feedings. No relationship exists between feedings and characteristics of stools and urine. If feedings are ineffective, this should be noted before there is any change in the child's weight.

6. The answer is (3). Children with celiac disease cannot tolerate or digest gluten. Therefore, because of its gluten content, wheat and wheat-containing products must be avoided. Rice, milk, and chicken do not contain gluten and need not be avoided.

7. The answer is (3). Episodes of celiac crises are precipitated by infections, ingestion of gluten, prolonged fasting, or exposure to anticholinergic drugs. Celiac crisis is typically characterized by severe watery diarrhea. Respiratory distress is unlikely in a routine upper respiratory infection. Irritability, rather than lethargy, is more likely. Because of the fluid loss associated with the severe watery diarrhea, the child's weight is more likely to be decreased.

8. The answer is (1). For the child with Hirschsprung disease, fever and explosive diarrhea indicate enterocolitis, a life-threatening situation. Therefore, the physician should be notified immediately. Generally, because of the intestinal obstruction and inadequate propulsive intestinal movement, antidiarrheals are not used to treat Hirschsprung disease. The child is acutely ill and requires intervention, with monitoring more frequently than every 30 minutes. Hirschsprung disease typically presents with chronic constipation.

9. The answer is (1). Failure to pass meconium within the first 24 hours after birth may be an indication of Hirschsprung disease, a congenital anomaly resulting in mechanical obstruction due to inadequate motility in an intestinal segment. Failure to pass meconium is not associated with celiac disease, intussusception, or abdominal wall defect.

10. The answer is (3). Because intussusception is not believed to have a familial tendency, obtaining a family history would provide the least amount of information. Stool inspection, pain pattern, and abdominal palpation would reveal possible indicators of intussusception. Currant, jelly-like stools containing blood and mucus are an indication of intussusception. Acute, episodic abdominal pain is characteristic of intussusception. A sausage-shaped mass may be palpated in the right upper quadrant.

11. The answer is (1). With a noncommunicating hydrocele, most commonly seen at birth, residual peritoneal fluid is trapped within the lower segment of the processus vaginalis (the tunica vaginalis). There is no communication with the peritoneal cavity and the fluid usually is absorbed during the first months after birth. A communicating hydrocele usually is associated with an inguinal hernia because the processus vaginalis remains open from the scrotum to the abdominal cavity. An inguinal hernia arises from the incomplete closure of the processus vaginalis leading to the descent of an intestinal portion. Incarceration occurs when the hernia becomes tightly caught in the hernia sac.

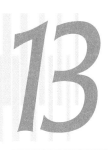

Hematologic Dysfunction

Structure and function of the hematologic system

A. Structure. Blood is composed of liquid plasma and formed cellular elements, which are formed in the red bone marrow—the major hemopoietic organ (Table 13-1).

1. **Plasma** is approximately 90% water and 10% solutes, chiefly albumin, electrolytes, and proteins. The proteins include clotting factors, globulins, circulating antibodies, and fibrinogen.

2. **Cellular elements** include white blood cells (WBCs), also called leukocytes; red blood cells (RBCs), also called erythrocytes; and platelets, also called thrombocytes.

B. Function

1. Plasma transports formed elements and helps maintain homeostasis.

2. The functions of the formed cellular elements include:

   a. **RBCs** primarily transport oxygen to, and carbon dioxide from, body tissues; this activity relies on hemoglobin, a component of the RBCs. RBCs also give blood its red color. The typical life span of RBCs is about 120 days.

   b. The primary function of **WBCs** is to protect the body against infection. Two types of WBCs exist—granulocytes and agranulocytes.

      (1) Granulocytes consist of neutrophils, which fight bacteria; basophils, which secrete heparin and speed fat removal; and eosinophils, which fight parasites and respond to allergens.

      (2) Agranulocytes consist of monocytes, which phagocytize large cells and have an important role in chronic infection; and lymphocytes, which are responsible for cell-mediated immunity (T lymphocytes) and humoral immunity (B lymphocytes).

   c. **Platelets**, the smallest blood cells, contain coagulation factors and help regulate hemostasis through a sequence of events known as the **coagulation process**.

      (1) Following blood vessel trauma, platelets adhere to the exposed vascular subendothelium, and subsequent platelet aggregation leads to the formation of a platelet plug at the site of the injury.

      (2) Platelet plugs are adequate to seal tiny vessels; however, clot formation is needed to seal injuries to larger vessels.

3. Various clotting factors and clot dissolution factors are found in plasma. After injury, the **clotting cascade** is activated. This cascade consists of an intrinsic pathway and an extrinsic pathway, and both of these lead to a common pathway that eventually results in clot formation at the injury site.

   a. The **intrinsic pathway** is activated by trauma to blood cells and exposure of the blood to the traumatized vascular wall: factor XII→factor XIIa (high-molecular-

TABLE 13-1
Development of the Hematologic System

AGE	STRUCTURE AND FUNCTION
Fetal development	Hematopoietic activity occurs by the second week of embryonic life, when blood islands arise from the yellow sac and liver. From the second to fifth month of gestation, the liver is the most active site of hematopoiesis. The spleen functions as an erythropoietic organ from the third to the fifth fetal months. Bone marrow becomes active around the fourth fetal month (within 2–3 weeks after birth, the bone marrow is the main site of hematopoietic activity).
Infant (0–1 year)	Red blood cell (RBC) and hemoglobin levels drop at 2–3 months. They gradually rise when erythropoiesis begins. White blood cell (WBC) levels are high at birth, then decline to adult levels.
Toddler/Preschooler (1–6 years)	RBCs are formed in the bone marrow of the ribs, sternum, and vertebrae, as they are in adulthood.
Schoolager (6–12 years)	No significant changes.
Adolescent (12–21 years)	Hemoglobin concentration and RBC mass increase due to hormone production. Hematocrit levels are high in boys; platelets, in girls. WBC counts decrease in both sexes. At end of adolescence, the blood volume in boys averages 5000 mL and in girls, 4200 mL.

weight kininogen, prekallikrein)→factor XI→factor XIa (calcium [factor IV])→factor IX→factor IXa (factor VIII, calcium [factor IV], platelet phospholipids)→common pathway (see c. for remaining part of the process).

b. The **extrinsic pathway** is activated by trauma to extravascular tissue and trauma to the vascular wall: release of tissue thromboplastin (factor III)→factor VII→factor VIIa (calcium [factor IV])→common pathway (see c. for remaining part of the process).

c. The **common pathway** flows from the combination of the intrinsic and extrinsic pathways resulting in: factor X→factor Xa (factor V, calcium [factor IV], phospholipids)→factor II (prothrombin)→thrombin→factor I (fibrinogen)→fibrin monomer→fibrin polymer (factor XIII, calcium [factor IV])→ stabilized clot.

 II. ## NURSING PROCESS OVERVIEW FOR
The Hematologic System

A. Assessment

   1. Health history

      a. Elicit a description of symptoms including onset, duration, location, and precipitation. **Cardinal signs and symptoms** can include:

         (1) Fatigue, headache, vertigo, irritability, and depression
         (2) Anorexia and weight loss
         (3) Bleeding or bruising tendency, including heavy menses and epistaxis
         (4) Frequent infections
         (5) Bone and joint pain

b. Explore prenatal, personal, and family history for **risk factors** for hematologic disorders.

    (1) Prenatal history risk factors include maternal-infant Rh or ABO incompatibility.

    (2) Personal history risk factors include prematurity, low birth weight, diet poor in iron sources or heavy in cow's milk (during infancy), bleeding (eg, heavy menses), dieting behaviors, or exposure to viral infections.

    (3) Family history risk factors include history of thalassemia, sickle cell anemia, or bleeding disorders.

2. Physical examination

a. **Vital signs.** Gross changes in vital signs are not a factor in most hematologic disorders. However, tachycardia and tachypnea may be noted.

b. **Inspection**

    (1) **Skin**. Pallor, flushing, jaundice, purpura, petechiae, ecchymoses, signs of pruritus (scratch marks), cyanosis, or a brownish discoloration may be seen.

    (2) **Eyes**. Jaundiced sclera, conjunctival pallor, retinal hemorrhage, or blurred vision may be seen.

    (3) **Mouth**. Gingival and mucosal pallor may be seen.

    (4) **Lymph nodes**. Lymphadenopathy may be seen.

    (5) **Pulmonary**. Tachypnea, orthopnea, or dyspnea may be seen.

    (6) **Neurologic**. Impaired thought processes or lethargy may be seen.

    (7) **Musculoskeletal**. Joint swelling may be seen.

    (8) **Genitourinary**. Blood in urine and abnormal or excessive menstrual bleeding may be seen.

c. **Palpation**

    (1) **Skin**. Decreased capillary refill time may be palpated.

    (2) **Lymph nodes**. Lymphadenopathy or tenderness may be palpated.

    (3) **Gastrointestinal**. Abdominal tenderness, hepatomegaly, or splenomegaly may be palpated.

    (4) **Musculoskeletal**. Decreased muscle mass or bone and joint tenderness may be palpated.

d. **Auscultation**

    (1) **Cardiac**. Murmurs may be auscultated.

    (2) **Pulmonary**. Adventitious sounds (if congestive heart failure [CHF] is present) may be auscultated.

3. Laboratory studies and diagnostic tests

a. A **complete blood count (CBC)** provides a fairly complete picture of the blood's formed elements. (See Appendix A for normal values.)

    (1) An **RBC count** determines the total number of RBCs found in a cubic centimeter of blood.

    (2) A **WBC count** is the measurement of the total number of circulating leukocytes.

    (3) A **differential WBC count** (granulocytes and agranulocytes) differentiates WBCs according to the five types of cells—neutrophils, eosinophils, and basophils (granulocytes), and lymphocytes and monocytes (agranulocytes).

    (4) **Hemoglobin (Hgb)** is assessed to determine anemia, its severity, and its response to treatment.

    (5) **Hematocrit (Hct)** determines the RBC mass by measuring space occupied by packed RBCs.

    (6) **Mean corpuscular volume (MCV)** is a measurement of individual RBC size.

    (7) **Mean corpuscular hemoglobin (MCH)** measures the average weight of hemoglobin in the RBCs.

(8) **Mean corpuscular hemoglobin concentration (MCHC)** measures the average concentration of hemoglobin in the RBCs.

(9) **Platelet count** measures the total number of circulating platelets to evaluate bleeding disorders.

b. **Reticulocyte count** helps to differentiate between the types of anemias.

c. **Coagulation** and **hemostasis studies** aid in differential diagnosis of hemorrhagic disorders.

d. **Total iron-binding capacity (TIBC), ferritin and iron, and transferrin** are used in the evaluation of anemia.

e. **Bone marrow aspiration** findings aid in the diagnosis of aplastic anemia, leukemia, and other disorders.

(1) Preparation for this test usually entails some form of sedation.

(2) The area must be closely monitored for bleeding and hematoma formation after the procedure is completed.

B. Nursing diagnoses

1. Fatigue
2. Activity intolerance
3. Risk for infection
4. Altered peripheral tissue perfusion
5. Risk for injury
6. Altered growth and development

C. Planning and outcome identification

1. The child will experience minimal fatigue and activity intolerance.
2. The child will not experience infection.
3. The child will experience minimal impairment of tissue oxygenation.
4. The child will experience minimal consequences from bleeding.
5. The child will not experience alterations in growth and development.

D. Implementation

1. **Minimize fatigue and activity intolerance**.
2. **Prevent infection**.
   a. Monitor for signs and symptoms of infection. Children on steroids are at increased risk for infection.
   b. Prevent infection through protective precautions and good hygiene.
   c. Help the child avoid known sources of infection.
   d. Promote adequate rest and good nutrition.
3. **Promote tissue oxygenation**.
   a. Assess skin color; in dark children, assess mucous membranes.
   b. Assess pulse and respiration rates at rest and during activity, during infections, or when there are other indications of decreased tissue perfusion.
   c. Promote tissue oxygenation by helping the child avoid overexertion and emotional stress, and by providing passive range-of-motion (ROM) exercises.
   d. Provide supplemental oxygen for severe tissue hypoxia.
   e. Administer blood transfusions, and observe for complications of transfusions.
4. **Prevent or minimize bleeding**.
   a. Observe for bleeding.
      (1) Check daily for new areas of petechiae and bruises.
      (2) Assess for abnormal bleeding tendencies (ie, perform dipstick test for blood in urine and guaiac test for blood in stools).

    b. Focus on safety when a bleeding disorder exists.
       (1) Enforce activity restrictions.
       (2) Avoid administering aspirin or aspirin-containing products.
       (3) Avoid taking rectal temperatures.
       (4) Avoid giving intramuscular injections.
    c. Handle the child gently when positioning.
    d. Pad the side rails.
    e. Teach the parents ways to minimize bleeding at home (Child and Family Teaching 13-1).
  5. Foster normal growth and development.
    a. Monitor height, weight, and developmental status because the child's growth may be delayed by severe anemia.
    b. Explain all procedures. Children with hematologic dysfunction commonly undergo a multitude of invasive tests, procedures, and treatments, which often leads to anxiety and stress.
    c. Promote self-care. These children typically depend on others for care and support and need the opportunity to perform as many self-care activities as possible to develop a normal sense of self-esteem and independence.

E. Outcome evaluation

  1. The child experiences minimal or no fatigue and activity intolerance.
  2. The child remains infection free.
  3. The child experiences optimal tissue oxygenation.
  4. The child does not experience consequences from bleeding.
  5. The child experiences optimal growth and development.

CHILD AND FAMILY TEACHING 13-1

Minimizing Bleeding at Home

- Provide information regarding the child's disorder and its severity.
- Identify common bleeding sites, such as the skin, nose, mouth, urinary tract, and muscles, and menstrual loss.
- Educate on measures to prevent bleeding:
  - Select daily activities that have a low risk for injury.
  - Follow sports guidelines for children with hemophilia.
  - Use protective equipment if necessary.
  - Avoid aspirin and aspirin-containing medications.
  - Avoid tobacco, alcohol, and drugs.
- Notify school personnel of the child's bleeding tendencies.
- Instruct the child and family on signs and symptoms of bleeding:
  - Tingling
  - Tenderness
  - Pain
  - Warmth
  - Swelling
  - Decreased mobility
- Discuss long-term consequences of bleeding.

III. Iron deficiency anemia

A. Description

1. Iron deficiency anemia is caused by an inadequate supply of iron for normal RBC formation. This results in smaller RBCs, depleted RBC mass, decreased hemoglobin concentration, and a decreased oxygen-carrying capacity of the blood.
2. Iron deficiency anemia is the most prevalent nutritional disorder in the United States.
   a. It is prominent in age groups that experience rapid growth (eg, toddlers and adolescents), and in pregnant and lactating women.
   b. In the United States, the incidence has decreased owing to improved nutrition and federal programs such as Women, Infants, and Children (WIC).
3. In children, it occurs most often between 6 months and 3 years of age; adolescents and premature infants also are at risk.

B. Etiology. Common causes of iron deficiency anemia include:

1. Inadequate dietary iron intake
2. Iron malabsorption
3. Low iron stores at birth
4. Significant blood loss

C. Pathophysiology. Iron deficiency anemia occurs in three stages.

1. **Stage 1** is characterized by depletion of hemosiderin, ferritin, and other iron storage compounds in the bone marrow, liver, and spleen.
2. **Stage 2** is characterized by a lack of transport iron resulting in the decrease of iron saturation of transferrin.
3. **Stage 3** is characterized by a marked deficit in transport iron, inhibiting the normal production of hemoglobin. Erythrocyte protoporphyrin increases, and transferrin receptors become more numerous in response to the iron-poor environment.

D. Assessment findings

1. **Clinical manifestations**. Although the child may be asymptomatic, the following are **common signs and symptoms** of iron deficiency anemia.
   a. Pale skin
   b. Fatigue
   c. Pica (eating nonfood items)
   d. Headaches, dizziness, and light-headedness
   e. Irritability
   f. Slowed thought processes, decreased attention span, apathy, and depression
2. **Laboratory and diagnostic study findings**
   a. CBC will reveal normal to slightly reduced RBCs, low hemoglobin and hematocrit, reduced MCV (microcytic), and reduced MCH (hypochromic).
   b. Erythrocyte protoporphyrin (EP) level will be greater than 35.
   c. Iron tests will reveal low serum iron capacity (SIC), decreased serum ferritin, and elevated TIBC.
   d. Reticulocyte count may be obtained 10 days after therapy is initiated to evaluate its effectiveness.

E. Nursing management

1. **Assess for fatigue, activity intolerance,** and other signs of impaired tissue oxygenation.
2. **Administer prescribed medications or therapy**. Usually treatment aims at correcting the underlying cause, if possible. Options may include:
   a. Oral iron (ferrous sulfate)

b. Parenteral iron (children with iron malabsorption or chronic hemoglobinuria)

c. Transfusions (for severe anemia, cases of severe infection, cardiac dysfunction, or surgical emergency)

3. **Promote an adequate intake of iron-rich foods** (eg, iron-fortified formula and cereals; lean meat; fish; dark, leafy green vegetables; beans; and whole-grain breads); discourage milk as the predominant food source.

4. **Provide child and family teaching**.

   a. Emphasize proper administration of oral iron supplements.

   (1) Give the supplements in two to three divided doses in a small amount of vitamin C-containing liquid (orange juice) between meals to enhance absorption and minimize side effects.

   (2) Administer iron with a dropper to an infant or through a straw to an older child.

   (3) Brush the child's teeth after administration to minimize staining.

   b. Explain the potential side effects of iron, which include nausea and vomiting, diarrhea or constipation, dark green or black stools, and tooth discoloration.

   c. Caution the parents about accidental ingestion because iron is toxic when overdosed. Give directions for storing iron supplements in a safe place out of children's reach.

   d. Discuss infection prevention measures through good hygiene, proper nutrition, and adequate rest.

IV. Sickle cell disease

A. **Description**

1. Sickle cell disease is a group of chronic, severe, genetic, hemolytic diseases associated with hemoglobin S (Hgb S), which transform RBCs into a sickle (crescent) shape when blood oxygenation is decreased.

2. Hemoglobin SS (sickle cell anemia) is the most common form of sickle cell disease.

3. Sickle cell anemia is found predominately in persons of African ancestry, but also in persons of Mediterranean, Caribbean, South and Central American, Arabian, and East Indian ancestry. Sickle cell anemia is the most common hemoglobinopathy in African Americans and occurs in approximately 1 of every 375 live births.

4. **Sickle cell trait** is the benign, carrier state of the disorder.

B. **Etiology**. Sickle cell disease is an autosomal recessive disorder. Therefore, there is a 25% chance of each child having sickle cell disease when both parents carry the trait.

C. **Pathophysiology**

1. Abnormal hemoglobin (Hgb S) replaces all or part of normal hemoglobin A; under conditions of increased oxygen tension and lowered pH, RBCs change from round to sickle or crescent shaped.

2. Sickle cells do not slide through vessels as normal cells do. Their angled shape causes clumping, thrombosis, arterial obstruction, increased blood viscosity, hemolysis, and eventually tissue ischemia and necrosis.

3. As sickling progresses, acute and chronic changes develop in various organs and structures.

D. **Assessment findings**

1. **Clinical manifestations**

   a. Clinical manifestations are varied; some characteristic signs and symptoms include:

   (1) Enlarged spleen from congestion with sickled cells

   (2) Enlarged and tender liver from blood stasis

       (3) Hematuria

       (4) Inability to concentrate urine

       (5) Enuresis

       (6) Nephrotic syndrome (occasionally)

       (7) Bone weakness

       (8) Dactylitis (symmetric swelling of the hands and feet)

   b. Other problems may include:

       (1) Cerebrovascular accident (CVA)

       (2) Myocardial infarction (MI)

       (3) Growth retardation

       (4) Delayed sexual maturation

       (5) Decreased fertility

       (6) Priapism

       (7) Recurrent severe infections (especially from pneumococcal and salmonella organisms)

   c. **Sickle cell crisis** is usually precipitated by infection, but possibly by dehydration, fever, cold exposure, hypoxia, strenuous exercise, extreme fatigue, or extreme changes in altitude.

   d. Sickle cell crisis may occur in different forms.

       (1) **Vaso-occlusive crisis** is the most common and painful form. Sickled cells obstruct blood vessels, causing fever, acute abdominal pain, dactylitis (hand–foot syndrome), priapism (unwanted painful erection), and arthralgia without exacerbation of anemia. Treatment includes hydration, electrolyte replacement, bed rest, and broad-spectrum antibiotics. Transfusions and oxygen are used to treat severe cases.

       (2) **Splenic sequestration** occurs when the spleen pools a large amount of blood, causing a severe drop in blood volume and shock. This condition is life-threatening, and symptoms include pallor, irritability, abdominal distention and pain, hypotension, and tachycardia. The chronic form is termed hypersplenism. Treatment includes transfusions and splenectomy.

       (3) **Aplastic crisis** occurs infrequently. It features diminished RBC production and is characterized by bone marrow failure. Symptoms include pallor, tachycardia, fever, and CHF. Treatment includes transfusion of packed RBCs.

       (4) **Hyperhemolytic crisis** is a rare event that causes an even greater rate of RBC destruction. This form of crisis suggests other coexisting problems such as viral illness or glucose-6-phosphate dehydrogenase (G6PD) deficiency.

       (5) **Megaloblastic anemia** probably results from an excessive nutritional need for folic acid, vitamin B_{12}, or both during periods of significant erythropoiesis.

       (6) A **stroke** can occur from sickle cells blocking major cerebral blood vessels, causing variable degrees of neurologic impairment.

       (7) **Chest syndrome** is believed to result from sickling in the small blood vessels of the lungs due to vaso-occlusive crisis or infection. Symptoms are similar to pneumonia.

       (8) **Overwhelming infections**, particularly from streptococcus pneumonia and hemophilus influenza type b, are a major cause of death in children younger than 5 years of age.

2. Laboratory and diagnostic studies. Hgb S is present from conception; however, fetal hemoglobin (Hgb F) inhibits sickling, making suspicions equivocal and diagnosis difficult, but not impossible, before 3 months of age.

   a. Sickledex screen, the most widely used test, will detect the presence of Hgb S but may yield false-negative results before the age range of 4 to 6 months.

b. If Sickledex findings are positive, hemoglobin electrophoresis is needed to distinguish between the sickle cell trait and the disease. Hemoglobin electrophoresis should be done at birth on all newborns.

c. Chorionic villus sampling (CVS) or analysis of fetal blood or cells may reveal sickle cell disease prenatally.

d. CBC will reveal a decreased RBC count and an elevated WBC and platelet counts.

e. Erythrocyte sedimentation rate (ESR) will be decreased.

f. Iron tests will reveal an increased serum iron level.

g. Serum RBC survival time will be decreased.

h. A reticulocyte count will reveal reticulocytosis.

E. Nursing management

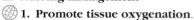 **1. Promote tissue oxygenation**.

2. Administer appropriate therapeutic measures.

a. Provide oral and intravenous (IV) hydration fluids to increase the fluid volume of blood and to help prevent sickling and thrombosis.

b. Administer electrolyte replacement to counter acidosis caused by hypoxia.

c. Deliver oxygen therapy to promote adequate oxygenation.

d. Institute bed rest and careful organization of the child's activities to minimize energy expenditure.

e. Administer and monitor transfusions to treat anemia and reduce the viscosity of the blood.

3. Relieve pain.

a. Provide a preventive schedule of medication around the clock.

b. Avoid administration of meperidine (Demerol) due to increased risk of seizures.

c. Reassure the family and child that analgesics are indicated, even high doses of opioids, and that addiction is rare.

d. Apply heat (soothing) to affected areas; avoid cold compresses, which will enhance vasoconstriction and sickling.

e. Monitor the effectiveness of all medications.

f. Use nonpharmacologic pain relief mechanisms.

g. Position the child for maximum comfort.

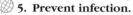 **4. Help ensure adequate hydration and a nutritionally balanced diet**.

5. Prevent infection.

6. Foster normal growth and development.

7. Support the child and family by allowing them to verbalize their fears, concerns, anger, and other feelings.

8. Provide child and family teaching.

a. Explain the disease process, genetic aspects, and early signs and symptoms of sickling crises.

b. Discuss home management measures for a mild crisis.

c. Identify ways to prevent sickling episodes by avoiding factors known to precipitate crises and by recognizing the early signs of infection.

d. Review the importance of regular health maintenance checkups, dental checkups, and eye examinations.

e. Emphasize the importance of maintaining as normal a lifestyle as possible.

f. Address the significance of genetic counseling.

g. Point out the importance of self-esteem and a positive body image.

Aplastic anemia

A. Description. Aplastic anemia is characterized by pancytopenia (anemia, granulocytopenia, and thrombocytopenia) and bone marrow hypoplasia.

B. Etiology

1. Aplastic anemia may be primary (congenital) or secondary (acquired).

2. Primary types include:

a. **Fanconi syndrome** is inherited as an autosomal recessive trait and is associated with cytopenia and multiple congenital anomalies.

b. **Blackfan-Diamond syndrome** (hypoplastic anemia), a rare condition, is characterized by destruction of RBCs and a slight decrease in WBCs and platelets; its transmission is unclear.

3. Common causes of acquired aplastic anemia include:

a. Idiopathic (no known cause)

b. Radiation therapy

c. Drugs, such as chloramphenicol, methicillin, sulfonamides, thiazides, and chemotherapeutic agents

d. Toxic agents, such as industrial and household chemicals, including dyes, glue, paint removers, insecticides, petroleum products, and benzenes

e. Infections, particularly hepatitis and sepsis

f. Infiltration and replacement of myeloid tissue (eg, leukemia and lymphoma)

g. Hemolytic deficiencies, such as sickle cell disease

h. Autoimmune or allergic states

C. Pathophysiology

1. In aplastic anemia, the decreased functional capacity of hypoplastic bone marrow results in pancytopenia.

2. Severe pancytopenia can produce massive bleeding or infection.

D. Assessment findings

1. Clinical manifestations

a. Whether aplastic anemia results from congenital or acquired factors, assessment findings are related to bone marrow failure as follows:

(1) A lack of RBCs is characterized by pallor, lethargy, tachycardia, and shortness of breath on exertion; in children, signs of anemia occur only when the hemoglobin level falls below 5 to 6 g/100 mL.

(2) A lack of WBCs is characterized by recurrent infections, including opportunistic infections.

(3) A lack of platelets is characterized by abnormal bleeding, petechiae, and bruising.

b. Children with Fanconi syndrome may have short stature, malformed kidneys and hearts, microcephaly, microphthalmos, dark pigmentation with café-au-lait spots, and congenitally absent radii and thumbs.

2. Laboratory and diagnostic study findings

a. Peripheral blood smear will reveal pancytopenia.

b. Bone marrow aspiration and biopsy are used to make a definitive diagnosis (ie, conversion of red bone marrow to yellow, fatty bone marrow with an almost complete absence of hematopoietic activity).

E. Nursing management. Nursing care is similar to that for children with leukemia (see the Implementation section under leukemia in Chap. 18).

1. Prevent infection.

2. **Assess for abnormal bleeding tendencies** (ie, perform a dipstick test for blood in urine and a guaiac test for blood in stools).
3. **Administer prescribed medications and blood products**.
   a. Antilymphocyte globulin (ALG) or antithymocyte globulin (ATG) are the treatments of choice. These drugs suppress T cell-dependent autoimmune responses without causing bone marrow suppression. Cyclosporine may be used for children who do not respond to ATG/ALG.
   b. Androgenic steroids (eg, testosterone) are used with corticosteroids to stimulate erythropoiesis. High-dose methylprednisolone has been used with success.
   c. Blood products such as RBCs, WBCs, and platelets, as well as antibiotics, are used as supportive therapy.
4. **Provide supportive treatment** to prevent or control infection; administer transfusions and steroid or hormone therapy.
5. **Monitor for complications of steroid therapy**, such as gastric irritation, infection, edema, weight gain, and hypertension.
6. **Monitor for complications of androgen therapy** signaled by abnormal liver function test results, weight gain, acne, increased hair growth, and deepening of the voice.
7. **Monitor for complications of ALG or ATG therapy**, which include fever, chills, rash, serum sickness, severe thrombocytopenia, and anaphylaxis.
8. **Provide information regarding bone marrow transplantation procedure and follow-up care**. Explain that early bone marrow transplantation is associated with a 3-year survival rate of 80%. (Bone marrow transplantation before blood transfusions decreases the likelihood of rejection.)
9. **Attempt to eliminate toxic agents from the child's environment**.
10. **Support the family** in coping with procedures and the uncertain prognosis and potential outcome of aplastic anemia.

Thalassemia

A. Description
1. Thalassemia is a group of inherited blood disorders characterized by a deficient synthesis of specific globulin chains of the hemoglobin molecule. For example, the most common type of thalassemia, β-thalassemia, is characterized by a deficient synthesis of beta chains.
2. It occurs in three major forms—thalassemia major, the homozygous form; thalassemia intermedia; and thalassemia minor, the heterozygous form.
3. Thalassemia major (ie, β-thalassemia, Cooley anemia) is the most severe form and usually is seen in children of Mediterranean (especially Italian and Greek) or Asian origins.

B. Etiology. Thalassemia is an autosomal recessive disorder.

C. Pathophysiology
1. There is a defect in the production of specific globulin chains (beta) in hemoglobin.
2. This defect results in a compensatory increase in hemoglobin production among other hemoglobin chains, which then become unbalanced, disintegrate, and destroy RBCs.
3. Compensatory increases in erythropoiesis cannot correct the severe anemia.

D. Assessment findings
1. **Clinical manifestations**
   a. **Thalassemia minor** commonly produces only mild to moderate anemia that may be asymptomatic and often goes undetected.

b. **Thalassemia major** commonly produces clinical manifestations around 6 months of age, after the protective effect of Hgb F diminishes.
   (1) **Early signs** are insidious onset, anemia, unexplained fever, poor feeding, poor weight gain, and a markedly enlarged spleen.
   (2) **Later signs** are chronic hypoxia; damage to liver, spleen, heart, pancreas, and lymph glands from hemochromatosis (damage caused by excess iron); slight jaundice or bronze skin color; thick cranial bones with prominent cheeks and a flat nose; growth retardation; and delayed sexual development.
   (3) **Long-term complications** result from hemochromatosis with resultant cellular damage leading to:
      (a) Splenomegaly (usually requiring splenectomy)
      (b) Skeletal complications, such as thickened cranial bones, enlarged head, prominent facial bones, malocclusion of the teeth, and susceptibility to spontaneous fractures
      (c) Cardiac complications, such as arrhythmias, pericarditis, CHF, and fibrosis of cardiac muscle fibers
      (d) Gallbladder disease, including gallstones (may require cholecystectomy [gallbladder removal])
      (f) Liver enlargement and subsequent cirrhosis
      (g) Skin changes, such as jaundice and brown pigmentation due to iron deposits
      (h) Growth retardation and endocrine complications (possibly caused by endocrine gland sensitivity to iron), such as delayed sexual maturation and diabetes mellitus

2. **Laboratory and diagnostic study findings**
   a. CBC will reveal microcytosis, hypochromia, anisocytosis (inequity in size), poikilocytosis (variation in shape), target cells (nonspecific enlarged RBCs), and basophilic stippling (spotted staining). In addition, hemoglobin and hematocrit values are decreased.
   b. Reticulocyte count will be decreased.
   c. Hemoglobin electrophoresis will reveal elevated Hgb F and Hgb A values because these do not depend on beta chains.
   d. CVS or analysis of fetal blood or cells will screen prenatally for thalassemia.

E. **Nursing management**
   1. **Assess for manifestations and complications of the disorder**.
   2. **Administer blood transfusions**, and **observe for complications of transfusions**; the most common problem is iron overload. Signs and symptoms of iron overload include:
      a. Abdominal pain
      b. Bloody diarrhea
      c. Emesis
      d. Decreased level of consciousness
      e. Shock
      f. Metabolic acidosis.
   3. **Implement iron chelation therapy** with desferoxamine (20–40 mg/kg/day), as prescribed, to eliminate excess iron and its side effects from deposition in tissues.
      a. Desferoxamine is administered during blood transfusion.
      b. Monitor vital signs, watching for hypotension.
      c. Be prepared for an allergic reaction.

    d. Check visual acuity (ocular toxic) and hearing (ototoxic).

    e. Monitor intake and output. The drug is excreted by the kidneys, and the urine may turn red.

4. Provide information and follow-up care if the patient requires a splenectomy.

    a. Explain that prophylactic antibiotics and vaccines are given to prevent complications from splenectomy.

    b. Explain that the child should avoid people with active infections.

5. Prepare for a bone marrow transplant when needed.

6. Prevent infection.

7. Prevent fractures by encouraging the child to avoid activities that may increase the risk for fractures.

8. Promote adequate rest by coordinating care.

9. Decrease dietary iron as much as possible.

10. Help the child cope with the illness by allowing him or her to verbalize concerns, by preparing for procedures, and by assisting him or her to develop coping skills.

11. Support the family by encouraging members to verbalize their feelings, by exploring feelings of guilt regarding the hereditary aspect of the disorder, and by encouraging the child to lead as normal a life as possible.

12. Refer the family to support groups, such as the Cooley's Anemia Foundation.

13. Provide child and family teaching.

    a. Discuss the nature of the disease and its management.

    b. Identify signs and symptoms of infection, iron overload, and other potential complications to watch for and report.

    c. Provide instructions for home chelation therapy.

    d. Review activity restrictions, including avoidance of activities that increase the risk of fractures.

    e. Outline dietary restrictions.

VII. Hemophilia

A. Description

    1. Hemophilia is a group of hereditary bleeding disorders characterized by a deficiency in a blood-clotting factor.

    2. The two most common forms are factor VIII deficiency (classic hemophilia, hemophilia A) and factor IX deficiency (Christmas disease, hemophilia B). The classic form is the most common.

    3. Hemophilia is classified as mild, moderate, or severe, depending on the level of factor produced by the body.

B. Etiology

    1. Hemophilia is an X-linked recessive disorder transmitted by females and found predominantly in males.

    2. It may also be caused by a gene mutation.

C. Pathophysiology

    1. In hemophilia A, there is a deficiency of, or a defect in, factor VIII (antihemophilic factor [AHF]), which is necessary for the formation of thromboplastin.

    2. In hemophilia B, there is a defect or deficiency of factor IX.

    3. Clotting factor malfunction causes abnormal bleeding owing to impaired ability to form a fibrin clot.

D. Assessment findings

1. Clinical manifestations

a. Hemophilia is suspected in a newborn with excessive bleeding from the umbilical cord or after circumcision.

b. In **mild hemophilia**, characterized by a factor level of 5% to 50%, children have prolonged bleeding only when they have been injured.

c. In **moderate hemophilia**, characterized by a factor level of 1% to 5%, prolonged bleeding occurs with trauma or surgery, but there may be episodes of spontaneous bleeding as well.

d. In **severe hemophilia**, characterized by a factor level under 1%, prolonged bleeding occurs spontaneously without injury.

e. **Common manifestations** can include:

(1) Easy bruising

(2) Prolonged bleeding from wounds

(3) Spontaneous hematuria

(4) Epistaxis

(5) Hemarthrosis (hemorrhages in the joints causing pain, swelling, and limited movement)

f. **Complications** may include:

(1) Bone changes, osteoporosis, and muscle atrophy, resulting in crippling deformities as a consequence of hemarthrosis

(2) Intracranial bleeding

(3) Gastrointestinal hemorrhage, leading to intestinal obstruction

(4) Hematomas in the spinal cord, resulting in paralysis

(5) Airway obstruction due to bleeding into the neck, mouth, or thorax

2. Laboratory and diagnostic study findings

a. Coagulation studies will reveal normal prothrombin and bleeding times, normal fibrinogen levels, low factor VIII in hemophilia A, low factor IX in hemophilia B, and a prolonged partial thromboplastin time.

b. CBC will reveal a normal platelet count.

c. DNA testing for hemophilia A will detect carriers of the disease.

d. Amniocentesis will diagnose hemophilia prenatally.

E. Nursing management

1. Assess for acute or chronic bleeding.

a. The skin, joints, and muscles are assessment priorities.

b. Check vision, hearing, and neurologic development.

c. Check for hematuria and bleeding from the mouth, lips, gums, and rectum.

2. Administer the missing clotting factor (ie, factor VIII or factor IX concentrate).

a. Due to recombinant DNA technology, the risk of transmitting human immunodeficiency virus (HIV), hepatitis, and other viruses has been eliminated because recombinant factor VIII is not derived from human plasma.

b. Recombinant factor IX will soon be available.

3. Administer DDAVP (desmopressin) to children with mild to moderate hemophilia A.

a. DDAVP promotes the release of factor VIII.

b. It is not used in hemophilia B.

4. Prevent or minimize bleeding.

a. Assess home safety and teach about injury prevention (see Child and Family Teaching 13-1). Consider the child's developmental level to ask specific safety questions.

    b. Recommend using a soft toothbrush and point out the need for regular dental checkups.

    c. Major bleeding requires hospitalization with nursing management.

       (1) Monitor for bleeding and its consequences.

       (2) Provide joint care (exercise).

    d. Control bleeding by applying pressure and cold to the injury site and by elevating and immobilizing the injured area.

    e. Observe for swelling and tenderness in the joints, and prevent contractures. Prevent crippling effects of joint degeneration by implementing a physical therapy program.

    f. Monitor for signs of hypovolemia.

5. Provide support.

    a. Foster the child's self-esteem by encouraging him or her to express concerns and feelings and by promoting a positive self-image.

    b. Encourage family members to verbalize their feelings, especially about any guilt they may have due to the genetic nature of the disorder. Assist their coping efforts by providing information about the disease and its management.

    c. Refer the child and family to support groups such as the National Hemophilia Foundation.

6. Provide child and family teaching.

    a. Explain how to care for, administer, store, and reconstitute the replacement factor.

    b. Inform the child and family that superficial injuries are treated with ice and pressure.

    c. Identify signs of hemarthrosis and teach parents how to immobilize the joint, pack it in ice, and administer replacement factor.

    d. Assist the child and parents to recognize signs of major bleeding (central nervous system manifestations such as headache, blurred vision, vomiting, lethargy, confusion, and seizures).

    e. Explain the possible side effects of therapy.

    f. Demonstrate passive ROM exercises.

    g. Emphasize avoidance of aspirin and aspirin-containing compounds.

    h. Provide diet information because weight increases can impose further stress on joints.

 Idiopathic thrombocytopenic purpura (ITP)

A. Description

    1. ITP is an acquired hemorrhagic disorder in which the number of circulating platelets is reduced.

    2. It may be acute or chronic, and it occurs most frequently between 2 and 5 years of age but may occur at any age.

B. Etiology

    1. The etiology is unknown, but theories of autoimmune phenomenon are widely accepted.

    2. The acute form typically occurs after an upper respiratory infection or a childhood communicable disease (eg, measles, chickenpox, or fifth disease).

C. Pathophysiology

    1. The number of circulating platelets is reduced as a result of the action of antiplatelet antibody produced in the spleen.

    2. The disease results in bleeding into the tissues (purpura).

D. Assessment findings

1. **Clinical manifestations**. It is important to note that the child with ITP does not look sick. **Careful assessment is necessary to rule out child abuse.**
   a. Easy bruising and petechiae
   b. Bleeding from mucous membranes; blood in stool or urine
   c. Hematomas

2. **Laboratory and diagnostic study findings**
   a. CBC will reveal a platelet count that drops below 20,000/mm³.
   b. Coagulation studies, including tourniquet test, bleeding time, and clotting reaction, are abnormal.
   c. Bone marrow aspiration (and other similar tests) is performed to rule out other disorders such as leukemia. In a child with ITP, the aspirate is normal except for a high level of circulating megakaryocytes, the parent cells of platelets.

E. Nursing management

1. **Prevent or minimize bleeding.** Focus on safety until the platelet count returns to normal.

2. **Administer prescribed medications**, which may include prednisone, intravenous immune globulin (IVIG), and anti-D antibody when warranted. Treatment is usually supportive because the disorder is typically self-limiting.
   a. **Prednisone** decreases antiplatelet antibodies. Monitor child for side effects of steroids, including increased risk of infection.
   b. **IVIG** is effective for rapid elevation of the platelet count. It decreases hospitalization time and the likelihood of splenectomy.
   c. **Anti-D antibody** is a new treatment for ITP that can be given in one dose. It alleviates the need for bone marrow aspiration to rule out leukemia before administration of prednisone, and it is less expensive than IVIG.
      (1) Children must meet specific criteria for administration, which include:
         (a) Greater than 1 year old but less than 19 years old
         (b) Rh(D) positive blood type
         (c) Normal WBC and hemoglobin
         (d) No active mucosal bleeding
         (e) No prior history of reaction to plasma products
         (f) No known IgA deficiency
         (g) No concurrent infection
         (h) No Evans syndrome or collagen disease
      (2) Prior to administration, obtain baseline vital signs.
      (3) Reevaluate vital signs 5, 20, and 60 minutes after administration begins.
      (4) Monitor for fever, chills, and headache. If these occur, diphenhydramine (Benadryl) and hydrocortisone (Solu-Cortef) should be given, and the child should be observed for an additional hour.

STUDY QUESTIONS

1. Which of the following age groups would be inappropriate for a school nurse to monitor for iron deficiency anemia while performing a community assessment?
   (1) Toddlers
   (2) Adolescents
   (3) Pregnant women
   (4) School children

2. After being instructed on foods to encourage in the child's diet, which of the following if stated by the parents of a child with iron deficiency anemia would indicate the need for further instruction?
   (1) Lean meats
   (2) Whole-grain breads
   (3) Yellow vegetables
   (4) Fish

3. In children with sickle cell disease, tissue damage results from which of the following?
   (1) A general inflammatory response due to an autoimmune reaction from hypoxia
   (2) Air hunger and respiratory alkalosis due to deoxygenated red blood cells (RBCs)
   (3) Local tissue damage with ischemia and necrosis due to obstructed circulation
   (4) Hypersensitivity of the central nervous system due to elevated serum bilirubin levels

4. When planning a client education program for sickle cell disease, the nurse should include which of the following topics?
   (1) Proper handwashing and infection avoidance
   (2) A high-iron, high-protein diet
   (3) Fluid restriction to 1 quart per day
   (4) Aerobic exercises to increase oxygenation

5. Which of the following interventions would be included in the plan of care of a child with sickle cell disease?
   (1) Administration of anticoagulants to prevent sickling

   (2) Health teaching to help reduce sickling crises
   (3) Observation of imposed fluid restrictions
   (4) Avoidance of the use of narcotics

6. The long-term complications seen in thalassemia major are related to which of the following?
   (1) Hemochromatosis
   (2) Splenomegaly
   (3) Anemia
   (4) Growth retardation

7. The physician orders desferoxamine (Desferal) for a child with thalassemia. Which of the following should alert the nurse to notify the physician?
   (1) Decreased hearing
   (2) Vomiting
   (3) Red urine
   (4) Hypertension

8. Which of the following tests is most helpful in diagnosing hemophilia?
   (1) Bleeding time
   (2) Partial thromboplastin time
   (3) Platelet count
   (4) Complete blood count (CBC)

9. Which of the following actions would you instruct the parents of a child with hemophilia to avoid?
   (1) Applying pressure
   (2) Applying cold to area
   (3) Immobilizing joint
   (4) Lowering injured area

10. Which of the following medications should be avoided by children with idiopathic thrombocytopenia purpura?
    (1) Aspirin
    (2) Acetaminophen
    (3) Codeine
    (4) Morphine

11. When administering steroids to a child with idiopathic thrombocytopenia purpura, the nurse should monitor the child for which of the following?
    (1) Anemia
    (2) Bleeding
    (3) Bruising
    (4) Infection

ANSWER KEY

1. The answer is (4). Periods of rapid growth predispose a person to developing iron deficiency anemia. Because the school age period is not a period of rapid growth, iron deficiency anemia is not prevalent in schoolagers. Toddlerhood, adolescence, and pregnancy are periods of rapid growth. Therefore, individuals in these groups are more likely to experience iron deficiency anemia. The "picky appetites" of toddlers and adolescents may also predispose them to this condition.

2. The answer is (3). If the parents state that they should stress the intake of yellow vegetables, they need additional teaching because yellow vegetables are not good sources of iron. Lean meats, whole-grain breads, and fish are good food sources of iron and should be encouraged.

3. The answer is (3). Characteristic sickle cells tend to clump, which results in poor circulation to tissue, local tissue damage, and eventual ischemia and necrosis. In sickle cell anemia, damage is not due to an inflammatory response. Air hunger and respiratory alkalosis are not present. The central nervous system effects are due to ischemia.

4. The answer is (1). Prevention of infection is an important measure in the prevention of sickle cell crisis. A high-iron, high-protein diet would have no effect on the disease or prevention of a crisis. Proper hydration should be encouraged to prevent crisis secondary to dehydration. Strenuous exercise and activity should be avoided to reduce the risk of increased tissue ischemia.

5. The answer is (2). Because there is no cure for sickle cell disease, prevention is one of the main aims of therapeutic management. Thus, health teaching to help reduce sickling crises is key. Anticoagulants do not prevent sickling. Fluids are encouraged to increase the fluid volume and prevent sickling. Narcotics usually are needed for pain control.

6. The answer is (1). Long-term complications result from hemochromatosis, excessive iron deposits collecting in the tissues and causing destruction. Cellular damage from hemochromatosis may lead to splenomegaly, growth retardation, skeletal complications, cardiac problems, gallbladder disease, hepatomegaly, and skin changes. Anemia is a symptom of this disorder.

7. The answer is (1). Desferoxamine is ototoxic. Therefore, any hearing problem should be promptly reported. Vomiting is not an emergent issue with this drug. Red urine is an expected occurrence with desferoxamine. Hypotension, not hypertension, is a possible side effect.

8. The answer is (2). In hemophilia, partial thromboplastin time is abnormal. Thus, this test would be most helpful in diagnosing the disorder. Bleeding time and platelet count are normal in hemophilia. The CBC is not affected in hemophilia.

9. The answer is (4). Typically, with any bleeding area, but especially with hemophilia-associated bleeding, the injured area must be elevated, not lowered. Applying pressure or cold to the area and immobilizing the joint are appropriate measures to control bleeding.

10. The answer is (1). Aspirin exerts an antiplatelet action and therefore may increase platelet destruction in ITP. Acetaminophen, codeine, and morphine have no affect on platelets and, therefore, are not contraindicated.

11. The answer is (4). Steroids may promote immunosuppression, making the child more susceptible to infections. Anemia is not associated with the disorder or medication. Bleeding and bruising are seen as a result of the disorder, not the steroid therapy.

Cardiovascular
Dysfunction

I. Structure and function of the heart

A. Structure

1. The **heart** is composed of four **chambers**—the **right atrium** and **left atrium** are the upper two chambers; the **right ventricle** and **left ventricle** are the lower chambers; and the wall between the right and left chambers is called a **septum**.

2. **Great vessels**
   a. **Arteries** include the coronary arteries, the aorta, the brachiocephalic artery, subclavian arteries, and the pulmonary artery.
   b. **Veins** include the inferior vena cava (IVC), superior vena cava (SVC), and the pulmonary veins.

3. **The heart is composed of three layers of tissue**:
   a. **Myocardium**
   b. **Endocardium**
   c. **Pericardium,** which is composed of two layers—the serous pericardium, parietal layer, and the serous pericardium, visceral layer. There is a space between the two layers (pericardial space) that contains a few drops of fluid (pericardial fluid). The layers allow for frictionless movement of the heart muscle.

4. There are four **heart valves**—the **pulmonic valve**, the **aortic valve**, the **mitral valve**, and the **tricuspid valve**.

5. The **electrical conduction system** is composed of the **sinoatrial (SA) node**, the **atrioventricular (AV) node**, the **atrioventricular bundle (bundle of His)**, and **Purkinje fibers**. Table 14-1 provides information on the development of the cardiovascular system.

B. Function. The cardiovascular system's basic function is to pump oxygenated blood to tissues and remove metabolic waste products from tissues.

1. **Cardiac cycle**
   a. The cardiac cycle is comprised of sequential contraction (**systole**) and relaxation (**diastole**) of the atria and ventricles.
   b. The atria contract, ejecting blood into the ventricles.
   c. Then, while the atria relax, the ventricles contract, ejecting blood into the aorta and pulmonary artery. Blood enters the systemic circulation from the aorta and the lungs from the pulmonary artery.
   d. Blood then enters the atria, completing the cycle. Blood returns to the right atrium from the systemic circulation via the vena cava and to the left atrium from the pulmonary circulation via the pulmonary vein.
   e. Valves within the heart and pressure difference between the left and right atria and ventricles regulate blood flow through the heart into the systemic circulation.

TABLE 14-1
Development of the Cardiovascular System

AGE	BP/PULSE	STRUCTURE AND FUNCTION
Infant (0–1 year)	BP: 80/40 Pulse: 120–130	The heart lies higher in the chest. Heart rate slows from 120–160 at birth to 100–120, and sinus arrhythmia may be noted (pulse slows with inspiration). The heart still occupies over one half the width of the chest, but it becomes more efficient with its decreased pulse and slightly elevated blood pressure (80/40–100/60). The infant's heart doubles in size by the first birthday.
Toddler/ Preschooler (1–6 years)	BP: 80–100/64 Pulse: 80–105	The heart quadruples its weight by 5 years of age, corresponding to the decrease in pulse rate and increase in blood pressure. Sinus arrhythmia becomes more apparent during the preschool years, the physiologic split may be present for the first time, and functional murmurs may be heard.
Schoolager (6–12 years)	BP: 94–112/56–60 Pulse: 70–80	The heart reaches 10 times its birth weight by puberty. However, the schoolager's heart size is proportionately smaller to body size than at any other stage in life. This is one of the reasons why schoolagers tire easily. As the heart grows, it becomes more vertical in the thoracic cavity.
Adolescent (12–21 years)	BP: 100–120/50–70 Pulse: 60–68	The heart continues to grow in size, and the blood vessels lengthen and widen. However, heart growth is relatively greater than vessel growth, possibly causing young adolescents to experience transient chest pain after periods of activity.

2. **Cardiac output** is the volume of blood ejected by the ventricles during a given period (1 minute). Cardiac output varies as the metabolic needs of the body tissues change. For example, output increases during exercise. Cardiac output is derived by multiplying the heart rate by the stroke volume.
   a. **Heart rate** is the number of heartbeats per minute.
   b. Control of heart rate
      (1) Heart rate changes are performed by reflex controls mediated by the autonomic nervous system, including its parasympathetic and sympathetic divisions. Sympathetic fibers increase heart rate, parasympathetic fibers decrease heart rate. The balance between the two usually determines the heart rate.
      (2) Circulating hormones, especially catecholamines, can influence heart rate.
   c. The **stroke volume** is the volume of blood ejected by the heart during one contraction.
   d. Control of stroke volume is chiefly determined by intrinsic contractility of the heart, preload, and afterload.
      (1) **Contractility** is the ability of the heart muscle to act as an efficient pump. It is increased by circulating catecholamines, sympathetic neuronal activity, and certain medications such as digitalis. It is decreased by hypoxemia and acidosis.

(2) **Preload** is the volume of blood that returns to the heart.

(3) **Afterload** is the resistance against which the ventricles must pump when ejecting blood. Afterload is determined by several factors, including the relative resistances of the systemic circulation (systemic vascular resistance) and the pulmonary circulation (pulmonary vascular resistance).

3. Conduction system function

a. The SA node is the heart's pacemaker; it initiates an impulse. The impulse spreads from there throughout the atria to cause depolarization.

b. While the atria depolarize, impulses spread to the AV node to conduct to the ventricles.

c. The impulses then spread to the AV bundle (bundle of His) and the Purkinje fibers to cause simultaneous depolarization of the ventricles.

C. Fetal and postnatal circulation

1. Fetal heart development begins during the first month of gestation. At about 21 days of gestation, the fetal heart begins beating, and blood begins circulating.

2. Between the second and seventh weeks of gestation, the primitive fetal heart undergoes a series of changes that create the four-chambered heart and its great arteries.

3. During gestation, the lungs are nonfunctional and fetal oxygenation occurs via the placenta.

4. Key structures in fetal circulation (Fig. 14-1) include:

a. **Foramen ovale**, which is an opening between the atria that allows blood flow from the right atrium directly to the left atrium

b. **Ductus arteriosus,** which is a conduit between the pulmonary artery and the aorta that shunts blood away from pulmonary circulation

5. Important **circulatory changes** occurring during the transition to extrauterine life (Fig. 14-2) include:

a. Inspired oxygen dilates pulmonary vessels, decreasing pulmonary vascular resistance and increasing pulmonary blood flow, which facilitates lung expansion.

b. The foramen ovale closes functionally soon after birth due to the compression of the atrial septum.

c. The ductus arteriosus closes functionally by 48 hours after birth.

 NURSING PROCESS OVERVIEW FOR
The Cardiovascular System

A. Assessment

1. Health history

a. Elicit a description of symptoms including onset, duration, location, and precipitation. **Cardinal signs and symptoms** may include:

(1) Feeding problems, including fatigue or diaphoresis during feeding, and poor weight gain

(2) Respiratory difficulties, including tachypnea, dyspnea, shortness of breath, cyanosis, and frequent respiratory infections

(3) Chronic fatigue or exercise intolerance

b. Explore prenatal, personal, and family history for **risk factors** for cardiovascular disorders.

(1) Prenatal risk factors include maternal use of medications, tobacco, and alcohol; maternal exposure to radiation; maternal viral illnesses (eg, coxsackievirus, cytomegalovirus, influenza, mumps, or rubella); or maternal age over 40 years.

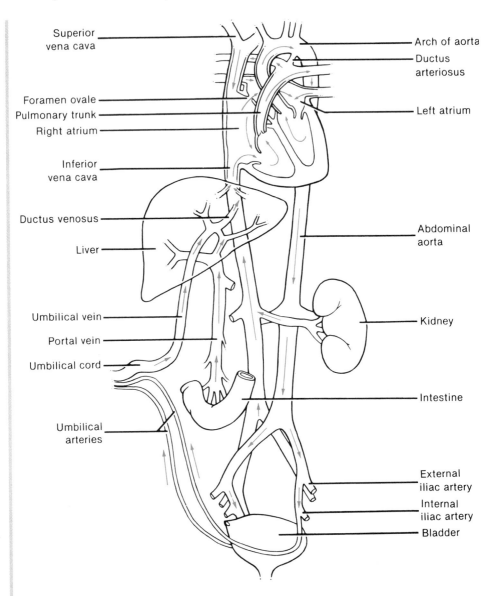

FIGURE 14-1
Fetal circulation shortly before birth; *arrows* indicate the course of blood.

    (2) Personal risk factors include chromosomal abnormalities, prematurity, infections, autoimmune disorders, obesity, tobacco and alcohol use, or medications such as corticosteroids, oral contraceptives, accutane, and anticonvulsants.

    (3) Family risk factors include congenital heart disease in sibling or parent, myocardial infarction before 55 years of age, or sudden death of unknown cause.

2. Physical examination

    a. **Vital signs**

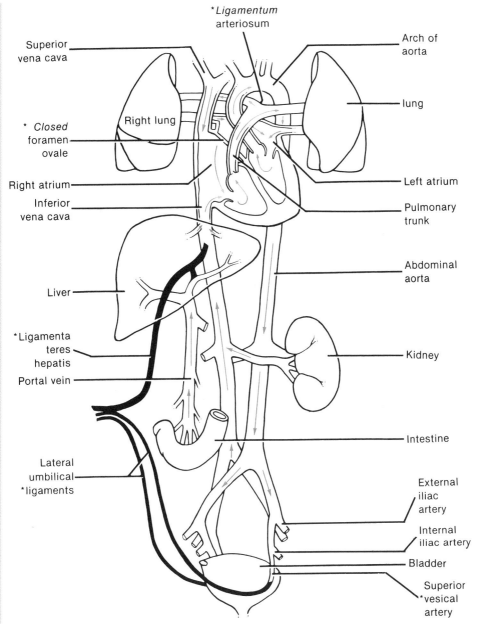

FIGURE 14-2
Neonatal circulation. Compare with fetal circulation (see Fig. 14-1).

(1) Monitor blood pressure for hypertension and hypotension. There should be no major difference between blood pressure of upper extremities and lower extremities. Table 14-1 gives normal blood pressures for various age groups.
(2) Monitor apical and peripheral pulses for rate, rhythm, and quality. There should be regular rate, rhythm, and quality in all pulses. Note tachycardia or

bradycardia, dysrhythmias, diminished peripheral pulses, thready pulse, and narrow or wide pulse pressures. Irregularities may suggest a cardiac disorder. Table 14-1 gives normal pulse rates for various age groups.

   (3) Monitor respirations for rate and effort. Rate should be normal for age and without effort. Tachypnea and dyspnea may suggest heart failure.

   (4) Monitor temperature for hyperthermia, which can suggest infection (eg, endocarditis).

   (5) Assess height and weight because growth failure can occur with severe cardiac disease.

  b. **Inspection**

   (1) Observe the skin for cyanosis, and periorbital and peripheral edema.

   (2) Inspect the neck for engorged neck veins.

   (3) Inspect the extremities for clubbing of the fingers and toes.

   (4) Inspect the abdomen for distention.

  c. **Palpation**

   (1) Palpate the extremities to note pitting.

   (2) Palpate the precordium for point of maximum impulse (PMI), thrills, lifts, and heaves.

   (3) Palpate the abdomen for hepatomegaly and splenomegaly.

  d. **Auscultation**

   (1) Auscultate the heart for normal heart sounds and extra heart sounds, including murmurs.

   (2) Auscultate the lungs for adventitious sounds.

 3. Laboratory studies and diagnostic tests (see Appendices A and B for normal findings and nursing considerations)

  a. A **complete blood count (CBC)** is performed to assess a compensatory increase in hematocrit, hemoglobin, and erythrocyte count (polycythemia).

  b. **Pulse oximetry** identifies the child's oxygen saturation level.

  c. **Coagulation studies** are performed to identify abnormalities in hemostasis (eg, thrombocytopenia), decreased platelet function, low prothrombin level, and decreased or absent clotting factors V, VII, or IX.

  d. **Electrocardiography (ECG)** helps evaluate cardiac musculature, cardiac rate and rhythm, and cardiac impulse conduction (Table 14-2).

  e. **Chest radiography** provides information on the size of the heart and its chambers and on the prominence and distribution of pulmonary blood flow.

  f. **Echocardiography** helps assess the thickness of the heart walls, the size of cardiac chambers, the motion of the valves and septa within the heart, and anatomic relationships of great vessels to various intracardiac structures.

  g. **Cardiac catheterization** provides information on oxygen saturation within heart chambers, pressures within chambers, changes in cardiac output or stroke volume, and anatomic abnormalities.

  h. **Transesophageal pacing/echocardiography** uses an esophageal probe to provide ultrasonic pictures or to pace the heart. It assesses both cardiac structure and function and aids in the identification of complex arrhythmias.

  i. **Angiography** is x-ray visualization of the anatomy of the heart chambers or blood vessels during or after the introduction of contrast medium.

B. Nursing diagnoses

  1. Decreased cardiac output

  2. Altered tissue perfusion

  3. Activity intolerance

TABLE 14-2
Commonly Measured ECG Components

COMPONENT	WHAT IT REPRESENTS	CORRELATION WITH CARDIAC CYCLE
P wave	Atrial depolarization	Contraction of the right atrium begins at the peak of the P wave; left atrial contraction follows.
T wave	Ventricular repolarization	Repolarization occurs while the ventricles are still contracting.
PR interval	Interval between the beginning of the P wave and the beginning of the QRS complex	This is the interval between the onset of atrial depolarization and the onset of ventricular depolarization (ie, the conduction time between the atria and the ventricles).
QT interval	Interval from the beginning of the QRS complex to the end of the T wave	This is the total time of ventricular depolarization and repolarization.
QRS complex	Wave of ventricular depolarization	Left ventricular contraction begins at the peak of the R wave; right ventricular contraction, shortly thereafter.

4. Altered nutrition: less than body requirements
5. Risk for infection
6. Altered growth and development
7. Risk for injury (postcardiac surgery)
8. Ineffective breathing pattern
9. Fluid volume excess
10. Altered family processes

C. **Planning and outcome identification**
   1. The child will maintain adequate oxygenation, as evidenced by normal color and improved blood gas values, and will exhibit minimal to no activity intolerance.
   2. The child will maintain adequate nutritional status.
   3. The child will remain infection free.
   4. The child will attain optimal growth and development.
   5. The child will remain free of postoperative complications.

D. **Implementation**
   1. **Promote adequate cardiac output and oxygenation**.
      a. Monitor vital signs; use a cardiac monitor as needed.
      b. Observe for hypoxia, which is manifested by tachypnea, cyanosis, bradycardia, tachycardia, restlessness, progressive limpness, and syncope.
      c. Manage hypoxia and respiratory distress by performing the following:
         (1) Place the child in the knee–chest position or in a position that eases respiratory distress.
         (2) Administer oxygen as needed.
         (3) Administer prescribed medications (Drug Chart 14-1).
      d. Observe for respiratory distress, which is manifested by tachypnea, tachycardia, retractions, grunting, nasal flaring, cough, and cyanosis.
      e. Monitor for signs and symptoms of thrombosis.
         (1) Signs and symptoms include irritability, restlessness, seizure activity, coma, paralysis, edema, hematuria, oliguria, and anuria.

DRUG CHART 14-1   **Medications Used in Cardiovascular Disorders**

Classifications	Used for	Selected Interventions

Potent vasopressors
    dopamine (Intropin)
    dobutamine (Dobutrex)
    epinephrine (Adrenaline)
    isoprotenerol (Isuprel)
	Used to increase blood pressure, cardiac output, heart rate, and renal and peripheral perfusion	Monitor vital signs and watch for infiltration to prevent burns.
		
		Monitor for side effects (arrhythmias, hypertension, vasoconstriction, tachycardia).

Angiotensin-converting enzyme (ACE) inhibitors
    enalapril (Vasotec)
    catopril (Capoten)
	Used for the treatment of hypertension and congestive heart failure	Instruct the family and child that the child should rise slowly from sitting to standing to minimize blood pressure drop.
		
		Monitor blood pressure.
		
		Monitor for side effects: tachycardia, proteinuria, rash, pruritus, cough, hyperkalemia.
		
		Administer 1 hour before or 2 hours after meals to increase absorption.
		
		Notify health care provider about dizziness, light-headedness, or fainting.

β-Adrenergic blocking agents propranolol (Inderal)	Used for hypertension and cardiac arrhythmias	Give oral medication with food to facilitate absorption. Monitor for side effects, which may include gastric pain, nausea, vomiting, bradycardia, arrhythmias, impotence, decreased libido, and decreased exercise tolerance. Monitor blood pressure and pulse. Provide comfort measures to help child cope with side effects.

Diuretics
    furosemide (Lasix)
    hydrochlorothiazide
        (Hydrodiuril)
    spironalactone (Aldactone)
	Used to manage edema in congestive heart failure and in conjunction with other medications to treat hypertension	Administer with food if GI upset occurs.
		
		Administer the drug in the morning.
		
		Monitor clinical status and lab values for hypokalemia/ hyperkalemia.
		
		Monitor for side effects, which may include dizziness, anorexia, dry mouth, constipation, polyuria, and electrolyte imbalance.
		
		Ensure ready access to the bathroom.
		
		Monitor intake and output and daily weight.

(continued)

DRUG CHART 14-1 Medications Used in Cardiovascular Disorders (Continued)

Classifications	Used for	Selected Interventions
Antiarrythmics digoxin (Lanoxin) (Others include: quinidine, lidocaine, propranolol, and verapamil)	Used for congestive heart failure and arrhythmias Used to strengthen cardiac contractility	Monitor apical pulse for 1 full minute prior to administration. Hold medication if heart rate <100 and notify health care provider. Prepare dosage carefully with a second nurse to check dosage amount. Monitor drug levels. Monitor for digitalis toxicity: early signs of toxicity are anorexia, nausea, and vomiting. Specific serum levels of digitalis and extreme bradycardia are cardinal signs of toxicity; withhold digoxin if the child's heart rate falls below the normal range for age (see Table 14-3), unless the physician specifies otherwise.
Antibiotics penicillin sulfadiazine	Prophylaxis for endocarditis Long-term prophylaxis for rheumatic fever	Encourage compliance with treatment. Monitor for penicillin side effects, which may include GI irritation, hypersensitivity, and superinfection. Monitor for sulfadiazine side effects, which may include GI irritation, headache, crystalluria, photosensitivity, and agranulocytosis. Encourage use of sunscreens and protective clothing. Encourage fluids.
Aspirin	Anti-inflammatory	Monitor for side effects such as GI disturbance, decreased platelet count, tinnitus, and headache. Warn parents to notify the physician if the child has signs of influenza or varicella due to the possibility of Reye syndrome when taking aspirin during these illnesses.
Corticosteroids	Anti-inflammatory	Monitor for side effects, including fluid retention, edema, hypokalemia, GI irritation, hyperglycemia, altered growth patterns, and Cushing syndrome.

GI, gastrointestinal.

(2) To reduce the risk of thrombosis, prevent dehydration (especially during acute illnesses).

f. Decrease cardiac workload.

(1) Schedule care to provide periods of uninterrupted rest.

(2) Prevent excessive crying in infants.

(3) Provide diversional activities that involve only limited energy expenditure in older children.

2. Promote adequate nutrition.

a. Evaluate food and fluid intake and weight gain daily.

b. Assess the child's food preferences.

c. Promote a well-balanced diet that is rich in iron and potassium and low in sodium.

d. Provide small, frequent feedings if the child tires easily.

e. Provide nipples that make it easier for an infant to suck and limit feedings to 45 minutes or less if the infant tires easily.

f. Prevent hypokalemia secondary to diuretic therapy by maintaining a high-potassium diet and administering potassium supplements when prescribed.

g. Prevent anemia by encouraging an iron-rich diet and by administering iron supplements as prescribed.

h. Confer with a nutritionist.

3. Prevent infection.

a. Prevent infection through careful handwashing, by avoiding contact with infected persons, and by providing adequate rest and nutrition.

b. Ensure that the child receives appropriate immunizations, including pneumococcal and influenza vaccines.

c. Observe for and assist in managing bacterial endocarditis, which is manifested by fever, pallor, petechiae, anorexia, and fatigue.

d. **Ensure administration of prophylactic antibiotics before dental work, surgery, certain invasive procedures, or laceration repair.** Bacterial endocarditis prophylaxis is required for the child with one or more of the following conditions:

(1) Most congenital heart defects

(2) Acquired valve abnormalities due to heart surgery, rheumatic fever, and heart disease

(3) Hypertrophic cardiomyopathy

(4) Mitral valve prolapse with regurgitation

(5) Persistent ventricular septal defect (VSD) despite surgery

(6) Prosthetic valves

(7) For the first 6 months after congenital heart defect (CHD) repair

4. Promote optimal growth and development.

a. Enhance the child's self-concept by encouraging him to express feelings about the defect, clarifying any misconceptions he expresses concerning the defect or its treatment, and supporting positive coping mechanisms.

b. Decrease the child's and family's anxiety and increase their understanding by providing developmentally appropriate explanations for medical and surgical treatments for the specific defect.

c. Assess for developmental delays. These are common in children with cardiovascular disorders, particularly in those with more severe cardiac disorders.

d. Allow the child sufficient time to complete tasks and activities. This is essential for nurturing a positive self-concept and promoting independence.

e. Limit activities only when essential. With many defects, an older child may be allowed to self-limit activities according to how he feels.

f. Encourage parental involvement in the child's care, as appropriate.

g. Provide parents with needed support and guidance in setting limits, providing discipline, and meeting their child's emotional needs.

h. Encourage the parents to treat the child as normally as possible.

i. Encourage the child to continue with schoolwork as appropriate.

5. Provide preoperative and postoperative care.

a. **Prepare the child and family preoperatively.**

(1) Discuss the purpose of surgery. Cardiac surgery is either an emergency or a planned procedure to correct defects or provide symptomatic relief.

    (a) **Open-heart surgery** involves incision of the myocardium to repair intracardiac structures. This type of surgery requires cardiopulmonary bypass.

    (b) **Closed-heart surgery** involves structures related to the heart but not the heart muscle itself. This type of surgery usually can be performed without cardiopulmonary bypass.

(2) Prepare the child and family emotionally.

    (a) Allow a visit to the intensive care unit.

    (b) Provide developmentally appropriate explanations of what to expect before, during, and after surgery.

    (c) Allow and encourage expression of feelings and questions.

(3) Perform a preoperative nursing assessment.

    (a) Health history should include history of cardiac, pulmonary, renal, hepatic, hematologic, and metabolic disorders and a medication history that includes allergies and adverse reactions.

    (b) Physical examination should include baseline assessments of height and weight, vital signs, sleep–wake patterns, elimination patterns, and fluid intake.

    (c) Laboratory studies should include CBC; serum electrolyte levels; clotting studies; urinalysis; nose, throat, and sputum cultures; antibody screen; renal and hepatic function tests; and radiographic and other diagnostic studies.

(4) Administer preoperative medications, which may include sedatives and antibiotics (see Drug Chart 14-1).

b. **Manage the child postoperatively**.

(1) Maintain optimal respiratory status.

    (a) Monitor respirations and provide good pulmonary hygiene.

    (b) If the child is intubated, monitor chest tube drainage and patency and blood gas values, and observe for signs of respiratory distress.

(2) Monitor cardiac status.

    (a) Heart rate and rhythm (count rate for 1 full minute and compare findings with the ECG monitor; document activity)

    (b) Blood pressure, including intra-arterial monitoring

    (c) Central venous pressure (CVP) and other hemodynamic parameters

    (d) Heart sounds

    (e) Peripheral pulses

    (f) Blood chemistry values

(3) Monitor lung sounds (decreased breath sounds may indicate atelectasis).

    (a) Suction only when needed (avoid vagal stimulation).

    (b) Monitor chest tubes and ventilator settings.

(4) Prevent postoperative hypothermia.

    (a) Provide external warmth.

    (b) Monitor for hyperthermia associated with infection.

    (5) Closely monitor fluid intake and output
      (a) Assess for signs of fluid overload, such as edema.
      (b) Maintain fluid restrictions, as prescribed.
      (c) Monitor intravenous (IV) lines, which includes peripheral line for fluids, a venous pressure line, and an atrial line.
    (6) Promote comfort.
      (a) Assess for pain.
      (b) Medicate as needed.
    (7) Maintain skin integrity.
      (a) Inspect all incision sites frequently.
      (b) Change the child's position frequently.
      (c) Provide skin care.
      (d) Change the child's dressings as prescribed.
      (e) Observe for infection.
    (8) Monitor for surgical complications.
      (a) Cardiac complications include congestive heart failure (CHF), hypoxia, low cardiac output syndrome, decreased peripheral perfusion, dysrhythmias, and cardiac tamponade.
      (b) Pulmonary complications include atelectasis, pneumothorax, pulmonary edema, and pleural effusion.
      (c) Neurologic complications include cerebral edema, brain damage, and seizure disorder.
      (d) Other complications include infection, acidosis, thromboembolism, electrolyte imbalance, and postpericardiotomy syndrome.
    (9) Prevent problems of sensory overload.
      (a) Orient the child to time, place, and person.
      (b) Prepare the child for all procedures.
      (c) Provide developmentally appropriate explanations.
      (d) Ensure adequate rest periods.
      (e) Observe for psychic disturbances and sleep deprivation.
  (10) During recovery, provide tactile stimulation for infants and diversions for older children.
  (11) Provide emotional support for children and parents by addressing concerns.
  (12) Refer family for community health nurse visits.
  (13) Provide child and family teaching (Child and Family Teaching 14-1).

E. Outcome evaluation
  1. The child maintains adequate oxygenation.
  2. The child maintains adequate nutritional status.
  3. The child remains infection free.
  4. The child attains optimal growth and development.
  5. The child is free of postoperative complications.

III. Congenital heart defects (CHDs)

A. Overview
  1. CHDs are structural defects of the heart, great vessels, or both that are present from birth. The incidence of CHD is 4 to 10/1000 live births.
  2. Children with CHD are more likely to have associated defects such as tracheoesophageal fistula.
  3. CHD is second only to prematurity as a cause of death in the first year of life.

CHILD AND FAMILY TEACHING 14-1

Postcardiac Surgery

Activity restrictions

- Young children tend to pace themselves and rest when tired.
- Older children are soon able to participate in normal activities.
- The sternum needs approximately 6 weeks to heal. During this time the child should avoid activities that may involve rough play, falls, or pressure to the chest.
- Avoid lifting child under the arms because this may cause pain at the operative site.

Incision site care

- Observe site for signs of infection (swelling, redness, and drainage).
- Keep the incision clean and dry. Wash with warm soap and water if it gets soiled.
- Leave steri-strips in place until the first office visit. Use a bandage if clothes irritate the wound.
- Sponge bath only for first week.

Medications

- Teach dosage, administration, and possible side effects of medications.

Diet and fluid restrictions

- Most children return to normal diets. Discuss restrictions for those who need them.

Infection prevention

- Teach infection control measures, including proper handwashing and avoidance of infected persons.
- Enforce the need for prophylaxis for bacterial endocarditis.

Pain

- Acetaminophen is usually prescribed.
- Teach the child and family nonpharmacologic pain relief methods.

Follow-up care

- Encourage the family to maintain follow-up appointments, including those for well child care, immunizations, and dental care.
- Teach family to monitor for complications and to contact health care provider if any of the following occur: tachycardia, fever, severe or persistent chest pain, labored breathing or tachypnea, feeding difficulties, decreased urination, and persistent swelling (edema).

B. Classifications. There are four classifications of CHD.

  1. Defects with increased pulmonary blood flow include patent ductus arteriosus (PDA), atrial septal defect (ASD), VSD, and atrioventricular canal defect (AV canal).

  2. Obstructive defects include coarctation of the aorta (COA), aortic stenosis (AS), and pulmonic stenosis (PS).

  3. Defects with decreased pulmonary blood flow include tricuspid atresia and tetralogy of Fallot (TOF).

  4. Mixed defects include transposition of the great vessels (TGV), truncus arteriosus, and hypoplastic left heart syndrome (HLHS).

C. Etiology

  1. In more than 90% of CHD cases, the exact etiology is unknown.

2. Factors associated with increased incidence of CHD include:

a. Fetal and maternal infection during the first trimester, especially rubella

b. Maternal alcoholism

c. Maternal use of other drugs with teratogenic effects

d. Maternal age over 40 years

e. Maternal dietary deficiencies

f. Maternal insulin-dependent induced diabetes

g. Sibling with CHD

h. Parent with CHD

i. A chromosomal abnormality, such as Down syndrome

D. Patent ductus arteriosus

1. Description. PDA results when the fetal ductus arteriosus fails to close completely after birth.

2. Pathophysiology. Blood flows from the aorta through the PDA and back to the pulmonary artery and lungs, causing increased left ventricular work load and increased pulmonary vascular congestion.

3. Assessment findings

a. **Clinical manifestations**

(1) If the defect is small, the child may be asymptomatic.

(2) A loud machine-like murmur is characteristic.

(3) Child may have frequent respiratory infections.

(4) Child may have CHF with poor feeding, fatigue, hepatosplenomegaly (HSM), poor weight gain, tachypnea, and irritability.   *enlargement of liver & spleen*

(5) Widened pulse pressure and bounding pulse rate may be detected.

b. **Laboratory and diagnostic study findings**

(1) The ECG is usually normal but may show ventricle enlargement if the shunt is large.

(2) Cardiac catheterization is usually not necessary.

4. Nursing management

a. **Provide family teaching** about treatment options for PDA.

(1) Some PDAs close spontaneously; others can be closed surgically or non-surgically.

(2) Surgical closure is accomplished by one of two methods.

(a) Left thoracotomy without pulmonary bypass

(b) Visual-assisted thorascopic surgery (VATS), which eliminates the need for thoracotomy.

(3) In premature infants, PDA sometimes can be closed using prostaglandin synthetase inhibitors (eg, indomethacin), which stimulate closure of the ductus arteriosus.

b. **Provide preoperative and postoperative care.**

E. Atrial septal defect

1. Description

a. An ASD is an abnormal communication between the two atria.

b. ASD results when the atrial septal tissue does not fuse properly during embryonic development.

2. Pathophysiology

a. Pressure is higher in the left atrium than the right, causing blood to shunt from the left to the right side of the heart.

b. The right ventricle and pulmonary artery enlarge because they are handling more blood.

3. Assessment findings

a. Clinical manifestations

(1) Most infants tend to be asymptomatic until early childhood and many defects close spontaneously by 5 years of age.

(2) Symptoms vary with the size of the defect; fatigue and dyspnea on exertion are the most common.

(3) Slow weight gain and frequent respiratory infections may occur.

(4) Systolic ejection murmur may be auscultated, usually most prominent at the second intercostal space.

b. Laboratory and diagnostic study findings

(1) Echocardiography with Doppler generally reveals the enlarged right side of the heart and the increased pulmonary circulation.

(2) Cardiac catheterization demonstrates the separation of the right atrial septum and the increased oxygen saturation in the right atrium.

4. Nursing management

a. Provide family teaching about treatment options for ASD.

(1) Defects are usually repaired in girls due to possibility of clot formation during child-bearing years.

(2) Small ASDs are left open in boys; larger ones are repaired.

(3) Surgical closure by suture or patch requires cardiopulmonary bypass and usually is performed during the school-age years.

(4) Closure via cardiac catheterization is on trial at some centers.

b. Provide preoperative and postoperative care.

F. Ventricular septal defect

1. Description

a. VSD, the most common CHD, is an abnormal opening between the right and left ventricles.

b. The degree of this defect may vary from a pinhole between the right and left ventricles to an absent septum.

2. Pathophysiology

a. Pressure from the left ventricle causes blood to flow through the defect to the right ventricle, resulting in increased pulmonary vascular resistance and right heart enlargement.

b. Right ventricular and pulmonary arterial pressures increase, leading eventually to obstructive pulmonary vascular disease.

3. Assessment findings

a. Clinical manifestations

(1) Symptoms vary with the size of the defect, age, and amount of resistance; usually the child is asymptomatic.

(2) Identifiable symptoms may be failure to thrive (FTT), excessive sweating, and fatigue.

(3) Child may be more susceptible to pulmonary infections.

(4) Child may exhibit signs and symptoms of CHF.

b. Laboratory and diagnostic study findings.

(1) Echocardiography with Doppler ultrasound or magnetic resonance imaging (MRI) reveals right ventricular hypertrophy and possible pulmonary artery dilatation from the increased blood flow.

(2) The ECG shows right ventricular hypertrophy.

4. Nursing management

a. **Provide family teaching about treatment options for VSD.**

(1) Some VSDs close spontaneously.

(2) Others are closed with a Dacron patch requiring cardiopulmonary bypass. This is recommended for children with large defects, pulmonary arterial hypertension, CHF, recurrent respiratory infections, and FTT.

(3) It is important to note that surgery is complex and that pulmonary artery banding may be done as a palliative procedure for infants who are poor surgical candidates.

b. **Provide preoperative and postoperative care.**

G. Atrioventricular canal defect

1. Description

a. An AV canal defect results from the incomplete fusion of endocardial cushions.

b. It consists of a low atrial septal defect that is continuous with a high ventricular septal defect and clefts of the mitral and tricuspid valves, creating a large central AV valve that allows blood to flow between all heart chambers.

2. Pathophysiology

a. Alterations in hemodynamics depend on the severity of the defect and the child's pulmonary vascular resistance, which is usually high in the newborn.

b. Once pulmonary vascular resistance drops, left-to-right shunting occurs, increasing pulmonary blood flow and resulting in pulmonary vascular engorgement and, possibly, CHF.

3. Assessment findings

a. **Clinical manifestations**

(1) Children usually have moderate to severe CHF.

(2) Child may have a mild cyanosis that increases with crying.

(3) A characteristic murmur exists.

b. **Laboratory and diagnostic study findings.** Echocardiography confirms the diagnosis.

4. Nursing management

a. **Provide family teaching about treatment options for AV canal defect.**

(1) Repair involves surgical patch closure of septal defects, possible mitral valve replacement, and reconstruction of AV valve tissue.

(2) Palliative repair, via pulmonary artery banding, may be necessary for symptomatic infants.

b. **Provide preoperative and postoperative care**.

H. Coarctation of the aorta

1. Description

a. COA is a defect that involves a localized narrowing of the aorta.

b. There are three types of COA, depending on location.

(1) Preductal COA is proximal to the insertion of the ductus arteriosus.

(2) Postductal COA is distal to the ductus arteriosus.

(3) Juxtaductal COA is at the insertion of the ductus arteriosus.

2. Pathophysiology

a. COA is characterized by increased pressure proximal to the defect and decreased pressure distal to it.

b. Restricted blood flow through the narrowed aorta increases the pressure on the left ventricle and causes dilation of the proximal aorta and left ventricular hypertrophy, which may lead to left ventricular failure.

c. Eventually, collateral vessels develop to bypass the coarctated segment and supply circulation to the lower extremities.

3. Assessment findings

a. Clinical manifestations

(1) The child may be asymptomatic or may experience the classic difference in blood pressure and pulse quality between the upper and lower extremities—the blood pressure is elevated in the upper extremities and decreased in the lower extremities while the pulse is bounding in the upper extremities and decreased or absent in the lower extremities. Thus, femoral pulses are weak or absent.

(2) Additional manifestations may include epistaxis, headaches, fainting, and lower leg muscle cramps.

(3) A systolic murmur may be heard over the left anterior chest and between the scapula posteriorly.

(4) Rib notching may be observed in an older child.

b. Laboratory and diagnostic study findings

(1) ECG, echocardiography, and chest radiography may reveal left-sided heart enlargement resulting from back pressure.

(2) The radiograph may also demonstrate rib notching from enlarged collateral vessels.

4. Nursing management

a. Provide family teaching about treatment options for COA.

(1) Repair involves surgical removal of the stenotic area; bypass surgery is not necessary because repair takes place outside of the heart.

(2) Nonsurgical repair via balloon angioplasty is performed in some centers.

b. Provide preoperative and postoperative care.

I. Aortic stenosis

1. Description. AS is a defect that primarily involves an obstruction to the left ventricular outflow of the valve.

2. Pathophysiology

a. Left ventricular pressure increases to overcome resistance of the obstructed valve and allow blood to flow into the aorta, eventually producing left ventricular hypertrophy.

b. Myocardial ischemia may develop as the increased oxygen demands of the hypertrophied left ventricle go unmet.

3. Assessment findings

a. Clinical manifestations

(1) The child with a severe defect may have a faint pulse, hypotension, tachycardia, and a poor feeding pattern.

(2) The child may experience signs of exercise intolerance, chest pain, and dizziness when standing for long periods.

(3) A systolic ejection murmur may be heard best at the second intercostal space.

b. Laboratory and diagnostic study findings

(1) ECG or echocardiography reveals left ventricular hypertrophy.

(2) Cardiac catheterization demonstrates the degree of the stenosis.

4. Nursing management

a. Provide family teaching about treatment options for AS.

(1) If the child's symptoms warrant, surgical aortic valvulotomy or prosthetic valve replacement is necessary.

(2) Balloon angioplasty can be used to dilate the narrow valve.

b. Provide preoperative and postoperative care.

J. Pulmonic stenosis

1. **Description.** PS is a defect that involves obstruction of blood flow from the right ventricle.

2. **Pathophysiology**
   a. As a result of right ventricular pressure increase, right ventricular hypertrophy may develop.
   b. Eventually, right ventricular failure may result.

3. **Assessment findings**
   a. **Clinical manifestations**
      (1) The child may be asymptomatic or may have mild cyanosis or CHF.
      (2) A systolic murmur may be heard over the pulmonic area; a thrill may be heard if stenosis is severe.
      (3) In severe cases, decreased exercise tolerance, dyspnea, precordial pain, and generalized cyanosis may occur.
   b. **Laboratory and diagnostic study findings**
      (1) ECG or echocardiography reveals right ventricular hypertrophy.
      (2) Cardiac catheterization demonstrates the degree of the stenosis.

4. **Nursing management**
   a. **Provide family teaching about treatment options for PS.**
      (1) Balloon angioplasty techniques are being widely used to treat PS.
      (2) Surgical valvulotomy may be performed (although the need for surgery is uncommon due to the widespread use of balloon angioplasty techniques).
   b. **Provide preoperative and postoperative care.**

K. Tricuspid atresia

1. **Description**
   a. Tricuspid atresia occurs when the tricuspid valve fails to develop.
   b. Without the tricuspid valve, there is no communication between the right atrium and the right ventricle.

2. **Pathophysiology**
   a. Often associated with PS and TGV, tricuspid atresia causes complete mixing of oxygenated and unoxygenated blood in the left side of the heart resulting in systemic desaturation and variable pulmonary obstruction.
   b. Blood flows through an associated ASD or patent foramen ovale to the left side of the heart and through an associated VSD to the right ventricle and to the lungs.

3. **Assessment findings**
   a. **Clinical manifestations**
      (1) Cyanosis is usually noted in the newborn. Tachycardia and dyspnea may be noted.
      (2) Older children have signs of chronic hypoxia, including clubbing.
   b. **Laboratory and diagnostic study findings.** Echocardiography reveals the defect.

4. **Nursing management**
   a. **Provide family teaching about treatment options for tricuspid atresia.**
      (1) Palliative procedures, such as a pulmonary-to-systemic artery anastomosis, are performed on children with CHF.
      (2) Corrective surgery may be performed using the hemi-Fontan or Fontan procedure.
      (3) Surgical mortality varies and there are several postoperative complications, including arrhythmias, pleural effusion, and ventricular dysfunction.
   b. **Provide preoperative and postoperative care.**

L. Tetralogy of Fallot

1. **Description**. TOF consists of four major anomalies.

   a. VSD

   b. Right ventricular hypertrophy

   c. PS

   d. Aorta overriding the VSD

2. **Pathophysiology**

   a. PS impedes the flow of blood to the lungs, causing increased pressure in the right ventricle, forcing deoxygenated blood through the septal defect to the left ventricle.

   b. The increased workload on the right ventricle causes hypertrophy. The overriding aorta receives blood from both right and left ventricles.

3. **Assessment findings**

   a. **Clinical manifestations** vary, depending on the size of the VSD and the degree of PS.

      (1) Acute episodes of cyanosis ("tet spells") and transient cerebral ischemia. "Tet spells" are characterized by irritability, pallor, and blackouts or convulsions.

      (2) Cyanosis occurring at rest (as PS worsens)

      (3) Squatting (a characteristic posture of older children that serves to decrease the return of poorly oxygenated venous blood from the lower extremities and to increase systemic vascular resistance, which increases pulmonary blood flow and eases respiratory effort)

      (4) Slow weight gain

      (5) Clubbing, exertional dyspnea, fainting, or fatigue slowness due to hypoxia

      (6) A pansystolic murmur may be heard at the mid-lower left sternal border

   b. **Laboratory and diagnostic study findings**

      (1) Echocardiography and ECG show the enlarged chambers of the right side of the heart.

      (2) Echocardiography also demonstrates the decrease in the size of the pulmonary artery and the reduced blood flow through the lungs.

      (3) Cardiac catheterization and angiography allow definitive evaluation of the extent of the defect, particularly the PS and the VSD.

      (4) CBC reveals polycythemia.

      (5) Arterial blood gases (ABGs) demonstrate reduced oxygen saturation.

4. **Nursing management**

   a. **Provide family teaching about treatment options for TOF.**

      (1) Elective repair is usually performed during the infant's first year of life, but palliative repairs may be warranted for infants who cannot undergo primary repair.

      (2) Total repair involves VSD closure, infundibular stenosis resection, and pericardial patch to enlarge right ventricular outflow tract.

   b. **Provide preoperative and postoperative care.**

M. Transposition of the great vessels

1. **Description**

   a. In TGV, the pulmonary artery leaves the left ventricle and the aorta exits the right ventricle.

   b. There is no communication between the systemic and pulmonary circulations.

2. **Pathophysiology**

   a. This defect results in two separate circulatory patterns; the right heart manages systemic circulation and the left manages pulmonary circulation.

b. To sustain life, the child must have an associated defect. Associated defects, such as septal defects or a PDA, permit oxygenated blood into the systemic circulation, but cause increased cardiac workload.

c. Potential complications include CHF, infective endocarditis, brain abscess, and cerebral vascular accidents resulting from hypoxia or thrombosis.

3. Assessment findings

a. **Clinical manifestations** vary, depending on associated defects.

(1) In infants with minimal communication (no associated defects), severe respiratory depression and cyanosis will be evident at birth.

(2) In infants with associated defects, there is less cyanosis but the infant may have symptoms of CHF.

(3) Easily fatigued

(4) FTT

(5) No murmur or presence of a murmur that is characteristic of an associated defect

b. **Laboratory and diagnostic study findings**

(1) Echocardiography reveals an enlarged heart.

(2) Cardiac catheterization reveals low oxygen saturation resulting from the mixing of blood in the heart chambers.

4. Nursing management

a. **Provide family teaching about the treatment options for TGV.**

(1) Prostaglandin E is administered to maintain a PDA and further blood mixing.

(2) An arterial switch procedure within the first week of life is the surgical procedure of choice.

b. **Provide preoperative and postoperative care.**

N. Truncus arteriosus

1. Description

a. Truncus arteriosus is the failure of normal septation and division of the embryonic bulbar trunk into the pulmonary artery and aorta.

b. This results in a single vessel that overrides both ventricles.

2. Pathophysiology

a. Blood ejected from the ventricles enters the common artery and flows into either the lungs or the aortic arch.

b. Pressure in both ventricles is high and blood flow to the lungs is markedly increased.

3. Assessment findings

a. **Clinical manifestations**

(1) Neonates with this defect typically appear normal; however, as pulmonary vascular resistance decreases after birth, severe pulmonary edema and CHF commonly develop.

(2) Marked cyanosis, especially on exertion

(3) Signs and symptoms of CHF

(4) Left ventricular hypertrophy, dyspnea, marked activity intolerance, and retarded growth

(5) Loud systolic murmur best heard at the lower left sternal border and radiating throughout the chest

b. **Laboratory and diagnostic study findings.** Echocardiography reveals the defect.

4. Nursing management

a. **Provide family teaching about the treatment options for truncus arteriosus.**

(1) Surgical repair is necessary in the first few months of life; the mortality rate associated with surgery is greater than 10%.

(2) Without surgery, children die within 1 year.

b. **Provide preoperative and postoperative care**.

O. Hypoplastic left heart syndrome

1. **Description**

a. HLHS is a disorder that results in underdevelopment of the left side of the heart and involves various left-sided defects, commonly including severe coarctation of the aorta, severe aortic valvular stenosis or atresia, and severe mitral valve stenosis or atresia.

b. The left ventricle, aortic valve, mitral valve, and ascending aorta usually are small or hypoplastic.

2. **Pathophysiology**

a. While the ductus arteriosus remains patent, there is systemic blood flow. This allows for possible survival.

b. When the ductus arteriosus closes (approximately 48 hours after birth), pulmonary edema and low cardiac output occur, leading to hypoxia, acidosis, and death.

3. **Assessment findings**

a. **Clinical manifestations** usually are evident by the first 2 weeks after birth.

(1) Signs and symptoms of CHF and pulmonary edema

(2) Single S_2

(3) Soft systolic ejection murmur

b. **Laboratory and diagnostic study findings.** Echocardiography reveals the defect.

4. **Nursing management. Provide family teaching about treatment options for HLHS.**

a. Surgical repair (Norwood procedure) is performed in stages and has a mortality risk greater than 25%.

b. Cardiac transplant has a mortality risk greater than 25%.

c. Without intervention, the defect is fatal; infants rarely survive longer than 1 month.

d. Infants are maintained on prostaglandin E_1, which will delay the closure of the ductus arteriosus, until a decision about treatment is reached.

IV. Congestive heart failure

A. Description

1. CHF is severe circulatory congestion due to decreased myocardial contractility, which results in the heart's inability to pump sufficient blood to meet the body's needs.

2. About 80% of CHF cases occur before 1 year of age.

B. Etiology

1. The primary cause of CHF in the first 3 years of life is CHD.

2. Other causes in children include:

a. Other myocardial disorders, such as cardiomyopathies, arrhythmias, and hypertension

b. Pulmonary embolism or chronic lung disease

c. Severe hemorrhage or anemia

d. Adverse effects of anesthesia or surgery

e. Adverse effects of transfusions or infusions

f. Increased body demands resulting from conditions such as fever, infection, and arteriovenous fistula

g. Adverse effects of drugs, such as doxorubicin

h. Severe physical or emotional stress

i. Excessive sodium intake

3. In general, causes can be classified according to the following:

a. **Volume overload** may cause the right ventricle to hypertrophy to compensate for added volume.

b. **Pressure overload** usually results from an obstructive lesion, such as COA.

c. **Decreased contractility** can result from problems such as severe anemia, asphyxia, heart block, and acidemia.

d. **High cardiac output** demands occur when the body's need for oxygen exceeds the heart's output as seen in sepsis and hyperthyroidism.

C. Pathophysiology

1. Right ventricular failure occurs when the right ventricle is unable to pump blood into the pulmonary circulation. Less blood is oxygenated and pressure increases in the right atrium and systemic venous circulation, which results in edema of the extremities.

2. Left ventricular failure occurs when the left ventricle is unable to pump blood into systemic circulation. Pressure increases in the left atrium and pulmonary veins; then the lungs become congested with blood, causing elevated pulmonary pressure and pulmonary edema.

3. To compensate, the cardiac muscle hypertrophies eventually resulting in decreased ventricular compliance. Decreased compliance requires higher filling pressure to produce the same stroke volume. Increased muscle mass impedes oxygenation of the heart muscle, which leads to decreased contraction force and heart failure.

4. As cardiac output fails, stretch receptors and baroreceptors stimulate the sympathetic nervous system, releasing catecholamines that increase the force and rate of myocardial contraction.

5. This causes increased systemic resistance, increased venous return, and reduced blood flow to the limbs, viscera, and kidneys.

6. Sweating results from sympathetic cholinergic fibers, there is extra work for the heart muscle, and there is less systemic blood flow.

7. The renal system responds by releasing renin-angiotensin, which sets off a chain of events—vasoconstriction, leading to increased aldosterone release, causing sodium and water retention, and, in turn, increasing preload. Finally, sodium and water retention becomes excessive, resulting in signs of systemic venous congestion and fluid overload.

D. Assessment findings

1. Clinical manifestations

a. It is clinically difficult to differentiate right from left ventricular failure. Failure of one chamber causes reciprocal changes in the opposite chamber.

b. Weakness and fatigue

c. Poor feeding, resulting in weight loss

d. Developmental delays

e. Irritability

f. Pallor and cyanosis

g. Dyspnea, tachypnea, orthopnea, wheezing, cough, weak cry, grunting, mild cyanosis, and costal retractions

h. Tachycardia and gallop rhythm

i. Hepatomegaly

    j. Weight gain from edema, ascites, and pleural effusions

    k. Distended neck and peripheral veins

    l. Sweating

  2. Laboratory and diagnostic study findings

    a. Chest radiography reveals cardiomegaly and pulmonary congestion. *cH (Left ventricular failure)*

    b. CBC reveals dilution hyponatremia, hypochloremia, and hyperkalemia.

    c. ECG reveals ventricular hypertrophy.

E. Nursing management

  1. Monitor for signs of respiratory distress.

    a. Provide pulmonary hygiene as needed.

    b. Administer oxygen as prescribed.

    c. Keep the head of the bed elevated.

    d. Monitor ABG values.

  2. Monitor for signs of altered cardiac output, including:

    a. Pulmonary edema

    b. Arrhythmias, including extreme tachycardia and bradycardia

    c. Characteristic ECG and heart sound changes

  3. Evaluate fluid status.

    a. Maintain strict fluid intake and output measurements.

    b. Monitor daily weights.

    c. Assess for edema and severe diaphoresis.

    d. Monitor electrolyte values and hematocrit level.

    e. Maintain strict fluid restrictions, as prescribed.

  4. Administer prescribed medications (see Drug Chart 14-1), which may include:

    a. Antiarrhythmics (eg, digoxin), to increase cardiac performance

    b. Diuretics, to reduce venous and systemic congestion

    c. Iron and folic acid supplements, to improve nutritional status

 5. Prevent infection.

  6. Reduce cardiac demands.

    a. Keep the child warm.

    b. Schedule nursing interventions to allow for rest.

    c. Do not allow an infant to feed for more than 45 minutes at a time.

    d. Provide gavage feedings if the infant becomes fatigued before ingesting an adequate amount.

7. Promote adequate nutrition. Maintain a high-calorie, low-sodium diet, as prescribed.

8. Promote optimal growth and development.

  9. As appropriate, **refer the family to a community health nurse** for **follow-up care after discharge**.

V. Rheumatic fever (RF)

A. Description

  1. RF is a systemic inflammatory disease that occurs as a result of naturally acquired immunity to group A β-hemolytic streptococcal infection. There is cardiac involvement in about 50% of cases.

  2. It is the most common cause of acquired heart disease in children worldwide. Although the incidence has sharply decreased in the United States within the past, it seems to be reappearing in some parts of the country.

3. RF usually occurs in children between 6 and 15 years of age, with peak incidence at 8 years of age. There are more frequent outbreaks in late winter and early spring when streptococcal infections are most common.

B. Etiology

1. The onset of RF usually occurs 2 to 6 weeks after an untreated upper respiratory infection with group A β-hemolytic streptococci.

2. It is believed that a genetic susceptibility to RF is associated with a state of immune hyperactivity to the streptococcal antigens; however, the exact etiology of RF is unknown.

C. Pathophysiology

1. The child becomes infected with group A β-hemolytic streptococcal bacteria.

2. Antibodies formed against these bacteria begin to attack the connective tissue of the body, producing inflammation, which affects the heart, joints, central nervous system, and subcutaneous tissue.

3. Cardiac involvement is characterized by **carditis**.

   a. A type of lesion, called an Aschoff body (a proliferating, fibrin-like plaque), forms on the heart valve causing edema and inflammation.

   b. When the healed area becomes fibrous and scarred, the valve leaflets fuse (stenosis), causing inefficiency and leakage.

   c. The mitral and aortic valves are affected most often.

D. Assessment findings

1. Clinical manifestations vary and depend on the site of involvement, the severity of the attack, and the stage at which the child is first examined. The Jones criteria, which divides signs and symptoms into major and minor characteristics of the disease, is used when assessing the child with suspected RF.

   a. **Major characteristics** include carditis, polyarthritis, chorea, erythema marginatum, and subcutaneous nodules.

   (1) **Carditis** signs include tachycardia (higher than would be expected for fever), cardiomegaly, murmur, muffled heart sounds, precordial friction rub, precordial pain, and a prolonged PR interval. Carditis can lead to CHF, pericardial friction rubs, cardiomegaly, and aortic or mitral valve regurgitation. This is the most serious problem.

   (2) **Polyarthritis** consists of swollen, hot, painful joints (usually large joints). Polyarthritis is the most common presenting symptom and it occurs in about 75% of all cases of RF.

   (3) **Chorea** (also called Sydenham chorea or St. Vitus dance) is demonstrated by sudden aimless, irregular movements of the extremities; involuntary facial grimaces; speech disturbances; emotional lability; muscle weakness; and movements that increase with stress and decreased with rest. It occurs in about 10% of all cases.

   (4) **Erythema marginatum** consists of clear-centered, transitory, nonpruritic, macules, with defined borders. They are noted mostly on the trunk and proximal extremities. This occurs in about 5% of all cases.

   (5) **Subcutaneous nodules** are nontender lesions that may persist, then resolve. They are located over bony prominences. These rarely occur in RF.

   b. **Minor characteristics** include fever, arthralgia, and specific laboratory findings (see below).

2. Laboratory and diagnostic study findings

   a. Laboratory findings consistent with the Jones criteria include:

   (1) Erythrocyte sedimentation rate (ESR) is elevated.

(2) C-reactive protein (CRP) is elevated.

(3) Acute-phase reactants (rising antistreptolysin-O [ASLO, ASO]) **titer,** demonstrated by at least two tests, is elevated (elevations of > 333 Todd units indicate recent streptococcus infection in children).

b. CBC will reveal transient anemia and elevated white blood count (WBC).

c. Throat culture findings may be positive for streptococcal infection.

d. Chest radiography studies may disclose cardiac enlargement.

e. ECG may reveal a prolonged PR interval.

E. Nursing management

1. Assess and monitor cardiac, joint, skin, and neurologic status.

a. Note and report any changes.

b. Monitor for signs of CHF and provide interventions as appropriate.

2. Promote compliance with bed rest and activity restrictions.

a. Plan low-activity diversions, but allow the child some autonomy in selecting from among appropriate activities.

b. Inform the child and family that although she may feel well, the body has not yet healed adequately.

3. Promote rest by organizing nursing care to allow for adequate rest periods.

4. Alleviate discomfort of fever and arthralgia.

a. Administer prescribed medications.

b. Use alternative pain relief methods, such as relaxation and meditation when appropriate.

c. Use bed cradles and soft linens to decrease pressure on joints.

d. Be careful and supportive when moving affected joints. Manipulation, heat, cold, and massage may aggravate joint pain.

5. Prevent skin breakdown by providing good skin care and by protecting bony prominences.

6. Promote adequate nutrition. Provide a diet rich in protein and adequate calories.

7. Promote optimal growth and development.

8. Provide child and family teaching. Topics to cover include:

a. The disease and its treatment (stress that chorea is self-limiting)

b. The relationship of exercise to cardiac workload

c. Rationales, side effects, and dosages of prescribed medications; for example:

(1) Child may receive monthly injections of benzathine penicillin (1.2 million U), two daily oral doses of penicillin (200,000 U), or one daily dose of sulfadiazine (1 g) to prevent recurrent streptococcal infections (duration of long-term prophylaxis is uncertain).

(2) Due to the risk of bacterial endocarditis, prophylaxis is used as discussed in the general nursing implementation section.

(3) Aspirin and corticosteroids may be used to minimize inflammation. Side effects of aspirin therapy include gastrointestinal (GI) disturbance, decreased platelet count, tinnitus, and headaches. Side effects of steroidal therapy include fluid retention, edema, hypokalemia, GI irritation, hyperglycemia, altered growth patterns, and Cushing syndrome.

(4) Digoxin may be added to therapy to slow the heart rate and strengthen myocardial contractility. The child should be monitored for signs of toxicity (Table 14-3).

d. How to promote compliance with bed rest

e. Psychological and physical preparation for procedures

f. Minimizing contact with infected persons and importance of handwashing

TABLE 14-3
Selected Clinical Signs of Digitalis Toxicity in Children

AGE	HEART RATE	DRUG BLOOD LEVEL
Newborn	<100 beats/min	>2 ng/mL
Infants: 1 month to 1 year	<100 beats/min	>2 ng/mL
Infants: >1 year	<100 beats/min	>2 ng/mL
Young children	<80 beats/min	>2 ng/mL
Older children	<60 beats/min	>2 ng/mL

Toxicity can occur at therapeutic levels, especially in chronic users. Poor renal function, amiodarone (Cordarone), and quinidine increase digoxin level.

    g. Recognizing signs of recurrent streptococcal infection and promptly seeking medical attention for a sore throat

9. Promote prevention of RF by encouraging proper evaluation and treatment of streptococcal infections.

STUDY QUESTIONS

1. Which of the following disorders leads to cyanosis from deoxygenated blood entering the systemic arterial circulation?
   (1) Patent ductus arteriosus
   (2) Tetralogy of Fallot
   (3) Coarctation of the aorta
   (4) Aortic stenosis

2. While assessing a child with coarctation of the aorta, the nurse would expect to find which of the following?
   (1) Absent or diminished femoral pulses
   (2) Cyanotic ("tet") episodes
   (3) Squatting posture
   (4) Severe cyanosis at birth

3. Which of the following nursing interventions would be appropriate to promote optimal nutrition in an infant with congestive heart failure?
   (1) Offering formula that is high in sodium and calories
   (2) Providing large feedings evenly spaced every 4 hours
   (3) Replacing regular nipples with easy-to-suck ones
   (4) Allowing the infant to feed for at least 1 hour

4. When developing a teaching plan for the parents of a child with pulmonic stenosis, the nurse would keep in mind that this disorder involves which of the following?
   (1) Return of blood to the heart without entry into the left atrium
   (2) Obstruction of blood flow from the right ventricle
   (3) Obstruction of blood from the left ventricle
   (4) A single vessel arising from both ventricles

5. Which of the following represents an effective nursing intervention to reduce cardiac demands and decrease cardiac workload?
   (1) Scheduling care to provide for uninterrupted rest periods
   (2) Developing and implementing a consistent plan of care

   (3) Feeding the infant over long periods of time
   (4) Allowing the infant to have her way to avoid conflict

6. Which of the following are defects associated with tetralogy of Fallot?
   (1) Coarctation of the aorta, aortic valve stenosis, mitral valve stenosis, and patent ductus arteriosus
   (2) Ventricular septal defect, overriding aorta, pulmonic stenosis, and right ventricular hypertrophy
   (3) Tricuspid valve atresia, atrial septal defect, ventricular septal defect, and hypoplastic right ventricle
   (4) Aorta exits from the right ventricle, pulmonary artery exits from the left ventricle, and two noncommunicating circulations

7. Which of the following would the nurse expect to see as a cardinal sign of digoxin toxicity in a child with congestive heart failure who is receiving digoxin?
   (1) Respiratory distress
   (2) Extreme bradycardia
   (3) Constipation
   (4) Headache

8. Which of the following indicates that a child with CHF is carefully following the prescribed medical regimen?
   (1) Elevation in red blood cell (RBC) count
   (2) Normal weight for age
   (3) Pulse rate below 50 beats/min
   (4) Use of daily antibiotics

9. Which of the following instructions would the nurse include in a teaching plan that focuses on initial prevention of rheumatic fever (RF)?
   (1) Using corticosteroids to reduce inflammation
   (2) Treating streptococcal throat infections with antibiotics
   (3) Providing antibiotics before dental work
   (4) Giving penicillin to patients with RF

10. Which of the following statements by the parents of a child with Sydenham chorea would indicate the need for additional teaching?

(1) "The disorder is progressive and untreatable."

(2) "We should look for involuntary movements."

(3) "This disorder is a symptom of RF."

(4) "The condition worsens with stress."

ANSWER KEY

1. The answer is (2). Tetralogy of Fallot consists of four major anomalies: ventricular septal defect, right ventricular hypertrophy, pulmonic stenosis, aorta overriding the ventricular septal defect. Pulmonic stenosis impedes the flow of blood to the lungs, causing increased pressure in the right ventricle, forcing deoxygenated blood through the septal defect to the left ventricle. As a result of this decreased pulmonary blood flow, unoxygenated blood is shunted into the systemic circulation. The increased workload on the right ventricle causes hypertrophy. The overriding aorta receives blood from both right and left ventricles. This is the definition of defect with decreased pulmonary blood flow where unoxygenated blood is shunted into the systemic circulation. Tetralogy of Fallot is the only one in this category. With patent ductus arteriosus, blood flows from the aorta through the patent ductus arteriosus and back to the pulmonary artery and lungs (shunting of oxygenated blood to the pulmonary system), causing increased left ventricular workload and increased pulmonary vascular congestion. Coarctation of the aorta and aortic stenosis are obstructive defects where obstruction, not shunting, is the problem.

2. The answer is (1). Absent or diminished femoral pulse is a classic characteristic of coarctation of the aorta. Tet episodes and squatting are characteristic of tetralogy of Fallot. Severe cyanosis at birth is seen in defects such as transposition of the great vessels.

3. The answer is (3). Because the infant may tire easily with regular nipples and thus would not be able to suck adequately, the nurse should replace regular nipples with easy-to-suck ones. Typically, the infant receives a low-sodium, high-calorie diet. Also to prevent tiring, small frequent feedings lasting no more than 45 minutes, rather than large evenly spaced feedings or ones lasting longer than 1 hour, should be given.

4. The answer is (2). Pulmonic stenosis refers to an obstruction of blood flow from the right ventricle. Total anomalous pulmonary venous communications involve the return of blood to the heart without entry into the left atrium and obstruction of blood flow from the left ventricle. Truncus arteriosus involves a single vessel arising from both ventricles.

5. The answer is (1). Organizing nursing care to provide for uninterrupted periods of sleep reduces cardiac demands. Developing a consistent plan of care can be important, but it is not related to decreasing cardiac demands or workload. Feeding time should be restricted to a maximum of 45 minutes or discontinued sooner if the infant tires. In an attempt to get her own way, the child may cry. Excessive crying should be limited; however, appropriate limit setting should still be observed.

6. The answer is (2). The defects associated with tetralogy of Fallot include ventricular septal defect, overriding aorta, pulmonic stenosis, and right ventricular hypertrophy. Coarctation of the aorta and aortic and mitral valve stenosis are defects associated with triscuspid atresia. Severe coarctation of the aorta, severe aortic valvular stenosis or atresia, and severe mitral valve stenosis or atresia are defects associated with hypoplastic left heart syndrome. Also, the left ventricle, aortic valve, mitral valve, and ascending aorta usually are small or hypoplastic. The aorta exiting from the right ventricle and the pulmonary artery exiting from the left ventricle with no communication between the systemic and pulmonary circulations describes the defects associated with transposition of the great vessels.

7. The answer is (2). Extreme bradycardia is a cardinal symptom of digoxin toxicity. Respiratory distress, constipation, and headache are not related to digoxin toxicity.

8. The answer is (2). Adequate weight for height demonstrates adequate nutritional intake and lack of edema. An elevated RBC count demonstrates polycythemia. A pulse rate below 50, bradycardia, probably indicates digoxin toxicity. Daily antibiotics are not indicated in congestive heart failure.

9. The answer is (2). Rheumatic fever results from improperly treated group A β-hemolytic streptococcal infections, usually pharyngitis. Therefore, prompt treatment of streptococcal throat infections with antibiotics is a key preventative measure. Corticosteroids may be used to decrease inflammation but these agents are used during treatment of rheumatic fever, not as a preventive measure. Prophylactic antibiotics are given to children with cardiac disease to prevent carditis, not rheumatic fever. Initial prevention is not possible once the child has rheumatic fever. However, the child will be treated with penicillin to prevent a recurrence of streptococcal infections.

10. The answer is (1). Sydenham chorea or St. Vitus dance is a self-limiting problem that resolves with treatment of rheumatic fever. One of the major clinical manifestations of rheumatic fever, Sydenham chorea, is demonstrated by sudden aimless, irregular movements of the extremities; involuntary facial grimaces; speech disturbances; emotional lability; muscle weakness; and movements that increase with stress and decrease with rest. It occurs in about 10% of all cases.

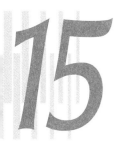

Genitourinary Dysfunction

I. Structure and function of the genitourinary (GU) system

A. Structure. The GU system is composed of the kidneys, ureters, bladder, and urethra. Development of the GU system is outlined in Table 15-1.

B. Function

1. The kidney's functional unit, the **nephron**, is composed of:
   a. **Glomeruli**, which filter water and solutes from the blood
   b. **Tubules**, which reabsorb needed substances (eg, water, protein, electrolytes, glucose, and amino acids) from filtrate and allow unneeded substances to leave the body in urine

2. Kidney functions include:
   a. **Regulating acid excretion** by renal excretion of acid that is bound to chemical buffers. Acid (H^+) is secreted by the renal tubular cells into the filtrate (fluid filtered through the walls of the glomerular capillary tufts) where it is buffered mostly by phosphate ions and ammonia.
   b. **Regulating electrolyte excretion**
      (1) Sodium. Most sodium chloride is reabsorbed by the kidneys. Water from filtrate follows the reabsorbed sodium to maintain osmotic balance. The remaining water and electrolytes are excreted in the urine. The regulation of sodium excretion depends on aldosterone, a hormone released by the adrenal cortex. If the blood aldosterone level is increased, less sodium is excreted because aldosterone fosters sodium reabsorption.
      (2) Potassium. Increased levels of blood aldosterone increase potassium excretion. Potassium retention is the most life-threatening effect of renal failure.
   c. **Regulating water excretion**
      (1) Osmolality. Osmolality reflects the number of particles dissolved in the urine; thus, it is the relative degree of dilution or concentration of the urine. As filtrate passes through the system, osmolality may vary from 50 to 1200 mOsm/L, reflecting the diluting and concentrating power of the kidneys.
      (2) Antidiuretic hormone (ADH). In the tubule, the varying amount of water that is reabsorbed in relation to electrolyte reabsorption regulates water excretion and urine concentration. ADH, secreted by the posterior part of the pituitary, controls the amount of water that is reabsorbed.
   d. **Production of hormones**
      (1) Renin helps regulate blood pressure.
      (2) Erythropoietin stimulates red blood cell production of bone marrow.

TABLE 15-1
Development of the Genitourinary System

AGE	STRUCTURE AND FUNCTION
Fetal development	Kidney development begins during the first few weeks of gestation but is not complete until the end of the first year after birth.
Infant (0–1 year)	Renal structures are present at birth. The bladder lies close to the abdominal wall, and the ureters are relatively short. The tubules reach adult-like proportions in size and shape by 5 months of age. Infants are unable to excrete water at the same rate as older children and adults. Renal function is not mature; thus, the child is unable to handle increased intake of protein. Sodium excretion is also reduced during infancy, and the kidneys are less adaptable to sodium deficiency or excess.
Toddler/Preschooler (1–6 years)	The bladder descends into the pelvis by 3 years of age. Renal function is mature as glomerular filtration and absorption reach adult capabilities between 1 and 2 years of age. However, under stress, water is conserved and urine is concentrated at an adult level.
Schoolager (6–12 years)	Bladder capacity increases, especially in girls. The kidneys double in size to accommodate increased metabolic functions between 5 and 10 years of age. Fluid and electrolyte balance becomes stable. Specific gravity and renal and urinary components are similar to those of the adult. However, some schoolagers have small amounts of albuminuria.
Adolescent (12–21 years)	Renal function is the same as an adult. Bladder capacity increases, and the adolescent voids up to 1500 mL daily.

(3) Metabolization of vitamin D to its active form is important in calcium metabolism.

3. Urine is formed in the nephron, then passes into the renal pelvis, through the ureter, into the bladder, and out of the body through the urethra.

II. NURSING PROCESS OVERVIEW FOR
The GU System

A. Assessment

1. **Health history**

    a. Elicit a description of symptoms including onset, duration, location, and precipitation. **Cardinal signs** may include:

    (1) Neonate signs include poor feeding, failure-to-thrive (FTT), frequent urination, crying on urination, dehydration, convulsions, and fever.

    (2) Infant signs include those seen in the neonate, plus persistent diaper rash, foul-smelling urine, and straining on urination.

    (3) Older children signs include poor appetite, vomiting, excessive thirst, enuresis, incontinence, frequent urination, urgency, dysuria, bloody urine, foul-smelling urine, fatigue, fever, and flank, abdominal, or back pain.

    b. Explore prenatal, personal, and family history for **risk factors** for GU disorders:

    (1) Prenatal risk factors include young maternal age, older maternal age, and multiparity.

    (2) Personal risk factors include recurring, afebrile urinary tract infections, indwelling catheter, incomplete toilet training, urinary retention, constipation,

diabetes, immunosuppression, increased sexual activity, and repeated strepto-coccal infections.

(3) Family risk factors include congenital or acquired renal disease, hypertension, and other problems related to renal dysfunction.

2. Physical examination

a. **Vital signs**

(1) Measure and plot height and weight for signs of growth retardation.

(2) Monitor temperature for hyperthermia.

(3) Monitor blood pressure for hypertension or hypotension.

(4) Monitor respiratory rate observing for abnormal rate and depth of respiration.

b. **Inspection**

(1) Observe for signs of circulatory congestion, including peripheral cyanosis, slow capillary refill time, pallor, and peripheral edema.

(2) Observe for abdominal distention.

(3) Observe for early signs of uremic encephalopathy, including lethargy, poor concentration, and confusion.

(4) Observe for signs of congenital anomalies, such as hypospadias, epispadias, ear abnormalities (ears and kidneys form at the same time in utero), prominent epicanthal folds, beaklike nose, and a small chin.

c. **Palpation**

(1) Palpate the kidneys for tenderness and enlargement.

(2) Palpate the bladder for distention.

3. Laboratory studies and diagnostic tests (see Appendices A and B for normal find-ings and nursing considerations).

a. **Urinalysis** is the most valuable laboratory test for determining renal function.

b. **Urine culture and sensitivity** determines the presence of bacterial pathogens. It demonstrates the type of pathogen, the colony count, and the effectiveness of var-ious antibiotics that will inhibit bacterial growth.

c. **Blood urea nitrogen (BUN)** represents a gross index of glomerular filtration rate; impaired renal function and rapid protein catabolism result in elevated BUN levels.

d. **Creatinine** is a by-product of energy metabolism. As long as muscle mass remains constant, creatinine levels are constant; renal disorders reducing creatinine excre-tion result in increased serum creatinine levels. Creatinine generally is a more sen-sitive indicator of acute renal failure than is BUN.

e. **Ultrasonography** is a nonradiographic, noninvasive examination of the urinary tract using ultrasonic technology.

f. **Voiding cystourethrography (VCU)** consists of serial x-rays of the bladder and urethra after intravesicular infusion of an iodine-bound contrast medium.

g. **Computed tomography (CT) scan** is a computerized calculation used to visual-ize horizontal or vertical cross sections of the kidney to determine the nature of tis-sue material. Iodine contrast may be used to enhance the image.

h. **Intravenous pyelography (IVP)** is the intravenous injection of a radiopaque con-trast medium followed by x-ray imaging of the kidneys and ureters as the contrast agent passes through.

i. **Cystoscopy** is the evaluation of the urinary tract using direct visualization via a metal tube or flexible sheath and fiberoptic technology.

j. **Renal biopsy** is the removal of renal tissue to obtain histologic and microscopic information. It can help distinguish types of nephrotic syndrome.

k. **Renal scan (radioisotope renogram)** involves the injection of radioactive mate-rial to allow visualization of kidney structures and function through serial films. **Dimercaptosuccinic acid (DMSA)** defines the parenchymal tissue and outlines defects in the cortex. **Diethylenetriamine acid (DTPA)** is used to evaluate renal function.

    l. **Urodynamics** is a series of tests that evaluates bladder and urethral function and innervation.

B. Nursing diagnoses

1. Risk for altered body temperature
2. Fatigue
3. Fluid volume excess
4. Altered growth and development
5. Hyperthermia
6. Incontinence
7. Risk for infection
8. Altered nutrition: less than body requirements
9. Pain
10. Risk for impaired skin integrity
11. Altered urinary elimination
12. urinary retention
13. Altered tissue perfusion (renal)
14. Anxiety

C. Planning and outcome identification

1. The child will maintain a fluid intake that approximates fluid output. The manifestations of altered urinary output are recognized early, and the child excretes 0.5 to 2.0 mL/kg/hour.
2. The child will not exhibit manifestations of fluid retention, or these manifestations are promptly recognized and treated.
3. The child will achieve and maintain a desired nutritional intake.
4. The child will not develop infection.
5. The child will not deviate from developmental norms due to illness.

D. Implementation

1. **Prevent altered urinary output**.
   a. Measure and record fluid intake, including oral and intravenous fluids and fluid output.
   b. Obtain daily weights.
   c. Encourage fluids (up to 1000 mL/day in older children) to dilute and remove endotoxins and debris. Water is the best fluid, but the child can have juice, soup, milk, gelatin, and ice pops. Chocolate and other caffeinated beverages should be avoided because they are bladder irritants. The benefits of cranberry juice have not been statistically supported; however, it can still be encouraged.
   d. Monitor for manifestations of dehydration, including poor skin turgor, dry mucous membranes, sunken fontanelle (infants), decreased output, and decreased perfusion.

2. **Prevent fluid overload**.
   a. Monitor fluid intake and output (I&O) and daily weight.
   b. Measure blood pressure because hypertension may result from fluid overload.
   c. Assess respiratory status, including tachypnea, retractions, and rales, because children with fluid excess can develop pulmonary edema.
   d. Limit fluid intake as ordered.
   e. Offer low-sodium diet if ordered.

3. **Promote desired nutritional intake**.
   a. Monitor daily weights and food intake.

b. Allow parents to bring foods from home, if these foods comply with dietary orders.

c. Offer small, frequent meals of preferred foods in a pleasant atmosphere to make mealtime pleasurable.

d. Consult with a nutritionist.

4. Prevent infection.

a. Use a good handwashing technique and instruct child and family on these techniques.

b. Instruct family to keep child away from persons with upper respiratory and other communicable infections.

c. Maintain adequate nutrition and rest.

d. Monitor the child for signs of infection.

e. Use proper technique for procedures, such as catheterization and dressing changes, to prevent infection.

f. Teach the family how to prevent urinary tract infections (UTIs). See Child and Family Teaching 15-1.

5. Promote normal growth and development.

a. **Infants.** After threatening procedures, the infant needs comforting and acceptance by family members to promote the development of a positive body image.

b. **Toddlers.** Problems of immobilization frustrate the toddler's drive for independence. Allowing the toddler to participate in care, as appropriate, may be helpful.

c. **Preschoolers.** Body image awareness is heightened, and the child's natural curiosity about the body may be stimulated by physical examinations. The child's rich fantasy life can contribute to fear of the simplest procedures; castration fears also are prominent at this age and may be heightened by procedures related to GU problems.

d. **Schoolagers.** Appearing different from peers is extremely anxiety producing, as are prohibitions on diet, sports, and other activities that focus on the child's differences from peers.

e. **Adolescents.** Because of the increased need for independence by adolescents, the enforced dependence imposed by rigorous therapeutic regimens can increase feelings of resentment and rebelliousness. Body image and sexuality concerns may also be heightened because of GU diagnoses, procedures, and treatment.

E. Outcome evaluation

1. The child has adequate urine output for age.

2. The child has no signs of fluid retention.

3. The child reaches and maintains preillness weight.

CHILD AND FAMILY TEACHING 15-1

Prevention of Urinary Tract Infections

- Provide good perineal hygiene (eg, cleaning a girl from the urethra back toward the anus).
- Avoid using irritants such as bubble bath and tight clothing.
- Wear cotton underwear instead of synthetics such as nylon.
- Maintain adequate fluid intake.
- Void regularly and completely empty the bladder with each urination.
- Maintain acidic urine by drinking beverages such as cranberry juice.
- Emphasize the importance of voiding both before and after sexual intercourse (for the sexually active adolescent).

4. The child shows no signs of infection (ie, maintains normal temperature and laboratory values and demonstrates no infectious manifestations).

5. The child does not deviate from developmental norms.

III.   Urinary tract infections (UTIs)

A. Description

1. UTIs are characterized by inflammation, usually of bacterial origin, of the urethra (urethritis), bladder (cystitis), ureters (ureteritis), or kidneys (pyelonephritis).

2. Peak incidence occurs between 2 and 6 years of age, with increased incidence also noted in adolescents who are sexually active.

3. Girls have a 10 to 30 times greater risk of developing UTIs than boys (except in neonates) because of their shorter urethral structure, which provides a quick pathway for organisms.

4. The recurrence rate in neonates is 25%; in older children, it is 30%.

B. Etiology

1. The gram-negative bacteria, *Escherichia coli,* accounts for 80% of all UTIs. The remaining 20% are caused by other gram-negative bacteria, such as *Proteus, Pseudomonas, Klebsiella, Haemophilus,* and coagulase-negative staphylococcus, and the gram-positive bacteria, *Staphylococcus aureus.*

2. In the neonate, the urinary tract may be infected via the bloodstream.

3. In older children, bacteria ascend the urethra, creating an increased incidence in girls. Contributing factors include:

a. Urinary stasis (the single most important host factor)

b. Urinary reflux

c. Inadequate fluid intake

d. Poor perineal hygiene

e. Constipation

f. Pregnancy

g. Noncircumcision

h. Indwelling catheter placement

i. Antimicrobial agents that alter normal urinary tract flora

j. Tight clothes or diapers

k. Local inflammation (eg, from vaginitis), which increases the risk of ascending infection

l. Sexual intercourse; improper use of diaphragm

m. Bubble bath

C. Pathophysiology

1. In an **uncomplicated UTI**, inflammation usually is confined to the lower urinary tract. Recurrent cystitis, however, may produce anatomic changes in the ureter that lead to vesicoureteral valve incompetence and resultant urine reflux. This provides organisms with access to the upper urinary tract.

2. **Pyelonephritis** usually results from an ascending infection from the lower urinary tract. It can lead to acute and chronic inflammatory changes in the pelvis and medulla, with scarring and loss of renal tissue.

3. **Recurrent or chronic infection** results in increased fibrotic tissue and kidney contraction.

D. Assessment findings. Characteristics vary with age and location of infection. About 40% of UTIs are asymptomatic.

   1. Clinical manifestations

   a. Infants may exhibit irritability, constant squirming, fever or hypothermia, jaundice, weight loss, FTT, vomiting and diarrhea, diaper rash, and an abnormal urinary stream.

   b. Older children exhibit manifestations according to where the infection is located.

   (1) Foul-smelling urine, hematuria (possibly), dysuria, increased frequency, increased urgency, incontinence, and abdominal pain are seen with lower UTIs.

   (2) Fever, costovertebral abdominal (CVA) tenderness, chills, and flank pain are seen with pyelonephritis.

   2. Laboratory and diagnostic study findings

   a. Urinalysis may disclose hematuria, proteinuria, and pyuria. Urine may have a foul odor and appear cloudy with strands of mucus.

   b. Urine culture is used to confirm diagnosis through detection of bacteria in urine culture. Suprapubic taps and catheterization are frequently performed in infants and young children. Follow-up cultures are needed, and many children warrant further studies to rule out structural abnormalities.

   c. Ureteral catheterization, bladder washout procedures, and radioisotope renography may be needed to localize the infection.

   d. Renal ultrasound, IVP, VCU, and DSMA pyelogram may be performed after the infection subsides to rule out structural abnormalities. All children under 5 years of age should have a renal ultrasound, a VCU, and, if necessary, an IVP to rule out underlying pathology, such as vesicoureteral reflux (VUR).

E. Nursing management

   1. Assess urinary status.

   a. Assess the appearance and odor of urine.

   b. Note signs and symptoms such as frequency, burning, enuresis, urinary retention, or flank pain.

   2. Administer prescribed antibiotics (Drug Chart 15-1).

   3. Prevent infection.

   4. Provide comfort measures.

   a. Promote rest.

   b. Administer analgesics as needed and antipyretics as prescribed.

   c. Encourage increased fluid intake to reduce fever and dilute urine.

   d. Tub baths, sitz baths, and perineal rinses can provide relief from dysuria.

   5. Provide child and family teaching.

   a. Provide medication instructions, including dosage, administration, and side effects.

   b. Explain the need for surgical correction of anatomic abnormalities, if necessary, to prevent recurrent disease.

   c. Discuss the need for performing follow-up cultures. These will be typically scheduled at monthly intervals for 3 months, and then at 3-month intervals for 6 months.

   d. Detail preventive measures to avoid reinfection (see Child and Family Teaching 15-1).

DRUG CHART 15-1   Antibiotics Used for Urinary Tract Infections

Classification	Used for	Selected Interventions
Penicillin	Susceptible gram-negative and gram-positive bacteria.	*For all classifications:*
Sulfonamides (including the trimethoprim and sulfisoxazole combination [Bactrim, Septra])		Assess child for medication allergies and kidney dysfunction.
Cephalosporins		Obtain urine culture before beginning antibiotic therapy.
Nitrofurantoin (Macrodantin)		Increase fluid intake.
		Monitor for, and report, stomach upset, diarrhea, signs of superinfections, rash, unusual bleeding or bruising, and difficulty breathing.
		For specific classifications:
		Administer oral form of cephalosporins, sulfonamides, and nitrofurantoin with food to minimize gastrointestinal upset.
		Use sunscreen and protective clothing when taking sulfonamides.
		Sulfonamides may turn urine yellow-orange.

 Enuresis

A. Definition

1. Enuresis is the repeated involuntary (usually nocturnal) urination in a child who should have already established bladder control (usually by 4 or 5 years of age).
2. Primary enuresis is the term used for wetting that occurs in children who have never attained dryness.
3. Secondary enuresis is the term used for wetting that occurs in children who have attained urinary continence.
4. The incidence at 5 years of age is about 7% for boys and 3% for girls.

B. Etiology

1. No clear etiology has been established.
2. Predictive factors include longer duration of sleep during infancy, a positive family history, and a slower rate of physical development in children up to 3 years of age.
3. Enuresis may have a genetic component. About 75% of all children with enuresis have a first-degree relative who has or had the disorder.

C. Pathophysiology. Enuresis is primarily a problem of delayed or incomplete neuromuscular maturation of the bladder. The condition is benign and self-limiting.

D. Assessment findings

1. **Associated findings**. A complete physical and psychosocial evaluation is performed to rule out pathology such as urinary tract infections, sickle cell anemia, neurologic deficits, diabetes, and psychogenic problems.

2. Clinical manifestations
  a. Nocturnal bed wetting
  b. Urinary urgency, dysuria, restlessness, and possible frequency
3. Laboratory and diagnostic study findings
  a. Urinalysis may be performed to rule out UTI and diabetes.
  b. Sickle cell test may be performed to rule out sickle cell anemia.
E. Nursing management
  1. Promote dryness.
    a. Assist with therapeutic treatment plan, which may include:
      (1) Conditioning training, which involves having child awaken to urinate after a stimulus (typically an alarm) is used
      (2) Retention control training (RCT), whereby child drinks fluids and delays urination as long as tolerated to stretch the bladder for the purpose of accommodating larger amounts of urine
      (3) The waking schedule treatment, which is used to encourage the child to awaken at intervals to void
      (4) Medication therapy, which is being used with greater frequency
        (a) Imipramine (Tofranil) has an anticholinergic effect on the bladder.
        (b) Desmopressin (DDAVP) nasal spray reduces nighttime urine output.
  2. Promote a healthy self-esteem.
    a. Provide emotional support.
    b. Encourage parents and other caretakers to accept the child's problem and to avoid placing blame or adopting attitudes that may foster feelings of worthlessness and hopelessness in the child.

 Vesicoureteral reflux (VUR)

A. Description
  1. VUR is characterized by the backward flow of urine in the urinary tract when voiding.
  2. The prevalence of VUR in healthy children is estimated at less than 1%; however, it is found in 29% to 50% of children following UTIs and is the most common radiographic abnormality associated with UTIs in children.
  3. Between 30% and 60% of children with VUR have renal scarring and most reflux associated renal scarring occurs at a very young age. Few develop scarring after 5 to 6 years of age.
B. Etiology
  1. Genetics may play a role in the development of VUR; siblings are 10 times more likely to develop it than other children.
  2. Primary reflux results from congenital abnormalities in insertion of ureters into the bladder.
  3. Secondary reflux results from infection and ureterovesicular junction incompetency related to edema; it may also be related to neurogenic bladder or result from progressive dilation of ureters following surgical urinary diversion.
C. Pathophysiology
  1. VUR occurs when urine flows from the bladder back into the ureters and the renal pelvis, usually a result of an incompetent valvular mechanism at the ureterovesicular junction.
  2. VUR is graded according to the degree of reflux.
    a. Grade I is characterized by reflux into the lower ureter only.

    b. Grade II is characterized by ureteral and pelvic filling without calyceal dilation.

    c. Grade III is characterized by ureteral and pelvic filling with mild calyceal dilation.

    d. Grade IV is characterized by marked distention of pelvis, calyces, and ureter.

    e. Grade V is characterized by massive reflux associated with severe hydronephrosis.

  3. VUR is a major cause of renal damage; refluxed urine ascending into the collecting tubules of nephrons gives microorganisms access to the renal parenchyma, initiating renal scarring.

  4. If the amount of refluxed urine is large, the child feels an urge to void shortly after having voided. If the amount is small, it may remain in the bladder, causing urinary stasis and predisposing the child to infection.

D. Assessment findings

  1. Clinical manifestations

    a. Dysuria

    b. Urinary frequency, urgency, and hesitancy

    c. Urine retention

    d. Cloudy, dark, or blood-tinged urine

  2. Laboratory and diagnostic study findings

    a. Urinalysis may reveal red blood cells or pyuria.

    b. IVP, voiding cystourethrography, and cystoscopy may detect structural abnormalities.

E. Nursing management

  1. Administer or teach parents to administer **prescribed medications**, such as continuous low-dose antibiotics. In most cases, a continuous low-dose antibacterial therapy is effective. There is an 80% chance of remission for grades I and II VUR.

  2. Prevent altered urinary output. Assist the child in the development of a regular (3-hour) voiding plan.

  3. Prevent and relieve constipation with a high-fiber diet to facilitate muscular relaxation, thereby helping to reduce residual urine.

  4. Provide support to the family by answering questions and providing information about diagnosis, tests, and treatments.

    a. Explain that antireflux surgery, involving reimplantation of ureters, is indicated when necessary to prevent renal damage secondary to recurrent infections. Surgical correction may be needed for grades IV and V; grade III is managed nonoperatively unless there are complications. Major indications for surgery include:

      (1) Significant abnormality at the ureterovesicular junction

      (2) Recurrent UTIs

      (3) The higher grade VURs

      (4) Noncompliance with medical therapy

      (5) VUR after puberty in girls

  5. Provide preoperative and postoperative care after antireflux surgery:

    a. Monitor quantity and quality of urine output.

    b. Observe and protect urinary drainage tubes (eg, indwelling catheter, suprapubic catheter, and ureteral stents).

    c. Administer analgesics for pain and antispasmodics for bladder spasms, as prescribed.

    d. Provide routine postoperative care (eg, dressing changes, vital signs monitoring, progressive diet, and ambulation).

  6. Provide child and family teaching on prevention of UTIs (see Child and Family Teaching 15-1).

Nephrotic syndrome

A. Description

1. Nephrotic syndrome is a symptom complex characterized by proteinuria, hypoalbuminemia, hyperlipidemia, altered immunity, and edema; it is of idiopathic origin 95% of the time.
2. Prognosis usually is good for the most common type of nephrotic syndrome, minimal change nephrotic syndrome (MCNS), which is self-limiting and usually responds to steroidal therapy.
3. MCNS accounts for 80% of all cases in children between 2 and 6 years old, and it is more common in boys than girls.

B. Etiology

1. **MCNS** is idiopathic in origin. A nonspecific illness, typically a viral upper respiratory tract infection, frequently precedes clinical manifestations by 4 to 8 days. However, this is considered a precipitating factor rather than a cause.
2. **Secondary nephrotic syndrome** usually occurs after glomerular damage of known or presumed etiology (eg, systemic lupus erythematosus, diabetes mellitus, or sickle cell disease).
3. **Congenital nephrotic syndrome** (Finnish type) is caused by an autosomal recessive gene. This rare disorder does not respond to usual therapy and the infant usually dies in the first or second year of life.

C. Pathophysiology

1. The pathogenesis in MCNS is not clear, but there is increased permeability to protein, exceeding 2 g/day. Proteins leak through the glomerular membrane resulting in protein, especially albumin, in the urine.
2. Once the albumin is lost, colloidal osmotic pressure decreases, permitting fluid to escape from the intravascular spaces to the interstitial spaces. The volume decrease stimulates ADH to reabsorb water.

D. Assessment findings

1. Clinical manifestations

a. Anorexia
b. Fatigue
c. Pallor
d. Diarrhea
e. Abdominal pain
f. Decreased urine output. Urine may become foamy or frothy.
g. Periorbital (typically the first sign), pedal and pretibial edema to generalized edema (anasarca), weight increase, ascites, and pleural effusion. Labial or scrotal swelling may also be noted. With marked edema, the child may appear pale and have respiratory distress.
h. Shiny skin with prominent veins
i. Normal or slightly decreased blood pressure
j. Increased susceptibility to infection, especially pneumonia, peritonitis, cellulitis, and septicemia; the child is susceptible to secondary infection because immunoglobulin is lost in the urine.

2. Laboratory and diagnostic study findings

a. Urinalysis shows marked proteinuria, hyaline casts, few red blood cells, and high urine specific gravity.

b. Serum protein level is markedly decreased, especially albumin level.

c. Serum cholesterol can be as high as 450 to 1500 mg/dL.

d. Hemoglobin and hematocrit are normal or elevated.

e. Platelet count is high (500,000–1,000,000).

f. Serum sodium concentration is low (130–135 mEq/L).

g. Renal biopsy may be performed to provide information on glomerular status and the type of nephrotic syndrome, as well as the response to medication and the course of the disease.

E. Nursing management

1. **Assess for fluid volume deficit** by monitoring for increased edema and by measuring abdominal girth, weight, I&O, blood pressure, and pulse rate. Test the urine for protein and specific gravity.

2. **Prevent infection and monitor for signs of infection.**

3. **Administer prescribed medications**, which may include:

   a. Corticosteroids may be used for children without hematuria. The medication is given until the urine remains free of protein for 10 to 14 days.

   b. An oral alkylating agent may be used to reduce the relapse rate and induce long-term remission.

   c. Loop diuretics in combination with metolazone can be used for children who have edema that interferes with respiration or children with hypotension, hyponatremia, or evidence of skin breakdown.

4. **Promote skin integrity** by checking areas of edema for skin breakdown, ensuring frequent position changes, using scrotal supports for boys, and providing good skin care.

5. **Promote a desired nutritional intake**

   a. Provide a high-protein, high-calorie diet without added salt.

   b. Fluid restriction may be necessary for children with severe edema.

6. **Conserve the child's energy** by enforcing bed rest and encouraging quiet activities.

7. **Help improve the child's self-concept** by providing positive feedback, emphasizing strengths, and encouraging social interaction and pursuit of interests.

8. **Support the family** by answering questions and providing information on diagnosis, tests, and treatment.

9. **Provide child and family teaching**.

   a. List the signs and symptoms of relapse to watch for and report.

   b. Demonstrate how to test urine for albumin.

   c. Discuss medication regime (ie, dosage schedule, administration techniques, and side effects).

   d. Explain special dietary instructions.

   e. Explain infection prevention measures.

   f. Promote proper skin care to avoid breakdown (eg, frequent position changes, daily baths, lotion for dry skin, elevation of edematous extremities with pillows, and physical activity as tolerated to promote circulation).

   g. Explain that immunization with initial live vaccines, but not boosters, may cause relapse. Live vaccines should be held until the child enters school.

   h. Explain that hospitalization is usually warranted for the first episode as well as specific problems such as pleural effusion.

Acute glomerulonephritis (AGN)

A. Description

1. A number of distinct entities are classified as AGN, which may be a primary event or a manifestation of a systemic disorder. Recovery occurs in about 95% of cases.
2. Acute poststreptococcal glomerulonephritis (APSGN) is the most common form. It can occur at any age but is usually seen in schoolagers, peaking at 6 to 7 years of age. APSGN occurs more commonly in boys than girls (2:1).

B. Etiology

1. Postinfectious AGN, an immune complex disease that results from immune injury, was once thought to be secondary to streptococcus. Now other organisms are involved, including pneumococci and viruses.
2. Most streptococcal infections do not cause AGN. When they do, a latent period of 10 to 14 days occurs between the infection, usually of the skin (impetigo) or upper respiratory tract, and the onset of clinical manifestations.

C. Pathophysiology

1. Antibodies interact with antigens that remain in the glomeruli, leading to immune complex formation and tissue injury, filtration decreases, and excretion of less sodium and water. High blood pressure, edema, and heart failure may result.
2. The major complications include hypertensive encephalopathy, acute cardiac decompensation, and acute renal failure.

D. Assessment findings

1. **Associated findings**. History of infection about 10 to 14 days before the onset of symptoms
2. **Clinical manifestations**
   a. Irritability, fatigue, and lethargy
   b. Anorexia
   c. Pallor
   d. High blood pressure
   e. Periorbital and generalized edema, weight gain, and electrolyte imbalance
   f. Oliguria and hematuria (urine is brown [cola or tea colored] and cloudy)
   g. Costovertebral tenderness
3. **Laboratory and diagnostic study findings**
   a. Urinalysis reveals red blood cells, casts, white blood cells, and protein. Diuresis indicates resolution; child usually recovers in 2 weeks.
   b. Serum chemistry values reveal elevated BUN and creatinine levels.
   c. Erythrocyte sedimentation rate (ESR) is elevated, and the antistreptolysin-O (ASO) titer is elevated if the child was exposed to streptococci.

E. Nursing management

1. **Assess fluid status** by monitoring I&O, taking and recording daily weights, and observing for edema.
2. **Ensure early detection of complications** by closely monitoring blood pressure and respiratory rate.
3. **Administer prescribed medications**.
   a. Antihypertensive medications, such as calcium channel blockers, β-blockers, or angiotensin-converting enzyme (ACE) blockers, may be needed in severe cases.

    b. Anticonvulsants are needed for seizure activity associated with hypertensive encephalopathy.

    c. Antibiotics are used for children with evidence of persistent streptococcal infection.

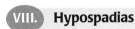**4. Promote desired nutritional intake.**

    a. Increase caloric intake to decrease protein breakdown, unless restricted. Impose sodium, potassium, or fluid restrictions, when prescribed.

    b. Dietary restrictions depend on the stage and severity. Normally, a regular diet is allowed, but sodium is limited (no added salt). Moderate sodium restriction is for children with hypertension or edema, and potassium-rich foods are limited during periods of oliguria. Protein is restricted only for those with severe azotemia.

5. Stimulate the child by providing quiet play activities.

6. Refer the child and family to a community health nurse for home visits, as needed, to help them adjust to home management.

7. Provide child and family teaching.

    a. Instruct about the need for medical evaluation and tissue culture of all sore throats.

    b. Discuss home care measures, including:

        (1) Urine testing

        (2) Blood pressure monitoring

        (3) Activity and diet instructions

        (4) Infection prevention measures

        (5) Signs and symptoms of potential complications to watch for and report (the child will require monthly urinalysis and blood pressure monitoring for 6 months and then every 3 to 6 months until she has been symptom free for 1 year)

    c. Explain all medications (ie, dosage, administration, and side effects).

    d. Discuss the possible need for peritoneal dialysis or hemodialysis if renal failure occurs.

VIII. Hypospadias

A. Description

1. Hypospadias is a condition in which the urethral opening is located below the glans penis or anywhere along the ventral surface (underside) of the penile shaft. The ventral foreskin is lacking, and the distal portion gives an appearance of a hood. In very mild cases, the meatus is just below the tip; in the most severe cases, the meatus is located on the perineum between the halves of the scrotum.

2. It occurs in approximately 1 of 500 male newborns and is the most common anomaly of the penis. Concurrent abnormalities include:

    a. Cryptorchidism (undescended testes)

    b. Chordee (ventral curve of the penis that results from the replacement of normal skin with a fibrotic band) usually accompanies more severe forms of hypospadias

    c. Inguinal hernias

B. Etiology

1. Genetic transmission is weakly correlated.

2. Exogenous factors include prenatal exposure to cocaine, alcohol, phenytoin, progestins, rubella, or gestational diabetes.

C. Pathophysiology

1. The abnormality results from a failure of the urethral folds to fuse completely over the urethral groove.

2. The abnormality can lead to infertility and psychological problems if unrepaired.

D. **Assessment findings**

 1. **Clinical manifestations.** Inappropriate location of urinary meatus should be evident at birth.
 2. **Diagnostic and laboratory study findings**. None, unless the presence of ambiguous genitalia needs to be ruled out or in cases when other abnormalities are suspected.

E. **Nursing management**

 1. **Inform the parents that early recognition is important so that circumcision is avoided**; the foreskin is used for the surgical repair.
 2. **Allow the parents to verbalize their feelings** about the child's structural problem.
 3. **Prepare the parents and child for the expected surgical procedures.** Surgical repair is performed to improve the child's ability to stand when urinating, to improve the appearance of the penis, and to preserve sexual adequacy. It is usually performed between 6 and 12 months of age with one- or two-stage repairs.
 4. **Explain expected cosmetic result**; the parents and child may feel great disappointment about this physical imperfection.
 5. **Monitor fluid I&O** and **urinary pattern, encourage fluids, maintain patency**, and **observe infection prevention measures if child is catheterized.**
 6. **Prepare parents and child for urinary diversion**, if necessary, while the new meatus is being constructed.
 7. **Teach parents how to care for an indwelling catheter**, if necessary.

STUDY QUESTIONS

1. When performing a procedure related to a genitourinary problem, the nurse would anticipate that which of the following age groups would find it especially stressful?
   (1) Infants
   (2) Toddlers
   (3) Preschoolers
   (4) Schoolagers

2. When developing a teaching plan for parents about contributing factors for urinary tract infections (UTIs), which of the following factors, if stated by the parents, would indicate the need for additional teaching?
   (1) Urinary stasis
   (2) Circumcision
   (3) Bubble baths
   (4) Indwelling catheters

3. Which of the following organisms is the most common cause of UTI in children?
   (1) *Staphylococcus*
   (2) *Klebsiella*
   (3) *Pseudomonas*
   (4) *Escherichia coli*

4. Which of the following would the nurse expect when assessing a child with cystitis?
   (1) High fever
   (2) Flank pain
   (3) Costovertebral tenderness
   (4) Dysuria

5. Which of the following instructions would be included in a sexually active adolescent's preventive teaching plan about UTIs?
   (1) Wiping back to front
   (2) Wearing nylon underwear
   (3) Avoiding urinating before intercourse
   (4) Drinking acidic juices

6. What is the most likely underlying pathophysiology of primary enuresis?

   (1) Urinary tract infection
   (2) Psychogenic stress
   (3) Vesicoureteral reflux
   (4) Delayed bladder maturation

7. Secondary vesicoureteral reflux (VUR) usually results from which of the following?
   (1) Congenital defects
   (2) Infection
   (3) Acidic urine
   (4) Hydronephrosis

8. Which of the following signs and symptoms are characteristic of minimal change nephrotic syndrome?
   (1) Gross hematuria, proteinuria, fever
   (2) Hypertension, edema, hematuria
   (3) Poor appetite, proteinuria, edema
   (4) Hypertension, edema, proteinuria

9. For a child with recurring nephrotic syndrome, which of the following areas of potential disturbances should be a prime consideration when planning ongoing nursing care?
   (1) Muscle coordination
   (2) Sexual maturation
   (3) Intellectual development
   (4) Body image

10. When teaching parents about known antecedent infections in acute glomerulonephritis, which of the following should the nurse cover?
    (1) Herpes simplex
    (2) Scabies
    (3) Varicella
    (4) Impetigo

11. Which of the following should be avoided if the child has hypospadias?
    (1) Circumcision
    (2) Catheterization
    (3) Surgery
    (4) Intravenous pyelography

ANSWER KEY

1. The answer is (3). In general, preschoolers have more fears in general because of their fantasies, contributing to fears of the simplest procedures. Castration fears also are prominent at this age and may be heightened by procedures related to GU problems. Typically, GU procedures do not create greater stress in the infant, toddler, and school-aged child age groups.

2. The answer is (2). Circumcision is not a contributing factor for the development of UTIs. However, children who are not circumcised have a greater risk for UTIs, especially if the area is not cleaned properly. Urinary stasis creates a medium for growth. Bubble baths cause irritation. Indwelling catheters provide an entry route for organisms.

3. The answer is (4). *Escherichia coli* is the most common organism associated with the development of UTI. Although *Staphylococcus, Klebsiella,* and *Pseudomonas* species may cause UTIs, the incidence of UTIs related to each is less than that for *E. coli.*

4. The answer is (4). Dysuria is a symptom of a lower UTI, such as cystitis. High fever, flank pain, and costovertebral tenderness are symptoms of pyelonephritis, an upper UTI.

5. The answer is (4). Drinking acidic juices, such as cranberry juice, helps keep the urine at its desired acid pH and decreases the chance of infection. The patient should wipe from front to back, wear cotton underwear, and void before and after intercourse.

6. The answer is (4). The most likely cause of primary enuresis is delayed or incomplete maturation of the bladder. UTIs may cause either primary or secondary enuresis, but they are not the leading cause of primary enuresis. Psychogenic stress may cause either primary or secondary enuresis, but it is not the leading cause of primary enuresis. Vesicoureteral reflux may cause either primary or secondary enuresis, but it is not the leading cause of primary enuresis.

7. The answer is (2). Infection is the most common cause of secondary VUR. Congenital defects cause primary VUR. Acidic urine is normal and helps to prevent infection. Hydronephrosis may result from VUR.

8. The answer is (3). Clinical manifestations of nephrotic syndrome include loss of appetite due to edema of intestinal mucosa, proteinuria, and edema. Gross hematuria is not associated with nephrotic syndrome. Fever would occur only if infection also existed. Hypertension alone or accompanied by hematuria is associated with glomerulonephritis.

9. The answer is (4). Because of the edema associated with nephrotic syndrome, potential self-concept and body image disturbances related to changes in appearance and social isolation should be considered. Muscle coordination, sexual maturation, and intellectual function are not affected.

10. The answer is (4). Impetigo, a bacterial infection of the skin, may be caused by streptococci and may precede acute glomerulonephritis. Although most streptococcal infections do not cause AGN, when they do, a latent period of 10 to 14 days occurs between the infection, usually of the skin (impetigo) or upper respiratory tract, and the onset of clinical manifestations. Herpes, scabies, and varicella are not associated with AGN.

11. The answer is (1). Hypospadias refers to a condition in which the urethral opening is located below the glans penis or anywhere along the ventral surface (underside) of the penile shaft. The ventral foreskin is lacking, and the distal portion gives an appearance of a hood. Early recognition is important so that circumcision is avoided; the foreskin is used for the surgical repair. Catheterization may be used to ensure urinary elimination. Surgery is the procedure of choice to improve the child's ability to stand when urinating, improve the appearance of the penis, and preserve sexual adequacy. Intravenous pyelography is contraindicated if the child has an allergy to iodine or shellfish.

Musculoskeletal and Neuromuscular Dysfunction

Structure and function of the musculoskeletal system

A. Structure

1. The musculoskeletal system is composed of bones, joints, muscles, tendons (fibrous tissue that connects muscle to bone), ligaments (fibrous bands that connect bones), and bursae (fluid-filled sacs found in connective tissue, usually at the joints).
2. The term neuromuscular pertains to nerves and muscles. Table 16-1 provides information on the development of the musculoskeletal system.

B. Function

1. The bony skeleton **supports** body structures.
2. The body's bony structure provides **protection** for vital organs.
3. Red bone marrow, located within bone cavities, produces white and red blood cells, a process called **hematopoiesis**.
4. The bone matrix **stores** fluoride, calcium, phosphorous, and magnesium. More than 99% of the body's total calcium is stored in bone.
5. Muscles and joints allow the body to **move**, as do tendons and ligaments. Bursa facilitate the gliding of muscles or tendons over bony or ligamentous surfaces.
6. Muscle contraction results in chemical action for **heat production** to maintain body temperature as well as movement.

C. Developmental differences in musculoskeletal response. Several significant differences in musculoskeletal function between children and adults have important implications for nursing care.

1. **Damage to the epiphyseal plate can disrupt bone growth**. The epiphyseal plate in children is an area of bone weakness that is susceptible to injury through fracture, crushing, or slippage.
2. Because a child is still growing, **some bony deformities due to injury can be remodeled or straightened over time**; conversely, this can also cause **some deformities to progress with growth**.
3. Because a child's bones are more pliable than an adult's bones, **more force is required to fracture a bone** and **specific forces may produce different types of fractures.**
4. **A child's bones generally heal much faster than those of an adult**, often greatly reducing the time required for immobilization after injury.
5. **Dislocations and sprains are less common in children than adults** because soft tissues are resilient.

TABLE 16-1
Development of the Musculoskeletal System

AGE	STRUCTURE AND FUNCTION
Fetal development	The musculoskeletal system arises from the embryonic mesodermal layer, which appears during the second week of gestation.
	By the eighth week of gestation, all major bones are present in the cartilaginous skeleton.
	Bone formation occurs by ossification, which begins as early as the eighth week of gestation and continues throughout gestation and childhood.
	Bone growth occurs in two dimensions—diameter and length. Growth in length occurs at the epiphyseal plate, a vascular area of active cell division. These cells are highly sensitive to the influence of growth hormone, estrogen, and testosterone.
Infant (0–1 year)	The skeletal system contains more cartilage than ossified bone at birth. However, the ossification process is quite rapid during the first year of life. The six skull bones are relatively soft and not joined.
	Muscular tissue is almost completely formed at birth. Growth results from the increasing size of already existing fibers influenced by growth hormone, thyroxine, and insulin. Strength increases as muscle size increases, and muscle fibers need consistent stimulation to develop.
Toddler/Preschooler (1–6 years)	Neuromuscular maturation and repetitive use of motor skills enhance development. Myelination is almost complete by 2 years of age, enabling the child to support most movement. Motor coordination increases.
Schoolager (6–12 years)	Myelination is complete, and the child moves from a clutzy 6-year-old to a coordinated 12-year-old. Bones continue to ossify, but mineralization is not complete until maturity, allowing children's bones to resist pressure and muscle pull less than adult bones.
Adolescent (12–21 years)	Growth occurs in skeletal size and muscle mass with the skeleton growing faster than the muscles; the hands and feet growing out of proportion to the body, and large muscles growing faster than small muscles. Ossification occurs later in boys than girls. Boys have more length in the arms and legs relative to trunk size, and they have greater shoulder width.

 II. **NURSING PROCESS OVERVIEW FOR**
The Musculoskeletal System

A. Assessment

1. **Health history**

   a. Elicit a description of symptoms including onset, duration, location, and precipitation. **Cardinal symptoms** may include:

      (1) Delayed walking or other motor developmental abnormalities

      (2) Pain, stiffness, or both

      (3) Physical limitation or lifestyle alterations imposed by immobility or limited range of motion (ROM)

   b. Explore prenatal, personal, and family history for **risk factors** for musculoskeletal disorders.

      (1) Prenatal risk factors include maternal infections, use of substances or medications, position in utero, or fetal hypoxia.

(2) Personal risk factors include multiple birth, type of delivery, genetic disorders, low birth weight, perinatal trauma, trauma, use of mobility aids, sports participation and safety measures used, obesity, use of steroids (prescription and anabolic), or delayed growth or puberty.

(3) Family risk factors include a history of musculoskeletal or neuromuscular disorders, such as osteogenesis imperfecta (OI), juvenile rheumatoid arthritis (JRA), or scoliosis.

2. Physical examination

a. **Vital signs.** Measure height and weight for signs of growth abnormalities.

b. **Inspection**
   (1) Inspect posture and gait.
   (2) Inspect the body for symmetry of shape and movement, including active ROM.
   (3) Observe for structural abnormalities, including asymmetrical limb lengths and spinal deformities (eg, clubfoot, hip dysplasia, leg-length discrepancy, or scoliosis).

c. **Palpation**
   (1) Palpate bony structures for tenderness, masses, and lesions.
   (2) Palpate the joints for ROM (passive), tenderness, and warmth (monitoring for signs of inflammation).
   (3) Palpate the spine to assess curvature (monitoring for scoliosis).
   (4) Assess muscle mass, tone, and strength.

3. Laboratory and diagnostic studies. See Appendices A and B for normal findings and nursing considerations.

a. **Radiographs** are the most common study to assess injury and healing, as well as to detect abnormalities and determine bone age. Bone appears whitish on an x-ray.

b. **Ultrasound** uses a Doppler probe to visualize tissue structure.

c. Blood studies include:
   (1) **Alkaline phosphatase (ALP)** is an enzyme that is elevated in bone disease and fractures.
   (2) **Creatinine kinase (CK)** is an enzyme that is elevated in trauma and muscular dystrophy.

d. **Arthroscopy** is used to visualize the inside of a joint for the diagnosis of major injury and to perform minor surgical repairs.

e. **Arthrography** is usually performed before arthroscopy and is used to evaluate suspected joint damage.

f. **Bone scans** use radioactive material to detect tumors, infection, and inflammation.

g. **Computed tomography (CT) scans** visualize anatomic details via a narrow beam x-ray and computerized process readings.

h. **Magnetic resonance imaging (MRI)** clearly defines marrow, bone and soft tissue tumors, muscle structures, ligaments, and bones. It uses magnetic and radio waves to create an energy field that can be transferred to a visual image.

i. In **joint aspiration** fluid is withdrawn to relieve pain or to detect infection.

B. Nursing diagnoses

1. Risk for neurovascular dysfunction
2. Risk for injury
3. Activity intolerance
4. Impaired skin integrity
5. Constipation
6. Altered urinary elimination
7. Ineffective breathing pattern

8. Risk for fluid volume deficit

9. Pain

10. Altered nutrition: less or more than body requirements

11. Altered growth and development

12. Sensory/perceptual alterations

13. Social isolation

C. Planning and outcome identification

1. The child will remain free of signs and symptoms of neurovascular compromise.

2. The child will remain free of injury and maintain muscle strength, endurance, and flexibility.

3. The child will maintain normal skin integrity.

4. The child will maintain normal elimination patterns.

5. The child will maintain normal cardiorespiratory patterns.

6. The child will remain pain free.

7. The child will remain well hydrated and well nourished.

8. The child will maintain age-appropriate autonomy, interact with peers and family, and express fears and concerns.

D. Implementation

1. Prevent neurovascular dysfunction.

a. Assess the neurovascular status of the affected extremity by monitoring color, temperature, pulse, mobility, sensation, and capillary refill.

b. Instruct the child to report numbness or a tingling or cold sensation.

c. Instruct the child to elevate casted extremities.

2. Prevent injury and maintain muscular strength and function. Most of the changes arise from decreased muscle strength and mass, decreased metabolism, and bone demineralization.

a. Assess for joint contracture and pain, muscular atony and weakness, fatigue, diminished reflexes, and delayed healing.

b. Assist with mobility to ensure safety.

c. Modify the environment as needed.

d. Implement developmentally appropriate safety measures.

e. Protect the child from injury by moving and positioning the child carefully and by monitoring physical activities closely; syncope and falling may result if child resumes normal activities too quickly.

f. Prevent contractures by maintaining proper body alignment and by performing ROM exercises.

3. Maintain skin integrity and prevent breakdown.

a. Monitor for early signs of breakdown, pressure ulcers, and sensory changes.

b. Turn the child frequently, unless contraindicated.

c. Place the child on a pressure-reducing surface (eg, sheepskin or alternate pressure mattress)

d. Protect pressure points.

e. Provide meticulous skin care. Massage only healthy skin with lotion.

f. Maintain integrity of casts and other appliances. Institute cast care intervention as follows:

(1) Inspect the skin underneath the cast. A foul odor, complaints of burning pain or "hot spots" on the cast may indicate infection.

(2) Prevent infection by keeping the cast clean and dry. Ensure that the child does not place crumbs or toys under the cast.

(3) Use a bed board or firm surface to support the cast.

(4) Place the cast on pillows to decrease edema and assist drying.

(5) Turn the wet cast with palms not fingertips to prevent creating pressure points.

(6) Splint upper extremity casts when dry.

(7) Check the cast for wetness (if a cast gets wet after drying initially, it will be gray, cold, musty, and dull to percussion), and petal the cast when dry.

(8) Initiate additional care for special casts, such as a spica cast.

    (a) Do not use the abduction bar as a handle to turn the child and never place plastic wrap around the genital area.

    (b) Tuck a disposable diaper under the edges of the perineal opening to keep excrement from running under the cast and to keep the perineum clean.

    (c) Turn the child every 2 hours when the cast is drying.

    (d) Institute measures to preserve the child's modesty.

    (e) Teach the child and parents how to care for the cast. Also tell them what to expect when the cast is removed (eg, noise from cast cutter, dry skin, and slight muscle atrophy).

4. Promote adequate bowel and bladder elimination. Restricted movement can cause functional and metabolic responses in most body systems.

  a. Assess for anorexia and constipation, renal calculi, urinary incontinence, or signs of urinary infection.

  b. Promote natural bowel elimination by encouraging fluids and a high-fiber diet. Administer stool softeners as prescribed.

  c. Promote urinary elimination.

    (1) Encourage fluids.

    (2) Monitor fluid intake and output (I&O).

    (3) Check for bladder distention.

    (4) Provide privacy.

  d. Help prevent urinary tract infections.

    (1) Keep the child well hydrated.

    (2) Promote frequent voiding.

    (3) Provide acid-ash foods, such as cereals, fish, poultry, cranberry or apple juice, and meats.

    (4) Limit calcium intake.

5. Promote optimal cardiorespiratory function.

  a. Assess for fatigue, orthostatic hypotension, signs and symptoms of thrombus formation, and shallow respirations.

  b. Prevent respiratory complications by keeping the child well hydrated, changing the child's position frequently, and encouraging deep-breathing exercises.

  c. Help maintain adequate cardiac output by changing the child's position frequently and by providing active and passive ROM exercises.

6. Promote comfort and relieve pain.

  a. Elevate affected area(s) to minimize edema.

  b. Anticipate the need for pain management and medicate the child as needed.

  c. Use nonpharmacologic methods of pain relief such as distraction and guided imagery.

  d. Change the child's position frequently.

  e. Use pads and pillows for support.

7. Provide adequate fluid and nutritional intake.

  a. Assess fluid and food intake.

  b. Promote adequate hydration by offering the child's favorite juices.

  c. Promote good nutrition by offering high-protein, high-calorie foods in small, frequent amounts in a pleasant atmosphere.

8. **Promote normal growth and development.** Treatment for musculoskeletal problems often requires immobilization (eg, casts, traction, and body frames), which can be frightening and painful. Physical activity is essential for growth and development; therefore, immobilization may have a serious psychological effect on children.

   a. Promote as much normal activity as possible and provide age-appropriate diversions.

   b. Encourage self-care (eg, place grooming and food items within easy reach) and provide regular social contact and age-appropriate activities. Play, social interaction, and self-care help the immobilized child gain self-esteem and independence and promote normal growth and development.

   c. Promote effective coping by encouraging verbalization, providing play therapy, and providing the necessary teaching of procedures and treatments.

   d. Explain to parents that the child (preschooler) may view immobilization as punishment. Encourage parents to listen for, and correct, any misconceptions that the child may have.

   e. Provide child and family teaching regarding immobilization as noted in Child and Family Teaching 16-1.

CHILD AND FAMILY TEACHING 16-1

Immobilization

Teach child and family:

- The action and purpose of restraining devices, such as a cast or traction.
- The proper techniques for holding, moving, feeding, care of restrictive devices, positioning, and signs and symptoms of complications (eg, increased temperature, pain or blood on voiding, or difficulty breathing).
- Skin care
- Measures to prevent constipation and urinary stasis
- Proper nutritional intake
- Cast care, especially for spica casts:

  Explain signs and symptoms of circulatory impairment and infection, as well as complications of immobilization, to watch for and report.

  Demonstrate how to care for the cast and the child in the cast, including how to use correct body mechanics when lifting the child, how to avoid using the abduction bar for moving the child, which measures to implement to prevent physical and developmental deficits, and how to keep the cast clean and dry (eg, tucking a disposable diaper beneath the entire perineal opening in the cast). Also point out the importance of restraining the child when moving him.

  Offer feeding tips and techniques for an infant or small child in a cast, including positioning the child so that she feels safe; using pillows for support; cuddling the child in the arms; and supporting the child in a "football" hold or fashioning a tilt table, depending on the infant's size.
- Family activities to include the child; a child confined in a cast or brace can be held and transported to areas of activity.
- Ways to nurture the infant or young child through stroking, holding, and maintaining physical closeness

E. Outcome evaluation

1. The child's affected area is pink, warm, and mobile with palpable pulses and good sensation.
2. The child is free of injury and retains an optimal functional status.
3. The child maintains normal skin integrity.
4. The child maintains normal elimination patterns.
5. The child maintains normal cardiorespiratory patterns.
6. The child remains well hydrated and well nourished.
7. The child is pain free.
8. The child maintains optimal growth and development.

III. Osteogenesis imperfecta (OI)

A. Definition

1. OI is a group of four types of heterogenous inherited disorders characterized by connective tissue and bone defects.
2. Abnormal precollagen type I OI is the most common, and the mildest, form of the disease. Type II OI is the most severe form and is characterized by multiple intrauterine or perinatal fractures, severe deformity, and, often, early death.
3. OI is the most common genetic bone disease.

B. Etiology. OI usually demonstrates an autosomal dominant inheritance pattern, but it can be recessive. The exact etiology remains unclear.

C. Pathophysiology

1. A biochemical defect causes a reduction in the synthesis of collagen.
2. This affects all connective tissue, resulting in lax joints and weak muscles, which leads to an increase in fractures whenever stress is placed on the bone.
3. Deformities result from fractures, bowing, and growth pattern disturbances.

D. Assessment (type I)

1. **Clinical manifestations**
   a. Frequent fractures (the incidence of fractures decreases with puberty when hormone production strengthens the bones).
   b. Thin skin
   c. Hyperextensible ligaments
   d. Epistaxis
   e. Blue sclera
   f. Easy bruising
   g. Excess diaphoresis
   h. Mild hyperpyrexia
2. **Laboratory and diagnostic study findings**
   a. Radiographs demonstrate multiple normal callous formations at new fracture sites, generalized osteopenia, evidence of previous fractures, and skeletal deformities.
   b. Prenatal ultrasound can detect some types of OI.

E. Nursing management

1. **Assess for fractures and other injuries.**
2. **Prevent injury.** Handle the child carefully, even when changing the diaper.

   3. Discuss home care with the family that includes:
      a. Safety precautions for home and school
      b. Adoption of a reduced-calorie, low-fat, high-fiber diet to prevent obesity
      c. Providing good oral care because the teeth are frequently broken
      d. Performing adequate skin care to manage diaphoresis
      e. Injury management
   4. Provide support.
      a. OI is frequently confused with child abuse. Once a diagnosis is made, encourage the family to carry a letter of explanation to present to authorities whenever the child is injured.
      b. Children with OI undergo frequent surgeries to correct fractures and deformities. Allow children to verbalize their fears and concerns and provide adequate preparation.
   5. Refer the family to the OI Foundation.

IV. Developmental dysplasia of the hip (DDH)

A. Description
   1. DDH is a group of congenital abnormalities of the hip joints, which includes subluxation, dislocation, and preluxation.
   2. Of the types of congenital hip abnormalities, subluxation is the most common.
   3. DDH typically is seen with other problems, such as neural tube disorders.
   4. Uncorrected subluxation or dislocation may lead to a permanent disability.

B. Etiology. The etiology of DDH is unknown but it may result from one of the following:
   1. The effect of maternal estrogen on the fetus, causing relaxation of the ligaments
   2. Hip and leg positioning in utero
   3. Genetic factors

C. Pathophysiology
   1. In **preluxation** (acetabular dysplasia) there is an apparent delay in acetabular development, but the femoral head remains in the acetabulum.
   2. In **subluxation** there is incomplete dislocation; the femoral head remains in contact with the acetabulum, but a stretched capsule and ligament tears cause the head of the femur to be partially displaced.
   3. In **dislocation** the femoral head loses contact with the acetabulum and is displaced posteriorly and superiorly over the fibrocartilaginous rim.

D. Assessment findings
   1. Clinical manifestations. Characteristics vary with age.
      a. Characteristics seen in newborns include the Ortolani sign, the Barlow sign, asymmetrical gluteal folds, limited abduction of affected hip, and the Galeazzi sign.
      b. Characteristics seen in older children include limping, toe walking, and the Trendelenburg sign.
   2. Laboratory and diagnostic study findings
      a. Radiographic examination does not yield reliable data until after ossification of the femoral head when the infant is between 3 and 6 months of age.
      b. Ultrasonography detects slight subluxations and dislocations.
      c. A CT scan assesses the position of the femoral head.
      d. Arthrography confirms stability and is useful in evaluating reduction.

E. Nursing management

1. **Assess newborns and infants for signs of DDH** to allow for early detection and intervention.

2. **Prepare the family for treatment:**

a. **Newborn to 6 months**. The infant usually is placed in an abduction device, such as the Pavlik harness. This device centers the femoral head into the acetabulum in an attitude of flexion and deepens the acetabulum by pressure. The infant wears the device until the hip joint is clinically and radiographically stable. Usually by 3 to 6 months, the child may be transferred to a protective abduction brace.

b. **Infants, 6 to 18 months**. Traction is used for gradual reduction, followed by closed reduction with cast immobilization until the joint is stable. If the hip is not reducible, an open reduction is performed, followed by a spica cast for 4 to 6 months (Fig. 16-1); this is then replaced with an abduction splint.

c. **Older child**. Correction is difficult because secondary changes create complications. Surgical reduction is required. Successful reduction after 4 years of age is difficult; it is inadvisable after 6 years of age.

 3. **Prevent neurovascular dysfunction** (caused by a cast or an immobilizing device).

4. **Maintain skin integrity and prevent breakdown**.

5. **Promote comfort.**

6. **Provide child and family teaching** regarding home care for immobility (see Child and Family Teaching 16-1).

V. Fractures

A. Description

1. A fracture is a break in the continuity of the bone.

2. Common fracture sites include:

a. Clavicle

b. Humerus. In supracondylar fractures, which occur when child falls backward on hands with elbows straight, there is a high incidence of neurovascular complications due to the anatomic relationship of the brachial artery and nerves to the fracture site.

c. Radius and ulna

d. Femur (often associated with child abuse)

e. Epiphyseal plates (potential for growth deformity)

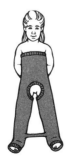
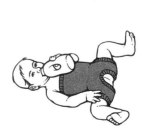

FIGURE 16-1
Hip spica casts.

B. Etiology

1. Fractures in children usually are the result of trauma from motor vehicle accidents, falls, or child abuse.
2. Because of the resilience of the soft tissue of children, fractures occur more often than soft tissue injuries.

C. Pathophysiology

1. Fractures occur when the resistance of bone against the stress being exerted yields to the stress force.
2. Fractures most commonly seen in children include:
   a. A **bend fracture** is characterized by the bone bending to the breaking point and not straightening without intervention.
   b. A **buckle fracture** results from compression failure of the bone, with the bone telescoping on itself.
   c. A **greenstick fracture** is an incomplete fracture.

D. Assessment findings

1. **Clinical manifestations**
   a. The five "Ps"—pain, pulse, pallor, paresthesia, and paralysis are seen with all types of fractures.
   b. Other characteristic findings include deformity, swelling, bruising, muscle spasms, tenderness, pain, impaired sensation, loss of function, abnormal mobility, crepitus, shock, or refusal to walk (in small children).
2. **Laboratory and diagnostic study findings**
   a. Radiographic examination reveals initial injury and subsequent healing progress. A comparison film of an opposite, unaffected extremity is often used to look for subtle changes in the affected extremity.
   b. Blood studies reveal bleeding (decreased hemoglobin and hematocrit) and muscle damage (elevated aspartate transaminase [AST] and lactic dehydrogenase [LDH]).

E. Nursing management

1. **Provide emergency management**, when the situation warrants, for a new fracture.
   a. Assess the five "Ps."
   b. Determine the mechanism of injury.
   c. Immobilize the part. Move injured parts as little as possible.
   d. Cover any open wounds with a sterile, or clean, dressing.
   e. Reassess the five "Ps."
   f. Apply traction if circulatory compromise is present.
   g. Elevate the injured limb, if possible.
   h. Apply cold to the injured area.
   i. Call emergency medical services.
2. **Assess for circulatory impairment** (cyanosis, coldness, mottling, decreased peripheral pulses, positive blanch sign, edema not relieved by elevation, pain, or cramping).
3. **Assess for neurologic impairment** (lack of sensation or movement, pain or tenderness, or numbness and tingling).
4. **Administer analgesic medications**.
5. **Explain fracture management to the child and family**. Depending on the type of break and its location, repair (by realignment or reduction) may be made by closed or open reduction followed by immobilization with a splint, traction, or a cast.
6. **Maintain skin integrity and prevent breakdown.** Institute appropriate measures for cast and appliance care.

7. **Prevent complications.**
    a. Prevent **circulatory impairment** by assessing pulses, color, and temperature, and by reporting changes immediately.
    b. Prevent **nerve compression syndromes** by testing sensation and motor function, including subjective symptoms of pain, muscular weakness, burning sensation, limited ROM, and altered sensation. Correct alignment to alleviate pressure if appropriate, and notify the health care provider.
    c. Prevent **compartment syndrome** by assessing for muscle weakness and pain out of proportion to injury. Early detection is critical to prevent tissue damage.
        (1) Causes of compartment syndrome include tight dressings or casts, hemorrhage, trauma, burns, and surgery.
        (2) Treatment entails pressure relief, which sometimes requires performing a fasciotomy.
    d. Prevent **infection**, including osteomyelitis, by using infection control measures.
    e. Prevent **renal calculi** by encouraging fluids, monitoring I&O, and mobilizing the child as much as possible.
    f. Prevent **pulmonary emboli** by carefully monitoring adolescents and children with multiple fractures. Emboli generally occur within the first 24 hours.

 VI. **Scoliosis**

A. **Description**
    1. Scoliosis is a spinal deformity that usually involves lateral curvature of the spine, spinal rotation, and thoracic hypokyphosis.
    2. It is the most common spinal deformity.
B. **Etiology**
    1. Scoliosis may result from leg-length discrepancy, hip or knee contractures, pain, neuromuscular disorders, or congenital malformations. However, it is usually idiopathic (IS).
    2. Evidence points to a probable genetic autosomal dominant trait with incomplete penetrance; or to multifactorial causes.
C. **Pathophysiology**
    1. Deformity progresses during periods of growth (adolescent growth spurt) and stabilizes when vertebral growth ceases.
    2. As the spine grows and the lateral curve develops, the vertebrae rotate, causing the ribs and spine to rotate toward the convex part of the spine. Spinous processes rotate toward the concavity of the curve.
    3. The child attempts to maintain an erect posture, resulting in a compensatory curve.
    4. Vertebrae become wedge shaped and vertebral disks undergo degenerative changes.
    5. Muscles and ligaments either shorten and thicken or lengthen and atrophy, depending on the concavity or convexity of the curve. A hump forms from the ribs rotating backward on the convex side of the curve.
    6. The thoracic cavity becomes asymmetrical, leading to severe ventilatory compensation.
    7. If significant scoliosis goes uncorrected, respiratory function is compromised and vital capacity is reduced; eventually, pulmonary hypertension, cor pulmonale, and respiratory acidosis may develop.

D. Assessment findings

1. Clinical manifestations

a. Scoliosis is asymptomatic most of the time and goes unrecognized until there is some degree of deformity.

b. The first signs of scoliosis include:

(1) Presence of a spinal curve

(2) Asymmetry of scapula and extremities

(3) Unequal distance between the arms and waist

2. Laboratory and diagnostic study findings

a. Radiographic examination reveals the degree and location of the curvature.

b. An MRI scan is used to evaluate the possibility of intraspinal pathology or other disease processes that can cause scoliosis.

E. Nursing management

1. Prevent physical and emotional trauma related to wearing a brace. The Boston brace and TLSO custom-molded jacket are the two most commonly used braces. The type of brace and wearing schedule (between 16 and 23 hours per day) are based on the age of the child, the nature of the curve, and any underlying condition associated with the curve.

a. Assess for and eliminate or minimize environmental hazards that may impede mobility.

b. Maintain skin integrity by properly applying braces and implementing corrective action to prevent and treat skin breakdown.

c. Promote a positive self-concept.

(1) Encourage verbalization of concerns and feelings.

(2) Assist the child in selecting clothing that will conceal the brace.

(3) Encourage positive aspects of wearing the brace, including improved posture and symptom relief.

(4) Assist the child and family in developing coping skills.

d. Promote normal growth and development by encouraging self-care activities and peer socialization.

e. Provide family support by referring parents to social services or an appropriate support group.

2. Evaluate the child's acceptance of the prescribed brace and exercise program to determine compliance level and the need for reinforced teaching. Supplemental exercises are used to prevent atrophy of spinal and abdominal muscles.

3. Prevent complications related to surgery. The surgical technique consists of realignment and straightening with internal fixation and instrumentation combined with bony fusion. Instrumentations include Harrington, Dwyer, Zielke, Luque, Cotrel-Dubouset, Isola, and Texas Scottish Right Hospital (TSRH).

a. Prevent neurologic deficit by monitoring motor, sensory, and neurologic status, particularly in extremities; prompt identification of neurologic deficit and correction can prevent permanent damage.

b. Detect impending hypoxia by monitoring blood gas values; notify health care provider if abnormal values are detected.

c. Assess for hypotension by monitoring I&O (will most likely have indwelling catheter) and vital signs, and observing skin color to assess tissue perfusion.

d. Maintain skin integrity and prevent breakdown.

e. Promote adequate bowel and bladder elimination.

(1) Prevent constipation by assessing bowel sounds.

(2) Prevent urinary complications by providing catheter care

4. Promote adequate fluid and nutritional intake. Maintain intravenous (IV) therapy until oral feedings are allowed.

5. Promote normal growth and development.

6. Promote comfort.

7. Provide the child and family with information about scoliosis and its treatment. Include information about the equipment used during treatment.

VII. Cerebral palsy (CP)

A. Description

1. CP is a group of disabilities caused by injury or insult to the brain either before or during birth, or in early infancy. CP is the most common permanent disability of childhood.

2. Classification of CP

   a. **Spastic CP** is the most common type and may involve one or both sides of the body.

      (1) Clinical hallmarks include hypertonicity with poor control of posture, balance, and coordinated movement, and impairment of fine and gross motor skills. Active attempts at motion increase the abnormal postures and lead to overflow of movement to other parts of the body.

      (2) Common types of spastic CP include:

         (a) Hemiparesis is when one side of the body is affected.

         (b) Quadriparesis (tetraparesis) is when all four extremities are affected.

         (c) Diplegia is when similar body parts are affected, such as both arms.

   b. The **dyskinetic/athetoid** type involves abnormal involuntary movements that disappear during sleep and increase with stress.

      (1) Major manifestations are athetosis (wormlike movement), dyskinetic movement of mouth, drooling, and dysarthria.

      (2) Movements may become choreoid (irregular, jerky) and dystonic (disordered muscle tone), especially when stressed and during the adolescent years.

   c. The **ataxic** type is manifested by a wide-based gait, rapid repetitive movements performed poorly, and disintegration of movements of the upper extremities when the child reaches for objects.

   d. The **mixed/dystonic** type is manifested by a combination of the characteristics of spastic and athetoid CP.

B. Etiology

1. CP commonly results from existing prenatal brain abnormalities.

2. Prematurity is the single most important determinant of CP.

3. Other prenatal or perinatal risk factors include asphyxia, ischemia, perinatal trauma, congenital and perinatal infections, and perinatal metabolic problems, such as hyperbilirubinemia and hypoglycemia.

4. Infection, trauma, and tumors can cause CP in early infancy.

5. Some cases (about 24%) of CP remain unexplained.

C. Pathophysiology

1. Disabilities usually result from injury to the cerebellum, the basal ganglia, or the motor cortex.

2. It is difficult to establish the precise location of neurologic lesions because there is no typical pathologic picture. In some cases, the brain has gross malformations; in others, vascular occlusion, atrophy, loss of neurons, and degeneration may be evident.

3. CP is nonprogressive but may become more apparent as the child grows older.

D. Assessment findings. The most common **clinical manifestation in all types of CP is delayed gross motor development** (delay in all motor accomplishments; delay becomes more profound as the child grows).

1. Additional manifestations include:
   a. Abnormal motor performance (eg, early dominant hand preference, abnormal and asymmetrical crawl, poor sucking, feeding problems, or persistent tongue thrust)
   b. Alterations of muscle tone (eg, increased or decreased resistance to passive movements, child feels stiff when handling or dressing, difficulty in diapering, or opisthotonos)
   c. Abnormal postures (eg, scissoring legs or persistent infantile posturing)
   d. Reflex abnormalities (eg, persistent primitive reflexes, such as tonic neck or hyperreflexia)
2. Disabilities associated with CP include mental retardation, seizures, attention deficit disorder, and sensory impairment.
3. Severe cases may be observed at birth; mild and moderate cases usually are not detected until the child is 1 or 2 years old. Failure to achieve milestones may be the first sign.
4. Diagnosis of CP is based on the following:
   a. Prenatal, birth, and postnatal history
   b. Neurologic examination
   c. Assessment of muscle tone, behavior, and abilities
   d. Other disorders, such as metabolic disorders, degenerative disorders and early, slow-growing brain tumors, are ruled out.
5. All infants should receive periodic developmental evaluations, especially those at risk.

E. Nursing management

1. **Prevent physical injury** by providing the child with a safe environment, appropriate toys, and protective gear (helmet, kneepads), if needed.
2. **Prevent physical deformity** by ensuring correct use of prescribed braces and other devices, and by performing ROM exercises.
3. **Promote mobility** by encouraging the child to perform age- and condition-appropriate motor activities.
4. **Promote adequate fluid and nutritional intake.**
5. **Foster relaxation and general health** by providing rest periods.
6. **Administer prescribed medications,** which may include sedatives, muscle relaxants, and anticonvulsants.
7. **Encourage self-care** by urging the child to participate in activities of daily living (ADLs) (eg, using utensils and implements that are appropriate for the child's age and condition).
8. **Facilitate communication.**
   a. Talk to the child deliberately and slowly, using pictures to reinforce speech when needed.
   b. Encourage early speech therapy to prevent poor or maladaptive communication habits.
   c. Provide a means of articulate speech such as sign language or a picture board.
   d. Technology, such as computer use, may help children with severe articulation problems.
9. As necessary, **seek referrals for corrective lenses and hearing devices** to decrease sensory deprivation related to vision and hearing losses.
10. **Help promote a positive self-image in the child.**
    a. Praise his accomplishments.

    b. Set realistic and attainable goals.

    c. Encourage an appealing physical appearance.

    d. Encourage his involvement with age- and condition-appropriate peer group activities.

11. Promote optimal family functioning.

    a. Encourage family members to express anxieties, frustrations, and concerns and to explore support networks.

    b. Provide emotional support and help with problem-solving, as necessary.

    c. Refer the family to support organizations, such as the United Cerebral Palsy Association.

12. Prepare the child and family for procedures, treatments, appliances, and surgeries, if needed.

13. Assist in multidisciplinary therapeutic measures designed to establish locomotion, communication, and self-help; gain optimal appearance and integration of motor functions; correct associated defects as effectively as possible; and provide educational opportunities based on the individual's needs and capabilities. Therapeutic measures include:

    a. Braces to help prevent or reduce deformities, increase energy of gait, and control alignment

    b. Motorized devices to permit self-propulsion

    c. Orthopedic surgery to correct deformities and decrease spasticity (medications are not helpful for spasticity)

    d. Medications to control possible seizure activity or attention deficit disorder

    e. Speech therapy and physical therapy

14. Inform parents that their child will need considerable help and patience in accomplishing each new task.

    a. Encourage them not to focus solely on the child's inability to accomplish certain tasks.

    b. Urge them to relax and demonstrate patience.

    c. Explain the importance of providing positive feedback.

15. Encourage the family to seek appropriate functional, adaptive, and vocational training for the child.

16. Encourage family members to achieve balance in their lives between caring for their disabled child and other family and personal matters.

VIII. Duchenne muscular dystrophy (MD)

A. Description

    1. MD is a group of disorders that cause progressive degeneration and weakness of skeletal muscles.

    2. Duchenne muscular dystrophy is the most common form of MD in children.

    3. In Duchenne MD, muscle weakness is progressive and leads to death, usually in adolescence, from infection or cardiopulmonary failure.

B. Etiology. Half of all cases are X-linked and boys are almost exclusively affected.

C. Pathophysiology

    1. Dystrophin, a protein product in skeletal muscle, is absent in the muscles of children with MD.

    2. There is a gradual degeneration of muscle fibers characterized by progressive weakness and muscle wasting.

D. Assessment findings

1. **Clinical manifestations.** Symptoms begin when the child is between 3 and 5 years old.
   a. Initial signs and symptoms include:
      (1) Weakness in the pelvic girdle
      (2) Delays in motor development
      (3) Difficulties in running, riding a bicycle, and climbing stairs
   b. Progressive signs and symptoms include:
      (1) Abnormal gait becomes apparent.
      (2) Walking ability ceases by the time the child is between 9 and 12 years old.
      (3) Gower sign. From a supine position, the child rolls over, kneels, and presses his hands against the ankles, shins, knees, and thighs in a "climbing" action to rise to a standing position.
      (4) Pseudohypertrophy of calf muscles
      (5) Cardiac problems
      (6) Delayed or impaired development (possibly)

2. **Laboratory and diagnostic study findings**
   a. Creatinine phosphokinase (CPK) is increased.
   b. Muscle biopsy discloses degeneration of muscle fibers.
   c. Electrocardiogram (ECG) and pulmonary function tests (PFTs) establish compromise of heart and lungs.
   d. Electromyography (EMG) findings show a decrease in amplitude and duration of motor unit potentials.

E. Nursing management

1. **Assess the child for signs of disorder progression** and for complications.
2. **Monitor temperature** because children with Duchenne type MD are at risk for malignant hyperthermia, a potential complication of anesthesia for children undergoing surgery.
3. **Maintain optimal physical mobility** by facilitating the maximal level of activity that the child can manage, by changing position every 2 hours, by ensuring proper body alignment, and by performing ROM exercises.
4. **Compensate for disuse syndrome**.
   a. Position the child to minimize the potential for contractures.
   b. Provide skin care and assess for skin breakdown.
   c. Encourage fluids.
   d. Provide chest physiotherapy.
   e. Assist in developing a bowel routine.
5. **Support the child and family in coping with this progressive disorder**.
   a. Encourage the family to verbalize their concerns.
   b. Assist them in developing coping strategies.
   c. Encourage participation in the child's care.
6. **Further assist family coping** by referring family members to support agencies such as the Muscular Dystrophy Association.
7. **Teach the family and child** about the following:
   a. Diagnosis of MD
   b. Treatment strategies
   c. Devices (braces, feeding devices)
   d. Complications associated with MD
   e. Prognosis of the disease
8. **Assist the family in obtaining genetic counseling**.

STUDY QUESTIONS

1. When a child injures the epiphyseal plate from a fracture, the damage may result in which of the following?
   (1) Bone growth disruption
   (2) Rheumatoid arthritis
   (3) Permanent nerve damage
   (4) Osteomyelitis

2. Which of the following statements by a 14-year-old girl who wears a brace for structural scoliosis indicates effective use of the brace?
   (1) "I wonder if I can take the brace off when I go to the homecoming dance."
   (2) "I'll look forward to taking this thing off to take my bath every day."
   (3) "I sure am glad that I only have to wear this awful thing at night."
   (4) "I'm really glad that I can take this thing off whenever I get tired."

3. Which of the following is the most common form of developmental dysplasia of the hip?
   (1) Preluxation
   (2) Subluxation
   (3) Acetabular dysplasia
   (4) Dislocation

4. When assessing a newborn for developmental dysplasia of the hip, the nurse would expect to assess which of the following?
   (1) Symmetrical gluteal folds
   (2) Trendelenburg sign
   (3) Ortolani sign
   (4) Characteristic limp

5. Which of the following would the nurse do to **best** assess a mother's ability to care for her child who requires the use of a Pavlik harness?
   (1) Have the mother verbalize the purpose for using the device.
   (2) Request a home health care nurse visit after discharge.
   (3) Have the mother remove and reapply the harness before discharge.
   (4) Demonstrate to the mother how to remove and reapply the device.

6. Which of the following is the **priority** nursing action for a child immediately following the application of a spica cast?
   (1) Perform neurovascular checks.
   (2) Elevate the cast.
   (3) Cover the perineal area.
   (4) Keep the cast clean and dry.

7. Which of the following is the **most common** permanent disability in childhood?
   (1) Developmental dysplasia of the hip
   (2) Cerebral palsy
   (3) Muscular dystrophy
   (4) Scoliosis

8. Which of the following statements made by the mother of a 4-month-old would indicate that the child may have cerebral palsy?
   (1) "I'm very worried because my baby has not rolled all the way over yet."
   (2) "My baby's left hip tilts when I pull him to a standing position."
   (3) "My baby won't lift her head up and look at me; she's so floppy."
   (4) "He holds his left leg so stiff that I have a hard time putting on his diapers."

9. Which of the following usually is the **first** indication of Duchenne muscular dystrophy?
   (1) Inability to suck in the newborn
   (2) Lateness in walking in the toddler
   (3) Difficulty running in the preschooler
   (4) Decreasing coordination in the schoolager

10. Besides assessing neurologic status immediately after Harrington rod instrumentation and spinal fusion for an adolescent with scoliosis, the nurse should be concerned with which of the following factors?
    (1) Understanding of the procedure
    (2) Comfort level
    (3) Physical therapy needs
    (4) Dietary tolerance

ANSWER KEY

1. The answer is (1). The epiphyseal plate is an important area of bone growth. Therefore, any disruption may result in limb shortening. Rheumatoid arthritis is a collagen disease with an autoimmune component with no relationship to fractures. Nerve damage and osteomyelitis may occur with any fracture, but growth disruption is a primary concern at the epiphyseal plate.

2. The answer is (2). The brace should be removed for only 1 hour of every 24-hour period for hygiene and skin care. Although physical appearance and social activities with peers are important, the brace should not be removed except for hygiene and skin care. Wearing the brace at night would be true only after radiologic studies indicate the spine has bone marrow maturity and the adolescent has been weaned from the brace over 1 to 2 years. Taking the brace off whenever tired indicates poor understanding of the brace.

3. The answer is (2). DDH is a group of congenital abnormalities of the hip joints, which includes subluxation, dislocation, and preluxation. Of the types of congenital hip abnormalities, subluxation is the most common. Preluxation, also known as acetabular dysplasia, is the mildest form. Dislocation is complete displacement of the femoral head out of the acetabulum.

4. The answer is (3). The Ortolani sign is felt and heard when the young infant's hip is flexed and abducted. Asymmetrical gluteal folds would be noted in congenital hip dysplasia. The Trendelenburg sign is noted in the weight-bearing child when the child stands on the affected hip and the pelvis tilts downward on the normal side instead of upward. A characteristic limp would be noted in the ambulatory child.

5. The answer is (3). Having the mother remove and reapply the harness before discharge allows the nurse to directly observe the mother's technique and comfort level. It also provides time for reinstruction if necessary. Verbalization is important to allow the nurse to assess the mother's understanding, but it does not permit evaluation of the mother's psychomotor skills. Requesting a home visit is further means of evaluation, but it does not provide immediate feedback. Although the nurse's demonstration is a good teaching technique, initially, it does not permit evaluation of the mother's technique.

6. The answer is (1). Neurovascular assessment is always a priority in the assessment of a freshly applied cast to ensure adequate circulation and neurologic function and prevent complications or injury. Elevating the cast to prevent or minimize edema, covering the perineal area to prevent wetness and soiling, and keeping the cast dry and clean are all important, but these are not the priority immediately following a cast application.

7. The answer is (2). CP is the most common permanent disability of childhood. CP is a group of disabilities caused by injury or insult to the brain either before or during birth, or in early infancy. Developmental dysplasia of the hip and scoliosis should not cause permanent disability. MD is a group of disorders that cause progressive degeneration and weakness of skeletal muscles.

8. The answer is (3). Hypotonia or floppy infant is an early manifestation of CP. Typically, the infant lifts head to a 90° angle by 4 months with only a partial head lag by 2 months. Rolling completely over usually does not occur until the infant is 6 months old. Tilting of the hip is an indication of developmental dysplasia of the hip. Although rigidity and tenseness are possible signs of cerebral palsy, a limitation in one leg suggests developmental dysplasia of the hip.

9. The answer is (3). Typically, signs and symptoms of Duchenne muscular dystrophy are not noticed until the ages of 3 to 5 years. Usually weakness starts with the pelvic girdle, evidenced as difficulty running in the preschooler. Duchenne muscular dystrophy usually is not diagnosed in the infant or toddler period and sucking is not affected. Diminished coordination is not the first sign of Duchenne muscular dystrophy.

10. The answer is (2). Instrumentation and spinal fusion cause considerable pain. Therefore, the adolescent needs vigorous pain management, which involves assessment, administration of pain medication, and evaluation of the response. In the immediate postoperative period, the child is conscious of sensation and surroundings. Assessment of understanding of procedure is a preoperative nursing responsibility. Physical therapy at this time is not an immediate postoperative goal. However, it may be appropriate later on in the postoperative period. Typically, immediately after surgery, the adolescent will not be receiving anything by mouth.

Neurologic and Cognitive Dysfunction

Structure and function of the nervous system

A. Structures

1. The neurologic system consists of two main divisions, the central nervous system (CNS) and the peripheral nervous system (PNS). The autonomic nervous system (ANS) is composed of both central and peripheral elements.

   a. The **CNS** is composed of the brain and spinal cord.

   b. The **PNS** is composed of the 12 pairs of the cranial nerves and the 31 pairs of the spinal nerves.

   c. The **ANS** is comprised of visceral efferent (motor) and visceral afferent (sensory) nuclei in the brain and spinal cord. Its peripheral division is made up of visceral efferent and afferent nerve fibers as well as autonomic and sensory ganglia.

2. The **brain** is covered by three membranes.

   a. The **dura mater** is a fibrous, connective tissue structure containing several blood vessels.

   b. The **arachnoid membrane** is a delicate serous membrane.

   c. The **pia mater** is a vascular membrane.

3. The **spinal cord** extends from the medulla oblongata to the lower border of the first lumbar vertebrae. It contains millions of nerve fibers, and it consists of 31 nerves— 8 cervical, 12 thoracic, 5 lumbar, and 5 sacral.

4. **Cerebrospinal fluid (CSF)** forms in the lateral ventricles in the choroid plexus of the pia mater. It flows through the foramen of Monro into the third ventricle, then through the aqueduct of Sylvius to the fourth ventricle. CSF exits the fourth ventricle by the foramen of Magendie and the two foramens of Luska. It then flows into the cisterna magna, and finally it circulates to the subarachnoid space of the spinal cord, bathing both the brain and the spinal cord. Fluid is absorbed by the arachnoid membrane. The development of the neurologic system is presented in Table 17-1.

B. Function

1. **CNS**

   a. **Brain**

      (1) The **cerebrum** is the center for consciousness, thought, memory, sensory input, and motor activity; it consists of two hemispheres (left and right) and four lobes, each with specific functions.

         (a) The **frontal lobe** controls voluntary muscle movements and contains motor areas, including the area for speech; it also contains the centers for personality, behavioral, autonomic, and intellectual functions and those for emotional and cardiac responses.

TABLE 17-1
Development of the Neurologic System

AGE	STRUCTURE AND FUNCTION
Fetal development	The CNS arises from the neural tube during embryonic development. By the fourth week of gestation, the neural tube has developed. Between weeks 8 and 12, the cerebrum and cerebellum begin to develop.
	Two periods of rapid nerve development occur—between the 15th and 20th weeks of gestation and from the 30th week of gestation through the first year of extrauterine life.
	In the first year of extrauterine life, the number of brain neurons increases rapidly. Normally accounting for 12% of the body weight at birth, the brain doubles its weight by the end of the first year of extrauterine life. CNS nerve myelinization, which enables progressive neuromuscular function, follows the cephalocaudal and proximodistal sequence; its rate accelerates rapidly after birth.
	The PNS arises from the neural crest, which originates from the neural tube during embryonic development.
Infant (0–1 year)	The neurologic system is incompletely integrated at birth. Most functions are primitive reflexes, and most primitive reflexes disappear by the time the infant is 12 months old. All cranial nerves are myelinated except the optic and olfactory nerves. The system remains immature during infancy, but grows at a rapid rate as evidenced by the infant's quickly changing development. However, stimulation is needed to promote neurologic development and skills.
Toddler/Preschooler (1–6 years)	The brain reaches 80% of adult size by 2 years of age. Myelinization is almost complete by 2 years of age, enabling the child to increase movement and to be toilet trained. A greater number of connections form between neurons, and the neurons increase in complexity.
	Specialization of the hemispheres is occurring, evidenced by hand preference. The right hemisphere matures faster in boys; the left, in girls, possibly accounting for the differences in spacial abilities in boys and language abilities in girls. The limbic system matures to better regulate sleep, wakefulness, and emotions.
Schoolager (6–12 years)	The brain reaches 90% of adult size by 7 years of age, after which brain growth slows and reaches adult size by 12 years of age. Myelinization is complete, and the child is better able to listen, remember, and make associations concerning stimuli. Nerve impulse transmission improves, which allows better balance and greater gross and fine motor development.
Adolescent (12–21 years)	Brain growth continues. The neurons do not increase in number, but there is an increase in the number of support cells that nourish them. There is expansion in cognitive development.

- (b) The **temporal lobe** is the center for taste, hearing and smell, and, in the brain's dominant hemisphere, the center for interpreting spoken language.
- (c) The **parietal lobe** coordinates and interprets sensory information from the opposite side of the body.
- (d) The **occipital lobe** interprets visual stimuli.
  - (2) The **thalamus** further organizes cerebral function by transmitting impulses to and from the cerebrum. It also is responsible for primitive emotional responses, such as fear, and for distinguishing between pleasant and unpleasant stimuli.
  - (3) Lying beneath the thalamus, the **hypothalamus** is an autonomic center that regulates blood pressure, temperature, libido, appetite, breathing, sleeping patterns, and peripheral nerve discharges associated with certain behavior and emotional expression. It also helps control pituitary secretion and stress reactions.
  - (4) The **cerebellum**, or hindbrain, controls smooth muscle movements, coordinates sensory impulses with muscle activity, and maintains muscle tone and equilibrium.
  - (5) The **brain stem**, which includes the mesencephalon, pons, and medulla oblongata, relays nerve impulses between the brain and spinal cord.
- b. The **spinal cord** forms a two-way conductor pathway between the brain stem and the PNS. It is also the reflex center for motor activities that do not involve brain control.
2. The **PNS** connects the CNS to remote body regions and conducts signals to and from these areas and the spinal cord.
3. The **ANS** regulates body functions such as digestion, respiration, and cardiovascular function. Supervised chiefly by the hypothalamus, the ANS contains two divisions:
- a. The **sympathetic nervous system** serves as an emergency preparedness system, the "flight-or-fight" response. Sympathetic impulses increase greatly when the body is under physical or emotional stress causing bronchiole dilation, dilation of the heart and voluntary muscle blood vessels, stronger and faster heart contractions, peripheral blood vessel constriction, decreased peristalsis, and increased perspiration. Sympathetic stimuli are mediated by norepinephrine.
- b. The **parasympathetic nervous system** is the dominant controller for most visceral effectors for most of the time. Parasympathetic impulses are mediated by acetylcholine.
C. **Differences in nervous system response.** The nervous system is one of the first systems to form in utero, but one of the last systems to develop during childhood.
1. Accuracy and completeness of a neurologic assessment is limited by the child's development.
2. The child's brain constantly undergoes organization in function and myelinization. Therefore, the full impact of insult may not be immediately apparent and may take years to manifest.
3. The peripheral nerves are not fully myelinated at birth. As myelinization progresses, so does the child's fine motor control and coordination.
4. Early signs of increased intracranial pressure (ICP) may not be apparent in infants because open sutures and fontanelles compensate to a limited extent.
5. The development of handedness before 1 year of age may signify a neurologic lesion.
6. Several primitive reflexes are present at birth, disappearing by 1 year of age. Absence, persistence, or asymmetry of reflexes may indicate pathology.
7. The spinal cord ends at L3 in the neonate, instead of L1–L2 where it terminates in the adult. This affects the site of lumbar puncture.
8. Children have 65 to 140 mL of CSF compared to 90 to 150 mL in the adult.

II. NURSING PROCESS OVERVIEW FOR
The Neurologic System

A. Assessment. Neurologic assessment of children must be based on the developmental level of the child and should attempt to determine if problems are acute or chronic, diffuse or focal, or stable or progressive.

1. Health history

a. Elicit a description of symptoms including onset, duration, location, and precipitation. **Cardinal symptoms** may include:

   (1) Headaches

   (2) Fainting and dizziness

   (3) Altered level of consciousness (LOC)

   (4) Abnormal gait, movements, or coordination

   (5) Developmental lags or loss of milestones

b. Explore prenatal, personal, and family history for **risk factors** for neurologic disorders.

   (1) Prenatal risk factors include maternal malnutrition, drug use (prescription, especially anticonvulsants, and illicit drugs), alcohol use, and illness (measles, varicella, human immunodeficiency virus/acquired immunodeficiency syndrome, toxoplasmosis, rubella, cytomegalovirus, herpes, syphilis, toxemia, and diabetes).

   (2) Personal risk factors include prematurity, perinatal hypoxia, birth trauma, delayed developmental milestones, head injury, near-drowning, toxic ingestion, including lead, meningitis, chronic illness, child abuse, chromosomal anomalies, and substance abuse.

   (3) Family risk factors include chromosomal anomalies, mental illness, neurologic disease, neurocutaneous disease, seizure disorders, mental retardation, learning problems, and neural tube defects.

2. Physical examination

a. **Vital signs**

   (1) Measure head circumference in all children under 2 years old and in older children when warranted (eg, suspected increased ICP).

   (2) Assess vital signs, because altered vital signs (hypertension, tachycardia leading to bradycardia, and apnea) are late signs of increased ICP.

b. **Inspection**

   (1) Assess LOC (full consciousness, confused, disoriented, lethargic, obtunded, stupor, or coma), general appearance, behavior, affect/mood, interactions, and speech. Behavioral change can be an early sign of a neurologic disorder. Note any memory loss, speech problems, or unusual habits.

   (2) Assess development, noting alterations in all areas (ie, cognitive, psychosocial, gross motor, and fine motor).

   (3) Assess cranial nerve function, such as pupillary response.

   (4) Assess taste, olfaction, and tactile sense, if needed.

   (5) Observe for clumsiness, abnormal movements such as tremors and tics, seizure activity, and sensory and motor problems.

   (6) Assess cerebellar status (ie, gait, balance, and coordination).

   (7) Assess reflexes, including infantile reflexes (see Table 1-5 in Chap. 1), later reflexes (eg, parachute), deep tendon reflexes, and superficial reflexes (Fig. 17-1).

c. **Palpation**

   (1) Palpate the fontanelles with infant in upright position. Fullness may indicate increased ICP.

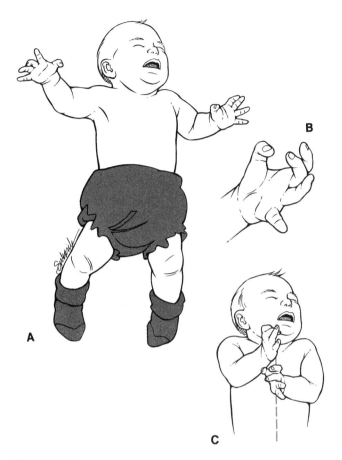

FIGURE 17-1
(A) An easily identified infantile reflex is the startle (or Moro) reflex in which the infant throws its arms out. **(B)** In the Moro reflex, the infant's hand assumes a classic "C" position. **(C)** During the startle reflex, the infant's arms return toward the body's midline. The startle reflex is never lost; however, the Moro reflex with the hand in a "C" position is indicative of a neurologic problem in an older child.

    (2) Assess muscle tone and strength.
    (3) Assess sensation and position sense.
    (4) Assess deep tendon and superficial reflexes.
  3. Laboratory studies and diagnostic tests (see Appendices A and B for normal findings and nursing considerations)
    a. **Blood studies** (eg, **complete blood count [CBC], blood culture**, and **lead test**) may be done to assess for infection, to detect toxic substances, and to monitor levels of seizure medication.
    b. **Urinalysis** may be performed to screen for toxicology.
    c. **Radiography** may be performed to detect fractures of the skull.
    d. **Electroencephalography (EEG)** may be performed to identify abnormal electrical brain discharges, as found in seizure disorders. The electric potential of the

brain is measured and recorded as electrodes placed on the scalp conduct and amplify electrical activity.

e. **Echoencephalography** records echoes from ultrasonic waves as they reflect off various surfaces of the skull. It identifies abnormal structure, position, and function. **Ultrasound** is also used to detect fetal defects, such as spina bifida.

f. **Computed tomographic (CT) scan** creates computerized images of horizontal and vertical cross-sections of the brain. It identifies abnormal tissue and structure, including tumors, bleeding, and hydrocephalus.

g. **Magnetic resonance imaging (MRI)** creates computerized images of the brain produced by radio frequency emissions from certain elements. MRI visualizes structures and tissue features at a level of detail not possible by other methods.

h. **Nuclear brain scan** identifies focal brain lesions and CSF pathways. The test measures abnormal uptake of radioactive contrast.

i. **A lumbar puncture** (LP, "spinal tap") involves the collection of CSF through a needle injected into the subarachnoid space of the spinal canal. The fluid is analyzed to measure pressure, assess chemistries, and detect infection. LP may also be used to administer medications.

B. Nursing diagnoses

1. Altered tissue perfusion
2. Risk for injury
3. Confusion
4. Altered thought processes
5. Risk for infection
6. Altered growth and development
7. Body image disturbance

C. Planning and outcome identification

1. The child will maintain or improve LOC and maintain normal ICP.
2. The child will maintain an optimal LOC and remain injury free.
3. The child will remain free of infection.
4. The child will perform at an optimal level of development.

D. Implementation

1. **Improve cerebral tissue performance**.

a. Assess neurologic status. In children with acute neurologic problems, perform neurologic checks of the following every 4 hours or more frequently.

(1) Vital sign assessment includes blood pressure, pulse, respiration, and temperature.

(2) LOC assessment includes Pediatric Coma Scale (assesses eye opening, verbal response, and motor response).

(3) Eye assessment includes pupil size, equality, and reaction to light; extraocular movements; corneal reflexes; and visual disturbances.

(4) Motor and sensory function assessment includes tone and movement in response to command and tactile or painful stimuli.

(5) Assess reflexes.

(6) Assess head circumference when appropriate.

(7) Assess fontanelles in infants.

b. Establish the child's baseline developmental level and assess for alterations.

c. Monitor the child's intake and output (I&O).

d. Administer medications, which may include those in Drug Chart 17-1.

e. Avoid placing the child in the prone position, in neck flexion, or in hip flexion. These positions can increase ICP.

DRUG CHART 17-1 Medications Used in Neurologic Disorders

Classification	Used for	Selected Interventions
Anticonvulsants—Long-term management	Seizure control	Monitor LOC and vital signs because many of these drugs cause sedation and respiratory depression.
carbamazepine (Tegretol)		Monitor for side effects, which include: Hepatic toxicity/failure, fatal cardiovascular complications, or potentially fatal hematologic complications.
valproic acid (Depakene)	Partial, generalized, and mixed seizures	Hepatic failure, thrombocytopenia, or hair loss
phenytoin (Dilantin)	Absence and multiple seizure types	Gum hyperplasia, hirsutism, ataxia, or depressed myocardial function
primidone (Mysoline)	Complex partial, generalized tonic-clonic	Vertigo, nystagmus, nausea, or vomiting
ethosuximide (Zarontin)		Rash, decreased leukocytes, irritability, anorexia, or abdominal pain
clonazepam (Klonopin)	Generalized tonic-clonic	Ataxia, weight gain, increased secretions, appetite changes, irritability
clorazepate (Tranxene)	Absence	Increased secretions
	Myoclonic, infantile spasms	
	Myoclonic	
Anticonvulsants—Short-term management	Status epilepticus	Monitor for side effects, which may include:
phenobarbital (Solfoton; can be used for long-term management)		Hyperactivity, GI upset, rash, or irritability
diazepam (Valium)		Respiratory arrest, slurred speech, or ataxia
fosphenytoin (Cerebyx)		Provide family teaching for all anticonvulsant use:
		Administer medications as directed. Do not stop without consulting health care provider.
		Monitor and report side effects.
		Provide mouth care as needed.
		Have blood levels monitored as directed.
		For adolescents:
		Adolescent must be seizure free for 1 year to obtain a driver's license.

(continued)

DRUG CHART 17-1   Medications Used in Neurologic Disorders (Continued)

Classification	Used for	Selected Interventions
		Anticonvulsants may decrease effectiveness of contraceptives.
		Anticonvulsants may increase acne; consult a dermatologist.
		Alcohol and drugs lower the seizure threshold and are best avoided.
Diuretics	Decrease ICP	Monitor vital signs (hypotension), respiratory status (pulmonary congestion), weight, and I&O.
		Monitor electrolytes.
		Monitor for other side effects:
mannitol (Osmitrol)		Dizziness, dry mouth, headache, or nausea
furosemide (Lasix)		Vertigo, weakness, rash, or muscle cramps
Neuromuscular blockers	Prevent agitation and resistance to mechanical ventilation	Monitor for prolongation of neuromuscular effects beyond the time needed by drug use.
pancuronium (Pavulon)		

GI, gastrointestinal; ICP, intracranial pressure; I&O, intake and output; LOC, level of consciousness.

    f. Raise the head of the bed (or use an infant seat) to a 35- to 45-degree angle because venous outflow drainage of the brain is facilitated by gravity.

    g. Keep emergency equipment near the bedside (eg, oxygen, suction, and a bag-valve mask).

2. Prevent injury.

    a. Institute seizure precautions.

      (1) If necessary, have the child wear a helmet, pad the bed's side rails, and have oxygen and suction equipment at the bedside.

      (2) During a seizure, *do not* restrain the child and *do not* place anything in her mouth.

      (3) During a seizure, remove harmful objects from the area, hyperextend the neck to maintain an airway, position the child on her side to allow secretions to flow from the mouth, loosen clothing, and observe the time and duration of the seizure.

    b. Orient the child to time, place, and person when appropriate for age.

    c. Maintain a safe environment by removing potential hazards.

    d. Ask a family member stay with the child, especially if the child is confused.

3. Prevent infection.

    a. Institute infection control measures.

    b. Minimize contact with infected persons.

    c. Ensure that the child is adequately immunized.

d. Use proper technique when caring for drainage tubes, dressings, and so on.

4. Promote optimal growth and development and minimize anxiety.

   a. Encourage and allow the child to participate in normal age-appropriate activities as much as possible.

   b. Explain all procedures and tests. Many of the specialized tests for neurologic function can be threatening to children.

      (1) Doll and puppet play is helpful for preschoolers.

      (2) Visual pictures of the machinery and explanations about the need to remain still during the scans are helpful to schoolagers.

   c. Allow young children to have transitional objects (eg, doll or blanket) with them during procedures.

   d. Encourage the child and family to verbalize their feelings. Neurologic deficits impede development and may cause significant psychosocial stress for the child and the family.

E. Outcome evaluation

   1. The child maintains or improves LOC.

   2. The child remains injury free.

   3. The child remains infection free.

   4. The child reaches an optimal level of development.

III. Increased intracranial pressure

A. Description. Increased ICP is excessive pressure within the rigid cranial vault that disrupts neurologic function.

B. Etiology

   1. Increased ICP can result from any alteration that increases tissue or fluid volume within the cranium, including:

      a. Tumors or other space-occupying lesions

      b. Accumulation of CSF in the ventricular system

      c. Intracranial bleeding

      d. Edema of the cerebral tissues

   2. Conditions that produce increased ICP include:

      a. Craniocerebral trauma

      b. Hydrocephalus

      c. Brain tumor

      d. Meningitis

      e. Encephalitis

      f. Intracerebral hemorrhage

C. Pathophysiology

   1. Normally, ICP remains relatively constant (within its normally fluctuating range) through a system of compensatory alterations among the cranium's contents (ie, brain tissue, meninges, CSF, and blood). Any increase in the volume of one component must be accompanied by a corresponding reduction in one or more of the others.

   2. After cranial sutures fuse and close, certain mechanisms can compensate for increasing intracranial volume—displacement of CSF to the spinal subarachnoid space and increased CSF absorption.

   3. An intracranial volume increase that exceeds the ability of the mechanisms to compensate produces signs and symptoms of increased ICP.

4. As ICP rises, it can trigger a cycle of decreasing perfusion, increasing edema, and further increased ICP. Left unchecked, this cycle can result in complete loss of cerebral arterial perfusion and brain cell death.

5. Brain stem compression secondary to herniation can cause life-threatening deterioration of vital functions.

D. Assessment findings

1. Clinical manifestations

a. Early signs and symptoms of increased ICP usually are subtle and include irritability, fatigue, and personality changes. Children with open fontanelles and sutures compensate by widening these spaces, but the compensation is limited.

b. Manifestations in infants and young children include:

(1) Tense, bulging anterior fontanelle

(2) High-pitched cry

(3) Increased occipital-frontal circumference (head circumference)

(4) "Setting sun" sign

(5) Macewen's sign ("cracked pot") in infants

(6) Irritability and restlessness

(7) Change in feeding habits

(8) Crying with cuddling and rocking

c. Manifestations in older children include:

(1) Headache

(2) Vomiting (usually projectile)

(3) Cognitive, personality, and behavioral changes (eg, indifference, declining school performance, diminished physical activity, and inability to follow simple commands)

(4) Diplopia and blurred vision

(5) Anorexia, nausea, and weight loss

(6) Seizures

d. Late manifestations of extremely high increased ICP include:

(1) Decreased LOC ranging from lethargy to coma

(2) Decreased motor response to commands

(3) Abnormal sensation to painful stimuli

(4) Decreased pupil size and reactivity

(5) Decerebrate (a sign of midbrain dysfunction manifested by rigid extension and pronation of the arms and legs) or decorticate (a sign of severe cerebral cortex dysfunction characterized by adduction of the arms at the shoulders, arms and wrists flexed over the chest, hands fisted, and legs extended and adducted) posturing

(6) Papilledema

(7) Abnormal breathing patterns, such as Cheyne-Stokes respirations (periods of hyperpnea alternating with apnea)

2. Laboratory and diagnostic study findings

a. Various devices (eg, intraventricular catheter with fibroscopic sensors attached to a monitoring system, subarachnoid bolt [Richmond screw], epidural sensor, or anterior fontanelle pressure monitor) will measure in-creased ICP.

b. CT scan and MRI are used to determine the underlying cause of increased ICP.

E. Nursing management

1. Assess for early changes in ICP by monitoring pressure range, vital signs, LOC, respiratory status, motor activity, behavior, and pupil size and reactivity.

2. **Administer prescribed medications**, which may include diuretics, corticosteroids, or both to control increased ICP (see Drug Chart 17-1).

3. **Keep head and neck neutral** in regard to the neck and shoulders by keeping the head elevated at 10° to 20°. Help the child avoid positions or activities that increase ICP, such as neck vein compression, flexion or extension of the neck, turning the head from side to side, and painful or stressful stimuli. Avoid performing respiratory suctioning or percussion because these may increase ICP.

4. **Assist with treatments and supportive measures**, such as those used to manage hyperventilation, provide mechanical ventilation, and prevent hypothermia.

5. **Prevent overhydration and underhydration** for adequate cerebral perfusion pressure; monitor I&O and impose fluid restrictions if needed.

6. **Promote normal bowel elimination** to prevent intra-abdominal pressure increase from straining at stool.

7. **Prevent weight loss**.
   a. Provide adequate nutrition in small, frequent feedings
   b. Administer intravenous (IV) nutrients if prescribed, or, possibly, through a gastrostomy tube if the child remains unconscious or is not sufficiently alert to take foods by mouth.

 8. **Promote optimal growth and development and minimize anxiety**. Do not overstimulate the child.

9. **Prevent skin breakdown** by placing the child on a sheepskin or other resilient mattress appliance.

10. As appropriate, **prepare the child for surgery** to relieve the increased ICP.

11. **Monitor for diabetes insipidus (DI) and syndrome of inappropriate antidiuretic hormone (SIADH)** which can occur as complications of increased ICP.
    a. DI characteristics include weight loss, hypotension, tachycardia, thirst, anxiety, depression, apathy, constipation, high urine output, low urine specific gravity, low urine osmolarity, high serum sodium, and a low volume of vascular fluid.
    b. SIADH characteristics include weight gain, hypertension, lethargy, coma, seizures, nausea, and vomiting, low urine output, high urine specific gravity, low serum sodium, and a high volume of vascular fluid.

IV. Seizure disorders

A. Description

1. Seizures are disturbances in normal brain function resulting from abnormal electrical discharges in the brain, which can cause loss of consciousness, uncontrolled body movements, changes in behaviors and sensation, and changes in the autonomic system.

2. The majority of seizures happen within the first years of life.

B. Etiology

1. There are many underlying possible causes such as prenatal or perinatal hypoxia, infections, congenital malformations, metabolic disturbances, lead poisoning, head injuries, drug abuse, alcohol misuse, tumors, medications, and toxins.

2. Many seizures are idiopathic.

3. There is some evidence of a genetic etiologic factor in which the seizure threshold is lowered in affected persons.

C. Pathophysiology

1. Seizures result from overly active and hypersensitive neurons in the brain that trigger excessive electrical discharges, causing a seizure.

2. The location of the abnormal cells and the pattern of discharges determine the clinical manifestations.

3. The three categories of seizures are generalized, partial, and unclassified.

   a. **Generalized seizures** involve both hemispheres of the brain, are bilateral and symmetrical, and may or may not involve prodromal syndromes.

   b. **Partial (focal) seizures** involve a limited area of the cerebral cortex; these may be simple or complex. Some children with complex partial seizures experience prodromes.

   c. Seizures may be termed **unclassified** when data are incomplete or inadequate. Neonatal seizures are considered unclassified.

D. Assessment findings

1. **Clinical manifestations**

   a. **Generalized seizures**

      (1) **Tonic-clonic (formerly grand mal) seizures** consist of tonic signs and symptoms—rigidity, extension of extremities, fixed jaw, respiratory cessation, and dilated pupils—and clonic signs and symptoms—rhythmic jerking of extremities, autonomic symptoms, and possible incontinence.

      (2) **Tonic seizures** are characterized by stiffening of the body.

      (3) **Clonic seizures** are characterized by clonic muscle activity.

      (4) **Atonic seizures** are characterized by a sudden loss of muscle tone followed by postictal confusion.

      (5) **Myoclonic seizures** are characterized by generalized short muscle contractions. The child will exhibit movements that are characteristic for her.

      (6) **Absence (formerly petite mal) seizures** are characterized by brief periods of unconsciousness or unawareness.

   b. **Partial seizures**

      (1) **Simple partial seizures** are characterized by maintenance of consciousness. They may also include a focal motor component (eg, abnormal movement of leg), a sensory component (eg, tingling, smell, sound, or taste), an autonomic component (eg, sweating), or a psychic component (eg, déjà vu or anger).

      (2) **Complex (psychomotor or temporal lobe) seizures** begin as simple and progress to unconsciousness. The child may stop whatever she is doing and engage in purposeless movement (eg, lip smacking or wandering), or may continue doing what she is doing but in an inappropriate manner.

   c. **Status epilepticus** involves recurrent or continuous, generalized seizure activity with the danger of cardiac arrest and brain damage.

   d. **Infantile spasm** refers to a rare disorder seen in the first few months of life that is characterized by signs such as brief flexion of the neck, trunk, or legs.

2. **Laboratory and diagnostic study findings**

   a. EEG will document abnormal activity.

   b. CBC and blood chemistries are used to assess for underlying disorders that may produce seizure activity, such as metabolic disturbances.

   c. Serum medication levels are used to monitor therapeutic levels of medications (if the child is taking anticonvulsant medications).

E. Nursing management

1. **Assess the child and obtain a thorough history** (eg, birth trauma, medications, injuries, illnesses, and family history).

2. **Administer prescribed medications**, which may include anticonvulsants (see Drug Chart 17-1).

3. **Prevent injury.**

4. Document all seizure activity, including:
 a. Apparent trigger factor, if known or suspected
 b. Behavior before the seizure; aura
 c. Time seizure began and ended
 d. Clinical manifestations of the seizure
 e. Postseizure behavior and symptoms
5. Help prevent seizures by preventing the child's exposure to known precipitants (eg, emotional stress or blinking lights).
6. Promote optimal growth and development and minimize the child's anxiety. Stay with the child during attacks and provide reassurance.
7. Prepare the family for alternative treatments when necessary.
 a. Surgery may be performed to remove a possible causative agent such as a tumor. Or, if seizures cannot be controlled by medications, surgery may be performed to remove the offending area of involvement, which can range from a lobe to a complete hemisphere, without causing further deficit.
 b. Vagus nerve stimulation may be performed by implanting a special device, which will reduce seizures in children who do not achieve adequate control with medications.
8. Provide child and family teaching, as discussed in Child and Family Teaching 17-1.

V. Neural tube defects (NTDs)

A. Description
 1. NTDs are a group of related defects of the CNS involving the cranium or spinal cord that vary from mildly to severely disabling. NTDs may be cystic or noncystic and include anencephaly, encephalocele, and spina bifida.
 2. NTDs are the largest group of congenital anomalies consistent with multifactorial inheritance.
 3. Many children with the myelomeningocele form of spina bifida have hydrocephalus.
B. Etiology
 1. Fifty percent of spina bifida cases are related to a nutritional deficiency, particularly a folic acid deficiency.
 2. The remaining cases are multifactorial.
C. Pathophysiology
 1. During the third to fourth week of gestation, the neural plate closes to form the neural tube that eventually forms the spinal cord and brain. The vertebral column develops along with the spinal cord.
 2. NTDs result from malformations of the neural tube during embryonic development.
 3. There are different types of NTDs.
 a. **Anencephaly** is a severe defect involving absence of the entire brain or cerebral hemispheres; the brain stem and cerebellum may be present. Total anencephaly is incompatible with life; many anencephalics are aborted or stillborn; living infants usually survive only a few hours.
 b. **Encephalocele** occurs when meningeal and cerebral tissue protrudes in a sac through a defect in the skull, with the occiput being the most common site. When possible, the brain is placed back in the skull. Many infants have hydrocephalus. In mild forms there is little or no residual neurologic impairment.
 c. **Spina bifida** is a defective closure of the vertebral column and is the most common defect of the CNS. Spina bifida may occur anywhere but usually occurs in the

Safety Measures for Children With Neurologic Impairments

- Be aware of the child's limitations, if any, and develop realistic goals.
- Foster healthy growth and development within the child's limitations. Promote as much self-care as possible, using assistive devices when needed.
- Avoid allowing the child to become over tired.
- Be familiar with the prescribed medication dose, administration, storage, and side effects. Be aware of the importance of not discontinuing the medication and of not switching to a different brand of the same medication.
- Understand the need for periodic reevaluation of medication effectiveness as well as close monitoring of blood cell counts, electrolyte levels, liver function, urinalysis, and vital signs.
- Fully understand how to use all of the child's medications, devices, and treatments.
- Make the home accessible to the child's mobility needs.
- Inform school personnel of the child's special needs.
- Prevent seizure activity:
  - Give medications as ordered.
  - Be aware of prodromal signs to watch for and steps to take if they occur.
  - Make sure the child avoids seizure-inducing activities, events, and stimuli.
  - Discourage the use of alcohol or illicit drugs.
- Report all side effects, even minor ones. Minor ones such as acne may cause noncompliance in adolescents.
- Have the child wear a medical alert bracelet or other identification alerting personnel to the seizure disorder.
- Teach the family how to manage seizures if they occur:
  Lie the child on side and stay with her.
  Loosen clothing and remove nearby hazardous objects, including eyeglasses.
  Allow the seizure to end without interference.
  Observe and document seizure activity, timing, precipitating event, and effects of the seizure (eg, loss of consciousness, paralysis, and so on).
  After the seizure ends, place the child in a side-lying position with the head midline.
  Call for medical assistance.
- Encourage adequate nutrition, rest, and exercise.

lumbosacral area. The three principal types of spina bifida are spina bifida occulta, meningocele, and myelomeningocele.

D. Assessment findings

1. Clinical manifestations

a. Manifestations vary with the degree of the defect. Defects other than spina bifida occulta are usually readily apparent on inspection. The degree of neurologic dysfunction is directly related to the anatomic level of the defect and, thus, to the nerves involved. Sensory disturbances usually parallel motor dysfunction.

b. Anencephaly is incompatible with life and most infants are stillborn.

c. Encephalocele symptoms are dependent on the presence of problems such as hydrocephalus and infection and the amount of neural tissue in the sac.

d. Spina bifida occulta usually does not affect the spinal cord. External signs may include dimpling of the skin, nevi, or hair tufts over a dermal sinus. It may go undetected, and most children do not display any neurologic signs. If they do occur, there usually is motor or sensory deficit of the lower extremities and involvement of the urinary and bladder sphincter.

 e. Meningocele is characterized by a sac, which contains meninges and CSF, protruding outside the vertebrae. The spinal cord is not involved and, therefore, there is usually little to no neurologic involvement.

 f. Myelomeningocele is similar to meningocele, but the spinal cord and accompanying nerve roots are involved. It is the most severe and most common type of spina bifida. Myelomeningocele involves sensorimotor deficits, urinary and bowel problems, and, possibly, in utero joint deformities such as congenital dislocation of the hip (CDH) and club foot. *— they cannot void and eliminate stool*

2. Laboratory and diagnostic study findings

 a. Assays of fetal amniotic fluid, ultrasonography, or maternal serum α-fetoprotein (MSAFP) concentrations will often detect the problem prenatally.

 b. Ultrasonography, CT, MRI, and myelography will evaluate the lesion, the amount of nerve involvement, and the degree of hydrocephalus in an infant born with myelomeningocele.

E. Nursing management

 1. Teach the family about the management required for the disorder.

  a. No treatment is indicated for spina bifida occulta unless there is neurologic damage. If a sinus is present, it may need to be closed.

  b. Meningocele requires closure as soon after birth as possible. The child should be monitored for hydrocephalus, meningitis, and spinal cord dysfunction.

  c. Myelomeningocele requires a multidisciplinary approach (ie, neurology, neurosurgery, pediatrics, urology, orthopedics, rehabilitation, and nursing). There is no cure. Closure is performed within 24 hours to minimize infection and prevent further damage to the spinal cord and roots; skin grafting may be necessary. Shunting is performed for hydrocephalus and antibiotics are initiated to prevent infection. The child will need correction of musculoskeletal deformities and management of urologic and bowel control problems.

 2. During the newborn period, assess and monitor vital signs, measure head circumference, and assess neurologic status, including signs of ICP.

 3. Monitor the child throughout childhood to detect the true extent of the disorder. Assess neurologic status, neuromuscular functioning, sensory perception, bowel and bladder control, sexual functioning, and psychosocial functioning.

 4. Administer prescribed medications. Antibiotics may be ordered to prevent infection; anticonvulsants may be ordered if seizures develop; and anticholinergics may be used for a neurogenic bladder (see Drug Chart 17-1).

 5. Prevent infection and injury.

  a. Preoperatively, apply a sterile dressing, constantly moistened with saline, to the lesion. Use protective devices and handle the infant with care.

  b. Preoperatively and postoperatively perform the following:

   (1) Maintain a sterile dressing.

   (2) Examine the dressing for leakage.

   (3) Avoid placing a diaper or other covering directly over the lesion (this could cause fecal contamination).

   (4) Monitor the child for signs of local infection and meningitis (eg, fever, irritability, and poor feeding).

  c. Position the infant in a prone or side-lying position to prevent contamination by stool or urine.

    d. Prevent hip subluxation by maintaining the legs in abduction with a pad between the knees and the feet in a neutral position with a roll under the ankles.

    e. Prevent skin breakdown by padding the bony prominences.

6. Prevent trauma from increased ICP because many children have associated hydrocephalus.

    a. Monitor head circumference and observe for signs of increased ICP.

    b. Minimize stress (increases ICP).

7. Prevent urinary complications.

    a. Assess urologic status.

    b. Instruct the child and family on self-catheterization.

    c. Prevent urinary tract infections (see Chap. 15).

    d. Maintain urinary diversion if the child has had this procedure.

8. Prevent trauma from latex allergy that results from repeated exposure to latex during surgeries and catheterizations.

    a. Screen for latex allergy.

    b. Administer antihistamines or steroids before surgery or procedures.

    c. Ensure that the child and family are aware of the child's allergy to latex and that they will inform medical and school personnel.

    d. Maintain a latex-free environment.

9. Prevent injury due to neuromuscular impairment.

    a. Carefully monitor the skin condition because the child may have decreased sensation in areas distal to the lesion, creating an increased chance for pressure sores.

    b. Promote mobility and turn the child frequently.

    c. Use caution in positioning the child because a lack of sensation makes the child unable to detect potential skin irritants (eg, wrinkled sheets, wheelchair belts, and so on).

10. Promote optimal bowel functioning because more than 90% of children with myelomeningocele have a neurogenic colon.

    a. Instruct the parents on colon training, which consists of timing, diet, exercise, posture, and rectal stimulation.

    b. Encourage a diet high in fiber and low in carbohydrates.

    c. Exercise the lower part of the body.

    d. Use the knee–chest position to put pressure on the abdomen and aid in bowel evacuation.

    e. Use rectal stimulation with digit (finger) or suppository.

11. Promote family coping.

    a. Explain the essentials of infant care, such as nutrition and elimination.

    b. Promote parent–infant relationship by encouraging parental participation with feeding, cuddling, and stimulation.

    c. Emphasize infection prevention and recognition of early signs and symptoms of infection and increased ICP. d/t hydrocephalus.

    d. Explain and demonstrate bladder and bowel management and skin care.

    e. Discuss the effects of immobilization and how to deal with them.

    f. Discuss the need for lifelong care.

    g. Encourage as much normalcy as possible. Most children suffer some degree of physical and cognitive impairment.

    f. Carefully assess the family's ability to care for the child and refer them for further assistance if needed.

    g. Encourage parents to verbalize their fears.

    h. Encourage parents to contact the Spinal Bifida Association of America.

12. Prevent the development of neural tube defects. Encourage women of child-bearing age to consume 0.4 mg of folic acid every day during the preconceptual period (recommended by the U.S. Department of Public Health). They should consult their primary care provider or pharmacist to ensure that their multivitamin contains this amount.

VI. Hydrocephalus

A. Description
1. Hydrocephalus is a condition caused by an imbalance in the production and absorption of CSF in the ventricular system. When production exceeds absorption, CSF accumulates, usually under pressure, producing dilation of the ventricles.
2. Hydrocephalus occurs with a number of anomalies, such as NTDs.

B. Etiology
1. Congenital hydrocephalus usually results from defects, such as Chairi malformations. It also is associated with spina bifida.
2. Acquired hydrocephalus usually results from space-occupying lesions, hemorrhage, intracranial infections, or dormant developmental defects.

C. Pathophysiology
1. The primary site of CSF formation is believed to be the choroid plexuses of the lateral ventricles. CSF flows from the lateral ventricles through the foramen of Monro to the third ventricle, then through the aqueduct of Sylvius into the fourth ventricle through the foramen of Luschka and the midline foramen of Magendie into the cisterna magna. From there it flows to the cerebral and cerebellar subarachnoid spaces where it is absorbed. How it is absorbed is not clear.
2. Causes of hydrocephalus are varied but result in either impaired absorption of CSF within the arachnoid space (formerly referred to as communicating hydrocephalus) or obstruction to the flow of CSF through the ventricular system (formerly referred to as noncommunicating hydrocephalus).
3. Most cases of obstruction are the result of developmental malformations; other causes include neoplasms, infection, and trauma. Obstruction to the normal flow can occur at any point in the CSF pathway, which produces increased pressure and dilation of the pathways proximal to the site of obstruction.
4. Impaired absorption can result from meningitis, prenatal maternal infections, meningeal malignancy (secondary to leukemia or lymphoma), an arachnoid cyst, and tuberculosis.

D. Assessment findings
1. **Clinical manifestations**
   a. Manifestations in infants include abnormal rate of head growth, bulging fontanelle, tense anterior fontanelle (often bulging and nonpulsatile), dilated scalp veins, Macewen's sign ("cracked pot"), frontal bossing, setting sun sign, sluggish and unequal pupils, irritability and lethargy with varying LOC, abnormal infantile reflexes, and possible cranial nerve damage.
   b. Manifestations in children include possible signs of increased ICP, which include headache on awakening with improvement following emesis, papilledema, strabismus, ataxia, irritability, lethargy, apathy, and confusion. *or diplopia*
2. **Laboratory and diagnostic study findings**
   a. Level II ultrasonography of the fetus will allow a prenatal diagnosis. (Transuterine placement of ventriculoamniotic shunts during late pregnancy is still being developed as a treatment modality.)
   b. CT scan will diagnose most cases postnatally.
   c. MRI can be used if a complex lesion is suspected.

E. Nursing management

1. Teach the family about the management required for the disorder.

a. Treatment is surgical by direct removal of the obstruction and insertion of shunts to provide primary drainage of the CSF to an extracranial compartment, usually the peritoneum (ventriculoperitoneal shunt).

(1) The major complications of shunts are infections and malfunction.

(2) Other complications include subdural hematoma caused by a too rapid reduction of CSF, peritonitis, abdominal abscess, perforation of organs, fistulas, hernias, and ileus.

b. A third ventriculostomy is a new nonshunting procedure used to treat children with hydrocephalus.

2. Provide preoperative nursing care.

a. Assess head circumference, fontanelles, cranial sutures, and LOC; check also for irritability, altered feeding habits, and a high-pitched cry.

b. Firmly support the head and neck when holding the child.

c. Provide skin care for the head to prevent breakdown.

d. Give small, frequent feedings to decrease the risk of vomiting.

e. Encourage parental-newborn bonding.

3. Provide postoperative nursing care (nursing interventions are the same as those for increased ICP).

a. Assess for signs of increased ICP and check the following: head circumference (daily), anterior fontanelle for size and fullness, and behavior.

b. Administer prescribed medications, which may include antibiotics to prevent infection and analgesics for pain.

c. Provide shunt care.

(1) Monitor for shunt infection and malfunction, which may be characterized by a rapid onset of vomiting, severe headache, irritability, lethargy, fever, redness along the shunt tract, and fluid around the shunt valve.

(2) Prevent infection (usually from *Staphylococcus epidermis* or *Staphylococcus aureus*).

(3) Monitor for shunt overdrainage (headache, dizziness, and nausea). Overdrainage may lead to slit ventricle syndrome whereby the ventricles become accustomed to a very small or slitlike configuration, limiting the buffering ability to increased ICP variations.

4. Teach home care.

a. Encourage the child to participate in age-appropriate activities as tolerated. Encourage the parents to provide as normal a lifestyle as possible. Remind both the child and parents that contact sports are prohibited.

b. Explain how to recognize signs and symptoms of increased ICP. Subtle signs include changes in school performance, intermittent headache, and mild behavioral changes.

c. Arrange for the child to have frequent developmental screenings and routine medical checkups.

VII. Reye's syndrome

A. Description

1. Reye's syndrome is an acute, multisystem disorder that follows a mild viral infection, usually influenza or varicella.

2. Early diagnosis and management are critical because the disorder has a rapid onset and can lead to death in hours.

B. Etiology

1. The cause remains unclear. However, three antecedents are frequently associated with its onset—respiratory infection, varicella, and diarrhea.
2. Salycilates, acetaminophen, toxins, and antidiarrheal drugs have all been linked to Reye's syndrome.
3. Warnings of the association between aspirin and Reye's syndrome have resulted in the decreased use of aspirin and a subsequent decrease in Reye's syndrome.

C. Pathophysiology

1. The disorder is characterized by encephalopathy and fatty degeneration of the liver.
2. Cell mitochondria are injured and become large and swollen causing cerebral edema and fatty infiltration of the liver, kidneys, and heart.
3. Hyperammonemia results from a reduction in the enzyme that converts ammonia to urea.

D. Assessment findings

1. **Clinical manifestations.** Although Reye's syndrome progresses in stages, deterioration can occur in 24 to 48 hours.
   a. **Stage I manifestations** include vomiting, lethargy, confusion, rhythmic slowing of EEG, and liver dysfunction.
   b. **Stage II manifestations** include disorientation, combativeness, hyperventilation, hallucinations, appropriate responses to painful stimuli, and liver dysfunction.
   c. **Stage III manifestations** include coma, decorticate rigidity, hyperventilation, and preservation of pupillary and ocular reflexes.
   d. **Stage IV manifestations** include deepened coma, decerebrate rigidity, loss of oculocephalic reflexes, large fixed pupils, and evidence of brain stem dysfunction.
   e. **Stage V manifestations** include seizures, flaccidity, respiratory arrest, and loss of deep tendon reflexes.
2. **Laboratory and diagnostic study findings**
   a. Liver function tests will detect elevated ammonia levels, elevated alanine aminotransferase (ALT; formerly serum glutamic oxaloacetic transaminase [SGOT]), aspartate aminotransferase (AST; formerly serum glutamate pyruvate transaminase [SGPT]), and lactic dehydrogenase (LDH) levels.
   b. Coagulation studies will detect prolonged prothrombin time.
   c. In children with hypoglycemia, arterial blood gasses will reveal a ventilatory and acid–base imbalance with respiratory alkalosis (increased pH, decreased $Paco_2$, and normal HCO_3) and metabolic acidosis (decreased pH, normal $Paco_2$, and decreased HCO_3).
   d. Liver biopsy is performed only if the diagnosis is unclear.

E. Nursing management. Management of increased ICP and fluid and electrolyte imbalance is a primary concern; children are treated in the intensive care setting, and an arterial line and a central venous line are inserted to monitor hemodynamic status.

1. **Monitor for increased ICP.**
   a. Inspect ICP monitor readings.
   b. Take regular arterial and venous pressures.
   c. Monitor blood gas levels. ↑$Paco_2$ ↓pH
   d. Check neurologic status.
2. **Administer prescribed medications.** A drug-induced coma may result when phenobarbital or pentobarbital with pancuronium (Pavulon) is given to paralyze skeletal muscles; hypoglycemia is controlled with hypertonic glucose and saline solution; vitamin K may be given to correct abnormal clotting.

3. **Maintain a patent airway.** The child is usually on a ventilator.
4. **Control increased ICP and monitor I&O.** Fluids may be restricted.
5. **Control hypothermia** with acetaminophen, tepid baths, and a hypothermia blanket.
6. **Prevent infection** in children who have an indwelling catheter.
7. **Monitor nasogastric output** for amount and character in children who have a nasogastric tube to prevent compression.
8. **Provide care for the child who is in a drug-induced coma and totally dependent on caregivers.**
   a. Satisfy all biologic needs.
   b. Provide sensory stimulation.
   c. Ensure adequate nutritional intake, usually IV or by nasogastric tube until the child can take food orally.
9. **Support family members.** Allow them to express their concerns and provide information on the disease process and treatment. Parents may feel guilty if they administered aspirin to their child.
10. **Promote prevention and early identification.** Teach parents not to give aspirin for viral syndromes, without the advice of their health care provider.

11. Decrease environmental stimuli
12. Check for jaundice

VIII. Head injury

A. Description

1. A head injury can be anything from a mild bump to severe damage to the head. The term encompasses everything from minor lacerations to diffuse brain injury.
2. Head injury is one of the most common causes of disability and death in children.
3. Major types of head injury include skull fractures, brain injury, and hematomas.
   a. Type, extent, and accompanying symptoms of **skull fractures** depend on the velocity, force, and mass of the object; on the area of skull involved; and on the age of the child. Fracture types include:
      (1) Linear fractures usually resemble a thin line. There usually are no other signs than those found on x-ray film. The child is observed for neurologic changes, and the fracture heals on its own.
      (2) Comminuted fractures have a "cracked eggshell" appearance. They also may be classified as depressed.
      (3) Depressed fractures show the skull indented at the point of impact, which may cause compression, shifting of the brain tissue, and intracranial damage. Symptoms depend on what area of the brain is damaged.
      (4) Basal fractures are the most serious and consist of a linear fracture through the base of the skull.
      (5) Diastatic fractures occur along a suture line. These usually do not occur at the site of impact and are frequently seen in newborns.
   b. Signs and symptoms of **brain injury** depend on the location and severity of the head injury.
   c. Epidural (between the skull and the dura) and subdural (between the dura and the arachnoid layer) **hematomas** are the most common types.

B. Etiology

1. Head injury usually is caused by motor vehicle accidents, abuse, falls, and birth trauma, with the etiology related to the child's age.

2. Factors that contribute to head injury include seizure disorders, gait instability, cognitive delays, poor judgment, and alcohol and drug use.

C. Pathophysiology

1. Pathophysiology is directly related to the force of the impact.

2. Intracranial contents are damaged when the force is too great to be absorbed by the skull.

D. Assessment findings

1. Clinical manifestations

    a. Specific signs and symptoms of a **basal fracture** are "raccoon eyes" (blood leakage into the frontal sinuses) and a "battle sign" (bruising behind the ear from bleeding into the mastoid sinus). Basal fractures may be accompanied by a CSF leak into the ears or nose and may cause cranial nerve damage.

    b. Post-traumatic syndromes (eg, seizures, hydrocephalus, or focal neurologic deficits) and metabolic complications (eg, diabetes insipidus, hyponatremia or hypernatremia, or hyperglycemic hyperosmolar states) of a **brain injury** may occur up to 2 years after the injury.

    c. An **epidural** hematoma is manifested by a rapid onset. It is life-threatening and characterized by rapid deterioration, headache, seizures, coma, and brain herniation with compression of the brain stem.

    d. A **subdural hematoma** occurs within 48 hours of injury and is characterized by headache, agitation, confusion, drowsiness, decreased LOC, and increased ICP. Chronic subdural hematomas may also occur.

    e. **General minor characteristics of head trauma**

        (1) Loss of consciousness (possible)

        (2) Transient confusion

        (3) Listlessness and irritability

        (4) Pallor and vomiting

    f. **Signs of injury progression**

        (1) Altered mental status

        (2) Increasing agitation

        (3) Development of focal signs

        (4) Marked changes in vital signs

        (5) Hyporesponsive, hyperresponsive, or nonexistent reflexes

2. Laboratory and diagnostic study findings

    a. Radiography may reveal fractures.

    b. CT or MRI is used to view brain injuries and hematomas.

    c. CBC, blood chemistries, toxicology screening, and a urinalysis may be ordered to test for associated factors and complications.

E. Nursing management

1. Promote prevention, especially of falls. Urge children to wear bike helmets, use seat belts, and practice safe driving (adolescents).

2. Perform the following neurologic assessments.

    a. Cerebral functioning (ie, alertness, orientation, memory, and speech)

    b. Vital signs (check for increased blood pressure and decreased pulse)

    c. Pupils

    d. Motor and sensory function (testing must be appropriate for the child's developmental stage)

3. Assess for other injuries, especially cervical injuries. Do not move the child until the possibility of cervical injury has been ruled out or managed. Raise the head of the bed to 30° if there is no cervical injury.

See NCLEX p. 379 Crit. Thinking

4. **Monitor for complications**, which can develop rapidly.
   a. Monitor vital signs and neurologic status frequently.
   b. Check for increased ICP.
   c. Check for drainage from the nose and ears (eg, CSF or blood). *fluid out from nose. CSF + (+) for glucose.*
5. **Use planning and intervention strategies for increased ICP.**
6. **Provide child and family teaching.**
   a. Teach signs of increased ICP. *★ check if fluid is (+) for gluco*
   b. When warranted, teach that seizures may occur for up to 2 years after the injury.
   c. When warranted, explain that the child may also have extensive damage requiring rehabilitation.
   d. Encourage the child and family to verbalize their concerns and refer them to the National Head Injury Foundation, if needed.

IX. Mental retardation

A. Description

1. Mental retardation is part of a broad category of developmental disability and defined by the American Association of Mental Deficiency as "... significantly subaverage, general intellectual functioning existing concurrently with deficits in adaptive behavior and manifested during the developmental period (18 years of age)."
2. Adaptive behaviors include communication, self-care, work, leisure, health, and safety.

B. Etiology

1. A diagnosis of mental retardation cannot be made on the basis of intellectual ability alone; there must be both intellectual and adaptive (personal independence and social responsibility) impairment.
2. Causes of mental retardation are genetic, biochemical, viral, and developmental.
   a. Prenatal infection and intoxication
   b. Trauma or physical agent (eg, lack of oxygen)
   c. Metabolic disturbance
   d. Inadequate prenatal nutrition
   e. Gross postnatal brain disease (eg, neurofibromatosis or tuberous sclerosis)
   f. Chromosomal abnormalities
   g. Prematurity
   h. Low birth weight
   i. Autism
   j. Environmental deprivation
3. Associated factors include:
   a. Maternal lifestyles (eg, poor nutrition, smoking, and substance abuse).
   b. Chromosomal disorders (most related to Down syndrome)
   c. Specific disorders, such as fetal alcohol syndrome
   d. Cerebral palsy, microcephaly, or infantile spasms

C. Pathophysiology

1. Pathophysiology depends on the cause; early diagnosis and prompt treatment may be particularly important in cases involving an identifiable and possibly correctable cause, such as phenylketonuria (PKU), malnutrition, or child abuse.
2. Diagnosis usually is made after a period of suspicion. Diagnosis may be made at birth from recognition of specific syndromes such as Down syndrome. Diagnosis and classification are based on standard IQ test scores.

D. Assessment findings
  1. **Clinical manifestations**. Findings vary depending on the classification or degree of retardation (ie, mild, moderate, severe, or profound).
    a. **Mild (50–70 IQ)**
      (1) Preschool. The child often is not noted as retarded, but is slow to walk, talk, and feed self.
      (2) School-age. The child can acquire practical skills, and learn to read and do arithmetic to sixth-grade level with special education classes. The child achieves a mental age of 8 to 12 years.
      (3) Adult. The adult can usually achieve social and vocational skills. Occasional guidance may be needed. The adult may handle marriage, but not child rearing.
    b. **Moderate (35–55 IQ)**
      (1) Preschool. Noticeable delays, especially in speech, are evident.
      (2) School-age. The child can learn simple communication, health, and safety habits, and simple manual skills. A mental age of 3 to 7 years is achieved.
      (3) Adult. The adult can perform simple tasks under sheltered conditions and can travel alone to familiar places. Help with self-maintenance is usually needed.
    c. **Severe (20–40 IQ)**
      (1) Preschool. The child exhibits marked motor delay and has little to no communication skills. The child may respond to training in elementary self-help, such as feeding.
      (2) School-age. The child usually walks with disability. Some understanding of speech and response is evident. The child can respond to habit training and has the mental age of a toddler.
      (3) Adult. The adult can conform to daily routines and repetitive activities, but needs constant direction and supervision in a protective environment.
    d. **Profound (below 20 IQ)**
      (1) Preschool. Gross retardation is evident. There is a capacity for function in sensorimotor areas, but the child needs total care.
      (2) School-age. There are obvious delays in all areas. The child shows basic emotional response and may respond to skillful training in the use of legs, hands, and jaws. The child needs close supervision and has the mental age of a young infant.
      (3) Adult. The adult may walk but needs complete custodial care. The adult will have primitive speech. Regular physical activity is beneficial.

E. Nursing management
  1. **Assess all children for signs of developmental delays.**
  2. **Administer prescribed medications** for associated problems such as anticonvulsants for seizure disorders, and methylphenidate (Ritalin) for attention deficit hyperactivity disorder (see Drug Chart 17-1).
  3. **Support the family at the time of initial diagnosis** by actively listening to their feelings and concerns and assessing their composite strengths.
  4. **Facilitate the child's self-care abilities** by encouraging the parents to enroll the child in an early stimulation program, establishing a self-feeding program, initiating independent toileting, and establishing an independent grooming program (all developmentally appropriate).

5. Promote optimal development by encouraging self-care goals and emphasizing the universal needs of children, such as play, social interaction, and parental limit setting.

6. Promote anticipatory guidance and problem solving by encouraging discussion regarding physical maturation and sexual behaviors.

7. Assist the family in planning for the child's future needs (eg, alternative to home care, especially as the parents near old age); refer them to community agencies.

8. Provide child and family teaching.

  a. Identify normal developmental milestones and appropriate stimulating activities, including play and socialization.

  b. Discuss the need for patience with the child's slow attainment of developmental milestones.

  c. Inform parents about stimulation, safety, and motivation.

  d. Supply information regarding normal speech development and how to accentuate nonverbal cues, such as facial expressions and body language, to help cue speech development.

  e. Explain the need for discipline that is simple, consistent, and appropriate to the child's development.

  f. Review an adolescent's need for simple, practical sexual information that includes anatomy, physical development, and conception.

  g. Demonstrate ways to foster learning other than verbal explanation because the child is better able to deal with concrete objects than abstract concepts.

  h. Point out the importance of positive self-esteem, built by accomplishing small successes, in motivating the child to accomplish other tasks.

9. Encourage the prevention of mental retardation.

  a. Encourage early and regular prenatal care.

  b. Provide support for high-risk infants.

  c. Administer immunizations, especially rubella immunization.

  d. Encourage genetic counseling when needed.

  e. Teach injury prevention—both intentional and unintentional.

X. Down syndrome

A. Description. Down syndrome, a disorder of chromosome 21, is the most common chromosomal abnormality.

B. Etiology

  1. The cause is unknown and multiple theories exist. The concept of multiple causality is most accepted.

  2. Cytogenetics of the disorder are well established.

  a. Approximately 92% to 95% of cases are attributed to an extra chromosome 21, hence the name trisomy 21.

  b. About 3% to 6% of cases may be caused by translocation of chromosomes 15 (and 21 or 22).

  c. From 1% to 3% of persons demonstrate mosaicism (cells with both normal and abnormal chromosomes).

  3. Children with Down syndrome are born to parents of all ages. Although there is a higher incidence among mothers over age 35, most are born to mothers under age 35 (80%).

C. **Pathophysiology**. The degree of cognitive and physical impairment is related to the percentage of cells with the abnormal chromosome makeup.

D. **Assessment findings**

1. **Clinical manifestations** include:
   a. Separated sagittal suture
   b. Oblique palpebral fissures
   c. Small nose
   d. Depressed nasal bridge
   e. High-arched palate
   f. Skin excess and laxity
   g. Wide space and plantar crease between the big and second toe
   h. Hyperextensible and lax joints
   i. Muscle weakness

2. Other **common findings** include a small penis, short, broad hands (transverse [simian] palmar crease), a protruding tongue, small ears, Brushfield spots, and dry skin.

3. **Associated problems and features** include:
   a. Intelligence varies from severely retarded to low normal but is usually in the mild to moderate range.
   b. Social development may be 2 to 3 years beyond mental age; temperament range is similar to normal children, with a trend toward the easy child.
   c. Congenital anomalies include congenital heart disease (especially septal defects), renal agenesis, duodenal atresia, Hirschsprung disease, tracheoesophageal fistula, and skeletal deformities.
   d. Sensory problems include strabismus, nystagmus, myopia, hyperopia, excessive tearing and cataracts, and conductive hearing loss.
   e. Other physical disorders include respiratory infections, leukemia, and thyroid dysfunction.
   f. Growth is reduced, and there is rapid weight gain.
   g. Sexual development may be delayed, incomplete, or both. Male genitalia and secondary characteristics are underdeveloped. Breast development is mild to moderate with menarche at appropriate age. Women may be fertile; men are infertile.

E. **Nursing management**

1. **Assess for associated problems.**
2. **Administer medications,** which may be prescribed for associated problems.
3. **Implement a plan of care** that is the same as for mental retardation. Include planning and intervention strategies for associated problems and features.
4. **Encourage genetic counseling**.
5. **Explain hypertonicity and joint hyperextensibility** to parents, and that the child's resultant lack of clinging is physiologic and not a sign of detachment.
6. **Prevent respiratory infections** by clearing the nose with a bulb syringe, using a cool mist vaporizer, performing chest physiotherapy when needed, providing good handwashing, and avoiding exposure to infection.
7. **When feeding infants and young children, use a small, straight-handled spoon to push food to the side and back of the mouth**. Feeding difficulties occur due to a protruding tongue and hypotonia.
8. **Encourage fluids and foods rich in fiber**. Constipation results from decreased muscle tone, which affects gastric motility.
9. **Provide good skin care** because the skin is dry and prone to infection.

XI. Lead poisoning (plumbism)

A. Definition

1. Lead poisoning is one of the most common pediatric problems in the United States. It results from ingesting or inhaling lead-containing substances.
2. The highest incidence of lead poisoning occurs in late infancy and toddlerhood.

B. Etiology

1. The child is exposed to, and can become poisoned with, lead by one of three ways—eating contaminated food or nonfood substances, breathing contaminated air, or drinking contaminated water.
2. Exposure to household dust or yard soil contaminated with lead is the predominant cause of lead poisoning. Lead poisoning can also occur when the infant or child is exposed to any of the following sources of lead—paint chips, powder from paint, gasoline, unglazed ceramic containers, lead crystal, water from lead pipes, batteries, folk remedies, fishing weights, furniture refinishing supplies, art supplies, cosmetics, and even certain industrial pollutants.

C. Pathophysiology

1. Lead, which is very slowly excreted through the kidney, gastrointestinal tract, and slightly through sweat, is stored chiefly in the bone. When the rate of absorption surpasses the rate of excretion, lead is deposited into soft tissues of the body and bone and attaches itself to red blood cells. In the erythrocytes, it interferes with the production of heme and the formation of hemoglobin, which results in a microcytic, hypochromic anemia.
2. Lead affects the kidneys by altering the permeability of the proximal tubules, resulting in increased urinary elimination of glucose and protein.
3. Lead deposits also increase vascular permeability, resulting in fluid shifts that lead to encephalopathy and increased ICP.

D. Assessment findings

1. **Associated finding**. A history of pica may be determined.
2. **Clinical manifestations**
   a. Hematologic manifestations include signs of anemia.
   b. Renal manifestations include glycosuria, proteinuria, ketonuria, and hyperphosphaturia.
   c. Gastrointestinal manifestations include acute crampy abdominal pain, vomiting, constipation, and anorexia.
   d. Musculoskeletal manifestations include short stature and lead lines in bones on x-ray films.
   e. Neurologic (CNS) manifestations
      (1) Low-dose lead exposure causes behavioral changes such as distractibility, hyperactivity, impulsivity, learning problems, hearing impairment, and mild intellectual deficits.
      (2) High-dose lead exposure causes lead encephalopathy, which is manifested by seizures, mental retardation, paralysis, blindness, coma, and death.
3. **Laboratory and diagnostic study findings**
   a. Lead tests will reveal a serum lead level exceeding 10 µg/dL (considered positive for lead poisoning).
   b. Traditionally, elevated erythrocyte protoporphyrin (EP) levels were considered positive for lead poisoning, but the Centers for Disease Control and Prevention (CDC)

currently suggests not using EP levels because they do not always detect elevated lead levels in children.

E. Nursing management

1. Minimize the consequences of lead exposure.
   a. Monitor the child for manifestations of lead toxicity.
   b. Administer chelation therapy, as prescribed.
      (1) Edetate calcium disodium (CaNa$_2$EDTA)
         (a) Carefully monitor renal functioning; appearance of sediment in urine may signal renal failure.
         (b) Give medication by IV route; if medication must be given intramuscularly (IM) (eg, if client has encephalopathy), administer with procaine.
         (c) Monitor for side effects, which include nephrotoxicity, headache, anorexia, vomiting, elevated liver function tests, and electrocardiographic (ECG) changes.
      (2) Dimercaprol (BAL)
         (a) Do not give this medication to children who are allergic to peanuts (medication contains peanut oil) or to children with glucose-6-phosphate dehydrogenase deficiency.
         (b) Because the medication forms a toxic compound with iron, start iron therapy at least 24 hours after BAL administration finishes. This medication must be administered deeply IM.
         (c) Monitor for side effects, which include increased blood pressure, tachycardia, nausea and vomiting, burning sensation in mouth area, muscle pain or weakness, mild conjunctivitis, and paresthesias.
      (3) Succimer (Chemet)
         (a) Administer succimer orally; the capsule can be opened and sprinkled on food.
         (b) Monitor for side effects, which include nausea, vomiting, diarrhea, elevated liver function tests, and neutropenia.
   c. Prepare the child and family for interventions, which vary according to lead level scores.
      (1) Rescreen for lead in 1 year when the lead level is less than 10 μg/dL.
      (2) Rescreen and provide family with lead education materials when the lead level is 10 to 14 μg/dL.
      (3) Rescreen, look for sources, and educate parents when the lead level is 15 to 19 μg/dL. If this lead level persists, initiate actions for a lead level of 20 to 44 μg/dL.
      (4) Conduct a medical examination; identify and eliminate sources of lead when the lead level is 20 to 44 μg/dL.
      (5) Begin treatment and environmental clearance in 48 hours when the lead level is 45 to 69 μg/dL.
      (6) Begin treatment and environmental clearance immediately when the lead level is 70 μg/dL and over.
   d. Encourage fluids to enhance lead excretion.
   e. Monitor fluid I&O to evaluate kidney function.
   f. Perform prescribed serial urine testing during chelation therapy to monitor kidney status and the rate and volume of lead excretion. Draw blood for analysis of serum lead. Additional routine analyses of serum blood urea nitrogen and creatine levels and urine protein concentration detect possible drug toxicity.

CHILD AND FAMILY TEACHING 17-2

Prevention of Lead Poisoning

- Ensure that your child does not have access to peeling paint or chewable surfaces that are coated with lead-based paint.
- Wash and dry your child's hands frequently.
- If soil is likely to be contaminated, plant grass or other ground cover.
- If you are remodeling an old home, follow correct procedures.
- Use only cold water from the tap for consumption, especially when preparing formula.
- Have your water and soil tested by a competent laboratory.
- Do not store food in opened cans.
- Do not use inadequately fired ceramic ware or pottery for food or drink.
- Do not store food or drink in lead crystal.
- Avoid folk remedies or cosmetics that may contain lead.
- Avoid home exposure to lead from occupations or hobbies.
- Make sure that your child eats regular meals and consumes adequate amounts of iron and calcium.

2. **Prevent further exposure to lead**.
   a. Provide child and family teaching regarding prevention of lead poisoning (Child and Family Teaching 17-2).
   b. Make a home referral for lead removal.

STUDY QUESTIONS

1. Which of the following would the nurse identify as normal when assessing infantile reflexes in a 9-month-old?
   (1) Robust Moro
   (2) Unilateral grasp
   (3) Persistent rooting
   (4) Bilateral parachute

2. When caring for a child with increased intracranial pressure, which of the following, if stated by the parents, would indicate a need to reexplain the purpose for elevating the head of the bed 10° to 20°?
   (1) Maintain a neutral position
   (2) Help alleviate headache
   (3) Reduce intra-abdominal pressure
   (4) Increase intrathoracic pressure

3. Early clinical manifestations of increased intracranial pressure (ICP) in older children include which of the following?
   (1) Macewen's sign
   (2) Setting sun sign
   (3) Papilledema
   (4) Diplopia

4. Which of the following would be the lowest priority for a child with a seizure disorder?
   (1) Teaching the family about anticonvulsant drug therapy
   (2) Assessing for signs and symptoms of increased ICP
   (3) Ensuring safety and protection from injury
   (4) Observing and recording all seizures

5. After teaching the parents about their child's unique psychological needs related to a seizure disorder and possible stressors, which of the following concerns voiced by them would indicate the need for additional teaching?
   (1) Poor self-image
   (2) Dependency
   (3) Feeling different from peers
   (4) Cognitive delays

6. Which of the following is the most useful tool in diagnosing seizure disorder?
   (1) Electroencephalography (EEG)
   (2) Lumbar puncture (LP)
   (3) Brain scan
   (4) Skull radiographs

7. Which of the following definitions **most** accurately describes meningocele?
   (1) Complete exposure of the spinal cord and meninges
   (2) Herniation of spinal cord and meninges into a sac
   (3) Sac formation containing meninges and spinal fluid
   (4) Spinal cord tumor containing nerve roots

8. The primary reason for surgical repair of a myelomeningocele is to do which of the following?
   (1) Correct the neurologic defect
   (2) Prevent hydrocephalus
   (3) Prevent seizure disorders
   (4) Decrease the risk of infection

9. Which of the following would not be a focus of a teaching plan for an adolescent with a seizure disorder?
   (1) Obtaining a driver's license
   (2) Increased risk for infections
   (3) Drug and alcohol use
   (4) Peer pressure

10. The development of Reye's syndrome has been associated with the use of aspirin and which of the following?
    (1) Varicella
    (2) Meningitis
    (3) Encephalitis
    (4) Strep throat

11. Signs of mild mental retardation would include which of the following?
    (1) Lateness in walking
    (2) Mental age of a toddler
    (3) Noticeable developmental delays
    (4) Few communication skills

12. Which of the following would the nurse expect to assess in a child with Down syndrome?
    (1) Large nose
    (2) Small tongue
    (3) Oblique palpebral fissures
    (4) Low-arched palate

13. The American Association of Mental Deficiency definition of mental retardation stresses which of the following?
(1) No responsiveness to contact
(2) Deficits in adaptive behavior with intellectual impairment
(3) Cognitive impairment occurring after age 22 years
(4) An IQ level that must be below 50

14. When teaching parents about the early signs and symptoms of lead poisoning, which of the following, if stated by the parents, would indicate the need for additional teaching?
(1) Anorexia
(2) Irritability
(3) Seizures
(4) Anemia

ANSWER KEY

1. The answer is (4). The parachute reflex appears at approximately 9 months of age and is normal. All of the following are considered abnormal when evaluating infantile reflexes: reflexes that are absent when they should be present (Moro), reflexes that are unilateral (grasp), and reflexes that persist after they should have disappeared (rooting).

2. The answer is (4). Head elevation decreases, not increases, intrathoracic pressure. Elevating the head of the bed in a child with increased ICP helps to maintain neutral position, alleviate headache, and reduce intra-abdominal pressure, which may contribute to increased ICP.

3. The answer is (4). Diplopia is an early sign of increased ICP in an older child. The Macewen's sign ("cracked pot" sign) and the setting sun appearance of the eyes are noted in infants with increased ICP. Papilledema is a late sign of increased ICP.

4. The answer is (2). Signs and symptoms of increased ICP are not associated with seizure activity and therefore would be the lowest priority. Improper administration of and incomplete compliance with anticonvulsant therapy can lead to status epilepticus; thus education is a priority. Safety is always a priority in the care of a child with a seizure disorder because seizures may occur at any given time. Careful observation and documentation of seizures provide valuable information to aid prevention and treatment.

5. The answer is (4). Children with seizure disorders do not necessarily have cognitive delays. Poor self-image, dependency, and feelings of being different from peers can put additional stress on a child trying to understand and manage chronic illness.

6. The answer is (1). The EEG detects abnormal electrical activity in the brain. The pattern of various spikes can aid in the diagnosis of specific seizure disorders. LP confirms problems related to CSF infection or trauma. Brain scans confirm space-occupying lesions. Skull radiographs can detect fractures and structural abnormalities.

7. The answer is (3). Meningocele is a sac formation containing meninges and CSF. Meningocele does not involve complete exposure of the spinal cord and meninges; this is a massive defect that is incompatible with life. Myelomeningocele is a herniation of the spinal cord, meninges, and CSF into a sac that protrudes through a defect in the vertebral arch. Tumor formation is not associated with this defect.

8. The answer is (4). Surgical closure decreases the risk of infection stemming from damage to the fragile sac, which can lead to meningitis. The neurologic deficit cannot be corrected. However, some surgeons believe that early surgery reduces the risk of stretching spinal nerves and preventing further damage. Surgical repair does not help relieve hydrocephalus. In fact, some researchers believe that repair exaggerates the Arnold-Chiari malformation and decreases the absorptive surface for CSF, leading to more rapid development of hydrocephalus. Surgical repair of the sac does not prevent seizure disorder, an impairment of the brain neuron tissue.

9. The answer is (2). Adolescents with seizure disorders are at no greater risk for infections than other adolescents. Obtaining a driver's license may be influenced by the adolescent's seizure history. Drug and alcohol use may interfere with or create side effects from anticonvulsant medications. Peer pressure may put the child at risk for increased risk-taking behaviors that may exacerbate seizure activity.

10. The answer is (1). Reye's syndrome has been associated with the ingestion of aspirin in children with viral infections such as varicella. The is no association between meningitis or bacterial infections such as strep throat and the development of Reye's syndrome. Encephalitis is a component of Reye's syndrome.

11. The answer is (1). Mild mental retardation is minimally noticeable in young children, with one of the signs being a delay in achieving developmental milestones, such as walking at a later age. Severe mental retardation is marked by the mental age of a toddler and little or no communication skills. Children with moderate mental retardation have noticeable developmental delays.

12. The answer is (3). Oblique palpebral fissure is another term for the "Mongolian slant" of the eyes, a common finding in children with Down syndrome. Children with Down syndrome have small noses with a wide nasal bridge, large protruding tongues, and high-arched palates.

13. The answer is (2). Mental retardation is part of a broad category of developmental disability and defined by the American Association of Mental Deficiency as "… significantly subaverage, general intellectual functioning existing concurrently with deficits in adaptive behavior and manifested during the developmental period (18 years of age)." Cognitive impairment is not part of the definition. However, the definition does states that the impairment or compromise must occur before age 18 years. IQ 70 or below is considered significant subaverage intellectual functioning.

14. The answer is (3). Seizures usually are associated with encephalopathy, a late sign of lead poisoning. Typically lead levels have already exceeded 70 μg/dL. Anorexia, irritability, and anemia are early signs.

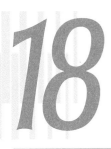

Endocrine Dysfunction

Structure and function of the endocrine system

A. Structure

1. The endocrine system is a network of six glands—pituitary, thyroid, parathyroids, adrenals, pancreas, and ovaries or testes.
2. Endocrine glands are ductless glands that secrete hormones (Table 18-1).

B. Function

1. The endocrine system regulates energy production, growth, fluid and electrolyte balance, response to stress, and sexual reproduction.
2. Hormonal regulation is based on a negative feedback system, and hormones stimulate or regulate the actions of other tissues called target tissues or organs.
3. The anterior pituitary or "master gland" is primarily responsible for stimulation and inhibition of target glandular secretions.
4. The endocrine glands function as follows.
   a. The pituitary gland consists of two portions.
      (1) The anterior (adenohypophysis) pituitary secretes growth hormone (GH), thyrotropin (thyroid-stimulating hormone [TSH]), adrenocorticotropic hormone (ACTH), gonadotropins, follicle-stimulating hormone (FSH), luteinizing hormone (LH), prolactin, and melanocyte-stimulating hormone (MSH).
      (2) The posterior (neurohypophysis) pituitary secretes antidiuretic hormone (ADH) and oxytocin.
   b. The thyroid gland secretes thyroxine (T_4), triiodothyronine (T_3), and calcitonin.
   c. Parathyroid glands secrete parathyroid hormone (PTH).
   d. Adrenal glands consist of two portions.
      (1) The adrenal cortex secretes mineralocorticoids (aldosterone), sex hormones (androgens, estrogens, progesterone), and glucocorticoids (cortisol, corticosterone).
      (2) The adrenal medulla secretes epinephrine and norepinephrine.
   e. The islets of Langerhans of the pancreas secrete insulin (beta cells), glucagon (alpha cells), and somatostatin.
   f. The ovaries secrete estrogen and progesterone.
   g. The testes secrete testosterone.
5. **Differences in endocrine response**. The endocrine is the least developed system at birth.
   a. The hormonal control of many body functions is lacking until 12 to 18 months of age. Thus, infants may exhibit imbalances in the concentration of fluids, electrolytes, amino acids, and trace substances.

TABLE 18-1

Development of the Endocrine System

AGE	STRUCTURE AND FUNCTION
Fetal development	Most endocrine glands and structures develop during the first trimester of gestation.
	The thyroid develops in three stages between weeks 7 and 14 of gestation.
	The parathyroid is recognizable between weeks 5 and 7 of gestation.
	The pancreas forms from two different cells that fuse to form a single organ at week 7 of gestation; insulin can be detected in beta cells several weeks later.
	The pituitary originates from fusion of two ectodermal processes.
	The primordia of anterior and posterior segments can be seen by the fourth week of gestation, and the gland takes its permanent shape and location in the sella turcica between the third and fourth month.
	The adrenal gland reaches its maximal size by the fourth month of gestation. The medulla arises from the ectoderm via the neural crest; the cortex, from the lateral plate of the embryonic mesoderm. Both corticosterone and aldosterone are secreted in utero.
Infant (0–1 year)	Maternal sex hormones are evident in the newborn as breasts can be engorged with secretion of milk (witch's milk) in both sexes; hypertrophy of the labia and pseudomenstruation can be noted in girls. The newborn endocrine system is structurally developed but functionally immature, and remains so throughout infancy. The posterior lobe of the pituitary produces limited amounts of antidiuretic hormone (ADH), or vasopressin, which inhibits diuresis, leaving the newborn very susceptible to dehydration. Corticotropin (ACTH) is produced in limited amounts, and the feedback mechanism between ACTH and the adrenal cortex is immature, making the infant less tolerant of stressful situations, affecting fluid and electrolyte balance, and the metabolism of carbohydrates, fats, and proteins. Blood sugar levels are labile, especially when stressed. The pituitary secretes growth hormone and thyroid-stimulating hormone.
Toddler/Preschooler (1–6 years)	Glucagon and insulin production remains labile and limited, causing blood sugar variations. Adrenal cortical secretions increase but remain limited. Insulin, growth hormone, and thyroxine remain important for regulating growth.
Schoolager (6–12 years)	The preadolescent growth spurt begins as early as 8 years old in girls. The average age is 10 years old, and the peak height velocity is reached at approximately 12 years old. The male spurt begins at about 12 years old and reaches its peak by 14 years old. In both sexes, the spurt begins in the hands and feet and progresses to the calves, forearms, hips, chest, and shoulders. The trunk is the last to demonstrate appreciable growth.
Adolescent (12–21 years)	All body systems grow rapidly.

    b. Normal hormone levels are related to age and stage of puberty. Evaluation of sexual development (Tanner's sexual maturation stages) is part of the diagnostic workup.

    c. Developmental assessment also is part of a diagnostic workup because delays can be associated with endocrine disorders.

II. NURSING PROCESS OVERVIEW FOR
The Endocrine System

A. Assessment

1. Health history

a. Elicit a description of symptoms including onset, duration, location, and precipitation. **Cardinal symptoms** may include:

   (1) Changes in growth (significant weight gain or loss, accelerated or delayed height velocity, and delayed or precocious puberty)

   (2) Changes in activity patterns (delayed developmental milestones and inability to keep up with peers)

   (3) Changes in appetite and thirst (thyroid disorders, diabetes mellitus, and diabetes insipidus)

   (4) Changes in elimination patterns (thyroid disorders, diabetes mellitus)

   (5) Visual disturbances (pituitary tumors and pancreatic disorders)

   (6) Fatigue (hypothyroidism)

   (7) Increased or decreased sweating; cold or heat intolerance (thyroid disorders)

   (8) Nausea and vomiting (parathyroid disorders and diabetes mellitus)

   (9) Mood changes; decreased libido (Cushing syndrome and adrenocortical insufficiency)

   (10) Changes in sleep patterns (thyroid disorders)

b. Explore prenatal, personal and family history for **risk factors** for endocrine disorders.

   (1) Prenatal risk factors include maternal illness, use of substances or medications, poor nutrition, and intrauterine growth retardation.

   (2) Personal risk factors include history of prematurity, positive screening on neonatal screening tests, viral illness, central nervous system trauma, infection or lesion, chromosomal abnormalities, and current medications.

   (3) Family risk factors include family history of endocrine disorders or disturbances in growth, development, or both.

2. Physical examination

a. **Vital signs**

   (1) Monitor and plot head circumference (children under 2 years old), height and weight for abnormal growth velocity (pituitary disorders), and weight loss (pituitary disorders, pancreatic disorders, and hyperthyroidism) or gain (adrenal disorders and hypothyroidism).

   (2) Monitor pulse. Pulse will decrease in hypothyroidism and increase in hyperthyroidism.

   (3) Monitor blood pressure for signs of hypotension (acute adrenocortical insufficiency) and hypertension (hyperthyroidism or Cushing syndrome).

   (4) Monitor for altered respiratory patterns. Dyspnea can occur during slight exertion in hyperthyroidism.

b. **Inspection**

   (1) Assess mental status for signs of lethargy, irritability, and confusion. Hypothyroidism is characterized by lethargy. Hyperthyroidism, diabetes insipidus, and syndrome of inappropriate antidiuretic hormone (SIADH) are characterized by irritability. Parathyroid disorders are characterized by confusion.

   (2) Inspect skin for color changes, hirsutism, easy bruising, and striae (pituitary disorders, adrenal disorders, and thyroid disorders).

   (3) Assess vision (pituitary tumors and pancreatic disorders).

(4) Assess face for abnormalities and deformities (Cushing syndrome and hypothyroidism).

(5) Inspect the mouth for abnormal odors and dentition delays. Fruity breath is noted in diabetic ketoacidosis. Dental delays are found in hypopituitarism.

(6) Assess for gait disturbances (hyperparathyroidism), hyperactivity (hyperthyroidism), and abnormal reflexes (hypocalcemia).

(7) Assess and stage sexual development, and assess genitalia for abnormalities. Gonadal disorders, thyroid disorders, hypopituitarism, and other problems can cause delays in development or abnormalities.

c. **Palpation**

(1) Palpate the hair and nails for brittleness (hypothyroidism).

(2) Palpate the skin to note dryness, coldness, and changes in texture (adrenal disorders and thyroid disorders).

(3) Assess muscle strength and tone. Weakness is noted in SIADH, hypothyroidism, and parathyroid disorders.

d. **Auscultation.** Auscultate the heart to note murmurs (hyperthyroidism).

3. **Laboratory studies and diagnostic tests**

a. Due to the nature of endocrine disorders, most diagnostics tests are very gland and disorder specific.

(1) **Thyroid function tests** (eg, **TSH** and **T_4 total**) are used to test thyroid function.

(2) **Growth hormone test** is used to evaluate GH deficiency. This is a time-specific test, so the specimen must be drawn accurately. The child is kept NPO and an agent such as insulin is administered to stimulate release of GH.

(3) **Blood glucose tests** are timed blood tests used to diagnose problems such as diabetes mellitus.

b. General studies may include:

(1) **Complete blood count (CBC)** is drawn to screen for systemic and chronic illnesses.

(2) **Serum chemistries** will determine calcium, phosphorus, alkaline phosphatase, and electrolyte levels.

(3) **Urine studies** will assess sodium, calcium, phosphorus, and glucose levels and specific gravity.

(4) **Radiographic studies** are done to evaluate bone age and density, as well as soft tissue calcification.

(5) **Computed tomography (CT) and magnetic resonance imaging (MRI) scans** and **ultrasound** may be used to determine structural abnormalities of endocrine glands and to identify problems such as tumors or cysts.

(6) **Genetic studies** may detect enzyme deficiencies (eg, congenital adrenal hypoplasia).

B. **Nursing diagnoses**

1. Altered growth and development

2. Impaired adjustment

C. **Planning and outcome identification**

1. The child's growth and development will progress in an age-appropriate manner within limits of the disorder.

2. The child and family will adjust and cope appropriately.

D. **Implementation**

1. **Promote normal growth and development.**

a. Encourage the child and family to participate in the therapeutic regimen, which may include measures to suppress, stimulate, or replace a specific hormone. See Drug Chart 18-1 for specific replacement hormones.
b. Provide adequate nutrition within the restrictions (if any) of the child's disorder.
c. Encourage the family to comply with the therapeutic follow-up plan.
d. Assist the family in setting realistic goals.
e. Help the parents promote their child's normal growth and development by teaching them about age-related developmental norms and by encouraging them to notify their primary care provider of abnormalities. Encourage parents to treat their child as "normal."

2. **Assist the child and family in adjusting to major lifestyle changes imposed by a chronic illness.**
   a. Be sensitive to developmental needs when preparing the child for invasive procedures and tests.
   b. Allow parents and children the needed opportunity to express their concerns and fears before and after diagnosis and throughout the course of treatment.
   c. Realistically reinforce the parents' and child's expectations of treatment and prospects for improvement.
   d. Allay the child's fears.
      (1) A young child may interpret therapy, such as daily or weekly hormonal injections, as punishment for wrongdoing. This child needs clear communication to help him distinguish between disease treatment and disciplinary measures.

DRUG CHART 18-1 Replacement Hormones

Hormone	Used for	Selected Interventions
Growth Hormone (GH)	Replace GH to increase rate of growth	Teach the parents correct dilution, administration, and storage.
		Monitor for side effects: local irritation at injection site.
Thyroid	Replacement for hypothyroidism	Administer at the same time every day.
		Monitor for side effects: hyperthyroidism, palpitations, sweating, and heat intolerance.
Insulin	Used in type 1 diabetes mellitus	Teach the child and family proper administration and storage.
		Teach the family how to monitor for hypoglycemia and how to manage it.
Glucagon	Used to treat severe hypoglycemic reactions	Arouse the child as soon as possible after injection to give oral carbohydrates.
		Teach the parents how and when to administer.

(2) Injections may be a source of fearful fantasies and may enhance a child's anxieties about body mutilation.

(3) Adolescents may have body image concerns, and they may fear rejection from peers because they are "different."

e. Help promote the child's self-esteem and a positive self-image by encouraging him to express feelings and concerns and to focus on personal strengths and assets.

f. Encourage the parents to emphasize their child's positive aspects and abilities, rather than dwell on their child's limitations.

g. Promote the child's social adjustment by encouraging interpersonal relationships with peers and involvement with special peer counseling groups.

h. Promote functional family coping by referring the parents and child to a support group composed of parents and children with similar disabilities.

E. Outcome evaluation

1. The child progresses in an age-appropriate, developmental manner.

2. The child and family adjust and cope appropriately.

III. Growth hormone deficiency (hypopituitarism)

A. Description. GH deficiency results from diminished or deficient secretion of GH from the pituitary.

B. Etiology

1. The cause is idiopathic in most cases.

2. Other causes include developmental defects (aplasia or hypoplasia), autoimmune hypophysitis, functional deficiency, tumors (craniopharyngioma, optic glioma, adenoma, astrocytoma, and germinosm), septic-optic dysplasia, empty sella (absent or small pituitary gland that does not fill the sella foramen), radiation therapy, and trauma.

C. Pathophysiology

1. GH deficiency produces varied effects, depending on the degree of dysfunction, including:

a. Decreased synthesis of somatomedin, resulting in decreased linear growth

b. Inhibited transport of protein-building amino acids into cells and increased protein catabolism, leading to decreased muscle mass, thin hair, poor skin quality, and delayed growth

c. Decreased fat catabolism and increased glucose uptake in muscles, which results in excessive subcutaneous fat and hypoglycemia

2. Associated deficiencies of other hormones, such as ACTH, TSH, LH, and FSH, produce effects related to the functions of these hormones.

D. Assessment findings

1. Clinical manifestations

a. The chief presenting complaint is short stature. Children generally grow during the first year, then follow a slow curve below the third percentile. Progressive growth slowing suggests idiopathic hypopituitarism, whereas sudden slowing suggests a tumor.

b. Partial GH deficiency presents with less dramatic growth retardation.

c. Height increase may be slower than weight gain, and the child may even become obese.

d. Skeletal proportions are normal, but children appear younger than their chronological age. Faces tend to be cherubic.

e. Sexual development usually is delayed, but normal.

f. Most children have normal intelligence, but appear precocious. Emotional problems are common. Academic problems also are common because many of these children are not encouraged to perform at their chronological age.

2. **Laboratory and diagnostic study findings**

a. **Bone age x-ray** may reveal a bone age younger than chronological age, but closely related to height age. The degree will depend on the duration of hormone deficiency.

b. **Overnight sleep studies of GH secretion** reveal fewer than three peaks of GH above 10 ng/mL.

c. **GH stimulation studies** using two or more GH stimulants, such as arginine, clonidine, glucagon, insulin, or levodopa/propranolol, reveal GH levels less than 10 ng/mL.

d. Insulin-like growth factor-1 (IGF-1) and IGF binding protein$_3$ (IGFBP$_3$) levels are usually below normal.

e. Blood glucose levels reveal hypoglycemia.

f. Renal, liver, and thyroid function tests are normal, as is the sedimentation rate.

g. CT scan and MRI of the head are normal.

E. **Nursing management**

1. **Assess for signs of growth delay,** and assist with diagnostic evaluation.

2. **Administer GH**, and teach parent proper reconstitution and administration techniques. Instruct on side effects, which include increased blood glucose, increased incidence of slipped capital femoral epiphysis, local infection at injection site, and pseudotumor. Leukemia has been reported as a rare finding in children taking GH.

3. **Provide nutritional teaching** to prevent obesity.

IV. Syndrome of inappropriate antidiuretic hormone

A. **Description**. SIADH results from the excessive production or release of ADH (vasopressin).

B. **Etiology**

1. SIADH usually occurs in childhood and is caused by disorders affecting the central nervous system, including infection, head trauma, and brain tumors.

2. Transient, but life-threatening, SIADH may occur after surgery for brain tumors.

C. **Pathophysiology**

1. Excessive ADH results in the kidneys reabsorbing too much water, causing decreased urine output and high urine osmolality.

2. The excess water causes an expanded fluid volume and a low serum sodium level. Once the sodium level falls below 125 mEq/L, the child becomes symptomatic.

D. **Assessment findings**

1. **Clinical manifestations**

a. Decreased urine output

b. Fluid retention

c. Weight gain

d. Hyponatremia

e. Weakness

f. Irritability, lethargy, and confusion, progressing to stupor and convulsions

g. Anorexia, nausea, vomiting, and abdominal cramps

2. **Laboratory and diagnostic study findings**

a. Serum chemistries demonstrate hyponatremia, hypochloremia, and low serum osmolality.

b. Urine studies reveal osmolality that is usually greater than serum osmolality, and a urine specific gravity greater than 1.030.

c. Further testing is performed to establish causation.

E. **Nursing management**

1. **Assess neurologic and hydration status** at least every 2 to 4 hours, **and closely monitor electrolyte levels**. Alert the health care provider to any change in status.

2. **Administer prescribed medications**, which may include intravenous solutions of sodium chloride, lithium, or demeclocycline.

3. **Enforce fluid restrictions and carefully monitor intake and output**.

4. **Provide frequent mouth care**.

5. **Include high-sodium foods in the diet**, but remember that salty foods may make the child thirsty.

6. **Implement seizure precautions**.

V. Precocious puberty

A. **Description**

1. Precocious puberty is the development of sexual characteristics before the typical age of the onset of puberty.

   a. In girls, it is breast development before 7.5 years of age.

   b. In boys, it is pubic hair development before 8.5 years of age.

2. In boys, secondary sexual characteristic development before 9 years of age is considered precocious.

B. **Etiology**

1. Gonadotropin-dependent precocious puberty may be caused by congenital anomalies, such as hydrocephalus, central nervous system tumors, inflammatory conditions, such as meningitis, and trauma. It may also be idiopathic.

2. Gonadotropin-independent precocious puberty may be caused by human chorionic gonadotropin (HCG)-secreting tumors, gonadal conditions, adrenal disorders, and exogenous ingestion or absorption of steroids.

3. Combined gonadotropin-dependent and gonadotropin-independent precocious puberty may be caused by congenital adrenal hyperplasia and an ovarian or adrenal tumor.

C. **Pathophysiology**

1. Gonadotropin-dependent precocious puberty is initiated by hypothalamic-pituitary activation, and it is similar to the mechanism seen in normal puberty. The hypothalamus secretes LH-releasing hormone (LHRH) in periodic bursts that stimulate the pituitary to release LH and FSH. LH and FSH stimulate the gonads to produce sex hormones causing sexual maturation.

2. Gonadotropin-independent precocious puberty is the result of the production of sex hormones by the adrenals or gonads, or from exposure to steroids.

3. Combination precocious puberty results from secondary activation of the hypothalamic-pituitary-gonadal axis by raised sex steroid levels from a peripheral source.

D. **Assessment findings**

1. **Associated findings**

   a. The history reveals early development of pubertal events, including breast buds, phallic enlargement, body hair, facial hair, acne, body odor, and voice deepening.

   b. The history may reveal head trauma, exposure to steroids or gonadotropins, or problems such as headache, visual disturbances, or motor incoordination.

    c. The family history may reveal precocious puberty, congenital adrenal hyperplasia, neurofibromatosis, and thyroid disease.

  2. Clinical manifestations

    a. Boys have obvious genital growth.

    b. Girls have breast growth and menses with little pubic hair.

    c. Behavioral changes include moodiness, irritability, or aggressiveness.

  3. Laboratory and diagnostic study findings. Findings depend on the type and underlying cause.

    a. Bone age x-ray may reveal that skeletal age is more advanced than chronological age.

    b. Gonadotropin-releasing hormone stimulation test may demonstrate elevated LH and FSH levels.

    c. CT or MRI may demonstrate pituitary or hypothalamic lesions.

    d. Ultrasonography may reveal adrenal or ovarian cysts.

E. Nursing management. Management depends on the underlying cause.

  1. Administer prescribed medications. For example, a synthetic analogue of LHRH is administered to children with precocious puberty of central (hypothalamic-pituitary) origin. This treatment allows the child to attain her predicted height.

  2. Provide support and guidance because these children have a high incidence of behavioral problems secondary to age and appearance dyssynchrony, and moodiness.

    a. Dress and activities should be appropriate to the child's chronological age.

    b. Instruct the parents that the child's mental age is congruent with the chronological age.

    c. Advise the parents that secondary sexual characteristics appear in their usual order.

VI. Hypothyroidism

A. Description

  1. Hypothyroidism is a chronic condition characterized by an inadequate amount of thyroid hormone necessary to meet metabolic needs.

  2. It may be congenital or acquired.

  3. Hypothyroidism is one of the most common endocrine problems in children.

B. Etiology

  1. The most common cause of **congenital hypothyroidism** is defective embryonic development of the gland. Another cause is maternal ingestion of goitrogens, such as antithyroid drugs or large amounts of iodine.

  2. Hashimoto or autoimmune thyroiditis is the most common cause of **acquired hypothyroidism** in children. Autoimmune thyroiditis is often associated with other endocrine disorders and chromosomal disorders.

  3. Other primary causes of acquired hypothyroidism are surgical thyroidectomy, radioactive iodine therapy, and radiation treatment.

  4. Secondary hypothyroidism is caused by a defect in either the hypothalamus or pituitary.

C. Pathophysiology

  1. In **congenital hypothyroidism**, the thyroid does not produce T_4, which is essential for growth and development, especially brain development. Left untreated, it results in mental retardation.

  2. In **acquired hypothyroidism**, there is an inadequate amount of T_4, and the adverse effects occurring after 2 to 3 years of age are often reversible.

D. Assessment findings

1. Clinical manifestations

a. Congenital hypothyroidism

(1) Prolonged jaundice

(2) Lethargy, excessive sleeping

(3) Constipation

(4) Feeding problems

(5) Cold to touch

(6) Umbilical hernia, distended abdomen

(7) Hypotonia and slow reflexes

(8) Large tongue

(9) Large fontanelle

(10) Hoarse cry

(11) Typical facies with depressed nasal bridge, short forehead, puffy eyelids, dull hair, and coarse cry

b. Acquired hypothyroidism

(1) Goiter

(2) Fatigue and tiredness; mental sluggishness

(3) Decreased growth

(4) Weight gain

(5) Dry, thick skin and coarse hair

(6) Cold intolerance

(7) Constipation

(8) Edema of face, hands, and eyes

(9) Irregular menses

2. Laboratory and diagnostic study findings

a. Low T4 level and TSH levels greater than 40 μU/mL in the newborn indicate congenital hypothyroidism.

b. Low T_4 levels and elevated TSH levels also indicate acquired hypothyroidism.

c. Circulating thyroid antibodies indicate thyroiditis.

E. Nursing management

1. **Assess and recognize the early signs of congenital and acquired hypothyroidism.**

2. **Administer replacement thyroid hormone.**

3. **Monitor the progress of growth and development.** Symptoms should resolve with adequate treatment.

4. **Instruct the parents on the importance of thyroid hormone replacement,** especially for congenital hypothyroidism, which is a chronic, lifelong disorder. In congenital hypothyroidism, frequently missed doses can lead to poor growth and developmental delays.

5. **Advise the parents of the importance of routine serum thyroid hormone monitoring and drug dosage adjustment.**

VII. Cushing syndrome

A. **Description.** Cushing syndrome is a cluster of clinical abnormalities resulting from excessive levels of adrenocortical hormones, particularly cortisol, and to a lesser extent, related corticosteroids, androgens, and aldosterone.

B. Etiology

    1. In infants and young children, the most common cause is an adrenocortical tumor.

    2. The common cause in older children is the result of side effects of steroids.

C. Pathophysiology

    1. Ineffectiveness of the normal feedback mechanisms that control adrenocortical function results in excessive secretion of cortisol from the adrenal cortex despite adequate levels in circulation.

    2. Clinical manifestations are the direct result of hormone excess (glucocorticoids, mineralocorticoids, and sex hormones); the predominant hormone excess—most commonly, glucocorticoids—determines the predominant manifestations.

    3. Depending on the underlying cause, treatment may involve surgical removal or irradiation of adrenal or pituitary tumors, or adrenalectomy to resect hyperplastic tumors.

    4. A child undergoing one of these treatments requires lifelong hormone replacement as prescribed therapy; specific agents depend on the nature of the procedure and on the particular deficiencies.

D. Assessment findings

    1. Clinical manifestations

        a. Centripetal fat distribution (truncal obesity and fat pads on the supraclavicular and neck areas ["buffalo hump"])

        b. Rounded or "moon" face, with reddened, oily skin

        c. Muscle wasting, thin extremities, and a pendulous abdomen

        d. Fragile, thin skin and subcutaneous tissue, acne, excessive bruising, and petechiae

        e. Reddish, purple abdominal striae

        f. Increased susceptibility to infection and poor wound healing

        g. Elevated blood pressure

        h. Compression fractures of vertebrae, kyphosis, backache, and osteoporosis

        i. Retarded linear growth

        j. Irritability, insomnia, euphoria or depression, and frank psychosis

        k. Precocious puberty in children

        l. Virilization in adolescent girls, marked by hirsutism, voice deepening, clitoral enlargement, breast atrophy, and amenorrhea

        m. Loss of libido, impotence, and gynecomastia in adolescent boys

    2. Laboratory and diagnostic study findings

        a. Adrenal function tests will reveal excessive plasma cortisol level.

        b. Glucose tolerance test will reveal hyperglycemia, glycosuria, and latent or overt diabetes.

        c. Serum chemistries will reveal hypokalemia, hypocalcemia, and alkalosis.

        d. Urine studies will reveal elevated urine levels of 17-hydroxycorticosteroid and 17-ketosteroid.

        e. Decreased ACTH production on dexamethasone (cortisone) suppression test helps to establish a more definitive diagnosis.

        f. CT scan, ultrasonography, or angiography may reveal an adrenal tumor.

        g. CT scan of the head may locate a pituitary tumor.

E. Nursing management

    1. Monitor vital signs for cardiac irregularities, bradycardia, and hypertension.

    2. Monitor for early signs of infection.

🖐 **3.** **If Cushing syndrome results from necessary steroid therapy, inform the child and family that the medication should never be abruptly stopped or a dose missed; either of these actions can precipitate an adrenal crisis.**
   a. Reinforce this information as necessary.
   b. Explain that cushingoid symptoms caused by steroid therapy may be relieved. The parents should consult with the physician who may recommend administering the steroids on an alternate-day basis and in the early morning.
4. Prevent infection by practicing good handwashing and limiting the child's exposure to persons with infections.
5. Help maintain skin integrity.
   a. Provide and promote good hygiene and skin care.
   b. Frequently change the child's position.
   c. Assess for redness and breakdown.
6. Provide a high-protein, low-sodium diet with potassium supplements.
7. Promote adequate rest to prevent fatigue.

VIII. Diabetes mellitus (DM)

A. Description
   1. DM is a chronic metabolic disorder that results from either a partial or complete deficiency of insulin.
   2. Type 1 DM is characterized by pancreatic beta cell destruction leading to absolute insulin deficiency.
   3. Type 2 DM usually results from insulin resistance.
   4. Type 1 DM (insulin requiring DM) is the most common endocrine disease of childhood.
   5. The primary long-term complications of DM are nephropathy, retinopathy, and neuropathy. Altered thyroid functioning is frequently noted in children with diabetes.
B. Etiology. Type 1 DM is an autoimmune disease that develops when a genetically predisposed child is exposed to a precipitating factor, such as a viral infection.
C. Pathophysiology
   1. Insulin is needed to support carbohydrate, protein, and fat metabolism, primarily to facilitate entry of these substances into cells.
   2. Destruction of 80% to 90% of the pancreatic beta cells results in a clinically significant drop in insulin secretion.
   3. This loss of insulin, the major anabolic hormone, leads to a catabolic state characterized by decreased glucose use, increased glucose production, and inability to store glycogen, eventually resulting in hyperglycemia.
   4. In a state of insulin deficiency, glucagon, epinephrine, GH, and cortisol levels increase, secondary to fat breakdown, stimulating lipolysis, fatty acid release, and ketone production.
   5. A persistent blood glucose concentration above 180 mg/dL (the renal threshold) results in glycosuria, leading to osmotic diuresis with polyuria and polydipsia.
   6. Excessive ketone production can cause diabetic ketoacidosis (DKA), an acutely life-threatening condition characterized by marked hyperglycemia, metabolic acidosis, dehydration, and altered level of consciousness ranging from lethargy to coma.
D. Assessment findings
   1. Clinical manifestations
      a. The classic symptoms of DM are polydipsia, polyuria, polyphagia, and fatigue.

b. Other symptoms include recent weight loss, dry skin, and blurred vision.

c. Signs of DKA include hyperglycemia, acidosis, glycosuria, and ketonuria.

d. Early signs of hypoglycemia include trembling, tachycardia, sweating, anxiety, hunger, pallor, and headache. Later signs include loss of coordination, personality and mood changes, slurred speech, sleepiness, nightmares, decreasing level of consciousness, and seizure activity.

2. Laboratory and diagnostic study findings. Blood glucose tests include:

a. Fasting blood glucose (FBG) will reveal a level above 120 mg/dL accompanied by a random blood glucose level above 200 mg/dL.

b. Oral glucose tolerance test (OGTT) will reveal blood glucose levels of 200 mg/dL or higher in a 2-hour sample.

E. Nursing management

1. Assess the child daily for signs of hypoglycemia, hyperglycemia, and complications.

2. Provide care during an acute phase, such as DKA.

a. Assess neurologic status by monitoring vital signs and noting any changes in level of consciousness.

b. Help prevent hypotension and convulsions by closely monitoring vital signs, cardiac status, and blood glucose levels.

c. Monitor electrolytes and cardiac status for signs of hypokalemia.

d. Promote adequate fluid volume by maintaining accurate and careful records of intravenous fluid infusion, blood glucose level, intake and output, and urine specific gravity.

e. Test urine for ketones every 3 hours when child is ill and whenever the blood glucose level is 240 mg/dL or higher.

f. Administer insulin, usually intravenously, to decrease elevated blood glucose levels.

3. Prevent injury related to insulin deficiency during daily management.

a. Monitor blood glucose levels regularly.

b. Administer appropriate insulin amounts based on the previous day's glucose monitoring.

(1) Conventional management consists of a twice-daily regimen consisting of rapid-acting (regular) and intermediate-acting (NPH or Lente) insulin drawn up in the same syringe and administered before breakfast and the evening meal.

(2) The insulin pump delivers fixed amounts of dilute solution of regular insulin continuously.

c. Encourage an adequate diet for age, using consistent menus and eating times, and complex carbohydrates.

d. Collaborate with a nutritionist or diabetic specialist for dietary instruction.

e. Encourage adequate rest and regular exercise.

4. Prevent injury related to hypoglycemia.

a. Recognize signs of hypoglycemia early, and be alert to when blood sugar levels are at their lowest (ie, during insulin peak times, during bursts of exercise, during the growth spurt, and when adequate food is not consumed).

b. Offer a readily absorbed carbohydrate, such as orange juice, to alleviate early symptoms. Follow up with a complex carbohydrate and protein snack, such as crackers with peanut butter.

c. Administer glucagon to the unconscious child. Position the child to minimize the risk of aspiration.

CHILD AND FAMILY TEACHING 18-1

Managing Diabetes

- Describe the disease process.
- Explain how to test blood glucose and urine ketones.
- Teach insulin administration and storage. Explain insulin therapy.
- Identify signs and symptoms of hypoglycemia and hyperglycemia, how to prevent them, and how to manage them.
- Discuss meal planning (adequate intake for age, consistent menus, complex carbohydrates, consistent eating times with use of snacks, and understanding carbohydrate counting), skin care, and special problems.
- Assist child in developing an exercise and rest/sleep plan.
- Encourage the child to wear identification, and inform school personnel of child's needs.
- Discuss the prevention of long-term complications.

5. **Provide child and family teaching** (Child and Family Teaching 18-1).
   a. Assess the child's and family's unique learning needs based on age, educational background, capacity to learn, and personal experience.
   b. Assess the child's and family's emotional and psychological state. Initial diagnosis may trigger shock and denial, which will hinder learning; acceptance of the disease is an important first step in learning to cope with long-term management.
   c. Create a positive learning environment, including a comfortable temperature; a quiet, unhurried atmosphere; and sufficient supplemental educational materials.
   d. If possible, limit teaching sessions to no longer than 15 or 20 minutes and teach one important skill at a time.
   e. Organize teaching to present simple information first followed by more complex information.
   f. Evaluate how well the child and family understand the information by having them perform return demonstrations and verbal explanations.
6. **Refer the family to an organization that can assist the family in coping with diabetes**, such as the Juvenile Diabetes Foundation International.
7. **Promote a sense of self-esteem in the child** by encouraging her to express feelings and concerns and to identify personal strengths and positive aspects of her situation.

STUDY QUESTIONS

1. Deficiency of which of the following causes poor linear growth and hypoglycemia?
   (1) Antidiuretic hormone
   (2) Melanocyte-stimulating hormone
   (3) Parathyroid hormone
   (4) Growth hormone

2. Short stature may result from which of the following?
   (1) Anterior pituitary gland hypofunction
   (2) Posterior pituitary gland hyperfunction
   (3) Parathyroid gland hyperfunction
   (4) Thyroid gland hyperfunction

3. A 12-year-old girl diagnosed with type 1 diabetes mellitus asks the nurse why she cannot take a pill instead of shots, like her grandfather does. Which of the following would be the nurse's **best** reply?
   (1) "The pills correct fat and protein metabolism, not carbohydrate metabolism."
   (2) "If your blood glucose levels are controlled, you can switch to using the pills."
   (3) "The pills only work on the adult pancreas, you can switch when you're 18."
   (4) "Your body does not make insulin, so the insulin injections help to replace it."

4. Which of the following phrases **best** describes hypopituitarism?
   (1) Normal growth for first 5 years, followed by progressive linear growth retardation
   (2) Growth retardation in which height and weight are equally affected
   (3) Linear growth retardation with skeletal proportions normal for chronological age
   (4) A completely normal growth pattern, but with the onset of precocious puberty

5. A 6-year-old boy is admitted to the hospital with height measured below the 3rd percentile and weight at the 40th percentile. His admitting diagnosis is idiopathic hypopituitarism. Which of the following would be the nurse's **first** action?
   (1) Place him in a room with a 2-year-old boy.
   (2) Arrange for a tutor for his precocious intellectual ability.
   (3) Plan for a dietitian to assess his caloric needs.
   (4) Suggest orthodontic referral for underdeveloped jaw.

6. The father of a 6-year-old boy with growth hormone (GH) deficiency shares with the nurse the child's desire to play baseball. However, the mother feels that the child will get hurt because he is so much smaller than the other children. In planning anticipatory guidance for these parents, the nurse should keep in mind which of the following?
   (1) The risk for fractures is increased because a GH deficiency results in fragile bones.
   (2) Activity could aggravate insulin sensitivity, causing hyperglycemia.
   (3) Activity would aggravate the child's joints, already overtasked by obesity.
   (4) The child should be allowed to participate as he can to foster healthy self-esteem.

7. When caring for a child with Cushing syndrome, which of the following nursing interventions would be **most** important?
   (1) Handling the child carefully to prevent bruising
   (2) Monitoring for signs and symptoms of hypoglycemia
   (3) Observing for signs and symptoms of metabolic acidosis
   (4) Monitoring vital signs for hypotension and tachycardia

8. Diabetic ketoacidosis (DKA) results from an excessive accumulation of which of the following?
   (1) Glucose from carbohydrate metabolism
   (2) Ketone bodies from fat metabolism
   (3) Potassium from cell death
   (4) Sodium bicarbonate from renal compensation

9. Which of the following is of **primary** importance when caring for a child who is admitted to the intensive care unit for DKA?
   (1) Restricting fluids to prevent aggravating cerebral edema
   (2) Administering intravenous NPH insulin in high doses
   (3) Monitoring the child's vital signs for hypertension
   (4) Assessing the child for cardiac irregularities

10. Which of the following actions should the nurse instruct the parents to take when the child with type 1 diabetes mellitus displays symptoms of hypoglycemia?
    (1) Give the child nothing by mouth.
    (2) Give the child a simple sugar, such as honey.
    (3) Give the child a complex sugar, such as milk.
    (4) Contact the physician before doing anything.

ANSWER KEY

1. The answer is (4). Growth hormone (GH) stimulates protein anabolism, promoting bone and soft tissue growth. A deficiency of GH would lead to decreased synthesis of somatomedin, resulting in decreased linear growth and decreased fat catabolism and increased glucose uptake in muscles, resulting in excessive subcutaneous fat and hypoglycemia. A deficiency of antidiuretic hormone (ADH) results in diabetes insipidus, marked by dehydration and hypernatremia. Deficiency of melanocyte-stimulating hormone causes diminished or absent skin pigmentation. Deficiency of parathyroid hormone causes hypocalcemia, marked by tetany, convulsions, and muscle spasms.

2. The answer is (1). Short stature usually results from diminished or deficient GH, which is released from the anterior pituitary gland. Posterior pituitary hyperfunction results in increased secretion of antidiuretic hormone (ADH) or oxytocin, leading to a syndrome of inappropriate ADH secretion, marked by fluid retention and hyponatremia. Parathyroid hypofunction leads to hypocalcemia. Thyroid hyperfunction causes increased secretion of T_4, T_3, and thyrocalcitonin, resulting in Graves' disease, marked by accelerated linear growth and early epiphyseal closure.

3. The answer is (4). The child has type 1 diabetes indicating a lack of functioning pancreatic beta cells and an absolute insulin deficiency. Oral hypoglycemic agents are only indicated for those with some functioning beta cells, as in type 2 diabetes. Therefore, injections are indicated to supply insulin that is lacking in type 1 diabetes. Oral hypoglycemics do not correct metabolism. A child with type 1 cannot substitute an oral hypoglycemic agent for insulin regardless of whether the blood glucose levels are controlled or age.

4. The answer is (3). Although linear growth retardation occurs in hypopituitarism, delayed epiphyseal maturation allows for normal skeletal proportions. Normal growth may occur for the first year, followed by linear growth thereafter. Height is affected more profoundly than weight, contributing to obesity. The child with hypopituitarism commonly experiences delayed sexual maturation.

5. The answer is (3). Because the child's weight is excessive for his height, he needs dietary assessment and planning to lose weight. Placing the child in a room with a toddler could contribute to poor self-esteem. Arranging for a school teacher to instruct him is an appropriate action, but the rationale is incorrect. Children with hypopituitarism often appear intellectually precocious because of the disparity between their size and their cognitive ability. They are usually of normal intelligence. An underdeveloped jaw is not normally a problem with hypopituitarism.

6. The answer is (4). Engaging in peer group activities can help foster a sense of belonging and a positive self-concept. T-ball is a good sport to choose because physical stature is not an important consideration in the ability to participate, unlike some other sports such as basketball and football. Hypopituitarism does not affect calcium and phosphorus homeostasis and demineralization of bone. So the risk for fractures is not increased. Although rare, physical activity without adequate carbohydrate intake can cause hypoglycemia, not hyperglycemia. Moderate physical activity increases caloric use and reduces weight without undue strain on weight-bearing joints.

7. The answer is (1). Cushing syndrome causes capillary fragility, resulting in easy bruising and calcium excretion, resulting in osteoporosis. Therefore, the nurse would handle the child carefully. Cushing syndrome causes hyperglycemia not hypoglycemia. It also causes increased excretion of potassium and hydrogen ions, resulting in alkalosis and increased water and sodium retention, and hypokalemia, resulting in a sluggish and irregular heart beat.

8. The answer is (2). Inability to use glucose causes lipolysis, fatty acid oxidation, and release of ketones, resulting in metabolic acidosis and coma. Inability to use glucose, not impaired carbohydrate metabolism, is the primary mechanism in diabetes mellitus. Potassium depletion, not potassium excess, occurs in DKA. Sodium bicarbonate administration is a treatment for DKA, not a cause.

9. The answer is (4). As the fluid volume deficit is corrected, total body potassium depletion may occur leaving the child vulnerable to hypokalemia and subsequently, cardiac arrest. The nurse should monitor the cardiac cycle for prolonged QT interval, low T wave, and depressed ST segment, which indicate weakened heart muscle and potential irregular heartbeat. Intravenous fluids should be given to correct dehydration. Regular insulin is the only insulin that can be given intravenously, NPH is an intermediate-acting insulin; continuous low-dose infusion of a rapid-acting insulin is preferred. Hypertension is more likely to occur secondary to dehydration.

10. The answer is (2). Prompt action is necessary. Thus, giving a little sugar temporarily corrects low serum glucose levels. Simple sugar is preferred because it is converted to glucose more quickly than a complex sugar. A hyperglycemic child needs fluids to prevent dehydration. Because complex sugars, such as milk, are absorbed more slowly, they do not provide an immediate response. Immediate action is necessary to prevent complications of hypoglycemia. Contacting the physician wastes valuable time during which emergency measures could be started to raise the child's glucose level.

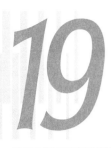

Children With Cancer

 Essential concepts of cancer in children

A. Overview

1. Cancer is the second leading cause of death in children between 1 and 14 years of age. Death from cancer is exceeded only by death from injury.
2. Leukemia is the most common type of cancer in children, followed by brain tumors, lymphoma, and kidney tumors. These types of cancer are covered in the text. Table 19-1 lists and describes other childhood cancers.
3. The prognosis for childhood cancer has improved over the years.
   a. More than 70% of children treated in major cancer centers survive longer than 5 years.
   b. Cancers with the greatest improvement in survival rates include acute leukemia, lymphomas, Wilms' tumor, rhabdomyosarcoma, osteosarcoma, and Ewing's sarcoma.
4. Criteria for cure of cancer include:
   a. Cessation of therapy
   b. Continuous freedom from clinical and laboratory evidence of cancer
   c. Minimal or no risk of relapse, as determined by previous experience with the disease
   d. Two- to 5-year time elapse

B. Etiology

1. The cause of cancer remains unknown.
2. The most enduring theory is that a genetic alteration results in unregulated proliferation of cells. Recent studies have demonstrated the existence of genes, activated in tumors, which are capable of causing uncontrolled cell proliferation when transmitted to normal cells.
3. Some childhood cancers may demonstrate patterns of inheritance that suggest a genetic basis for the disorder. These include Wilms' tumor, retinoblastoma, and neuroblastoma.
4. Children with immune disorders, such as human immunodeficiency virus/acquired immunodeficiency syndrome (HIV/AIDS) and Wiskott-Aldrich syndrome, and certain chromosomal disorders, such as Down syndrome and Klinefelter syndrome, are at greater risk for developing certain cancers.
5. Several environmental agents are considered carcinogenic, including radiation, toxic chemicals, electromagnetic fields, and chemotherapy. Viral illnesses have also been linked as causative factors.

TABLE 19-1
Other Childhood Cancers

CANCER	DESCRIPTION	ASSESSMENT FINDINGS
Osteogenic sarcoma	This is a malignant tumor of the long bone involving rapidly growing bone tissue (mesenchymal matrix-forming cells).	The child is usually taller than average. Pain and swelling occur at the tumor site. The area may be erythematous and warm to the touch. The child may have a history of recent trauma at the site.
Ewing sarcoma	This is a malignant tumor that occurs most often in the bone marrow of the diaphyseal area (midshaft) of long bones. Metastasis is usually present at the time of diagnosis, with the lungs and bones being the most common sites.	Pain occurs at the site of the tumor. It eventually becomes so severe that the child cannot sleep at night.
Neuroblastoma	These are tumors that arise from cells of the sympathetic nervous system. The cells are very undifferentiated and highly invasive. They occur most frequently in the abdomen near the adrenal glands or spinal ganglia.	Tumors are usually discovered during abdominal palpation. Anorexia, weight loss, abdominal pain, and constipation may be present. If tumor puts pressure on the adrenal glands, the child may exhibit excessive sweating, flushed face, and hypertension. If tumor puts pressure on spinal nerves or if it invades the intervertebral foramina, the child may exhibit loss of motor function in the lower extremities. If the tumor is in the chest, the child may exhibit dyspnea, difficulty swallowing, and neck and facial edema.

(continued)

6. Of major concern is the increased risk of secondary cancers in some children successfully treated for their primary malignancy.

C. **Characteristics of childhood cancers**

1. Childhood cancers are very different from those found in adults.
2. Most cancers arise from the mesodermal layer.
   a. In the fetus, the mesodermal layer becomes connective tissue, bone, muscle, cartilage, kidneys, blood, blood vessels, sex organs, lymphatics, and lymphoid organs.
   b. Therefore, 92% of childhood cancers are primitive embryonal tissue, sarcomas, leukemias, and lymphomas.
3. Other cancers arise from neuroectodermal tissue and give rise to central nervous system (CNS) tumors.

D. **Cancer staging**

1. Various staging criteria and terminology are used, depending on the specific tumor or treatment center, to describe and classify the extent of malignant neoplasms and their metastases.
2. The staging systems are used to guide therapy and evaluate progress.

TABLE 19-1
Other Childhood Cancers *(Continued)*

CANCER	DESCRIPTION	ASSESSMENT FINDINGS
Rhabdomyosarcoma	This is a tumor of the striated muscle that arises from the embryonic mesenchyme tissue that forms muscle, connective, and vascular tissue.	Symptoms depend on the site of the tumor. Orbit symptoms include proptosis and a visible and palpable conjunctival or eyelid mass. Nasopharynx symptoms include airway obstruction, epistaxis, dysphagia, and a visible mass in the nasal or nasopharygeal passages. Paranasal sinus symptoms include swelling, pain, nasal discharge, and epistaxis. Middle ear symptoms include pain, chronic otitis media, hearing loss, facial nerve palsy, and a mass protruding into the external ear canal. Neck symptoms include hoarseness, dysphagia, and a visible and palpable neck mass. Bladder and prostate symptoms include dysuria, urinary retention, hematuria, constipation, and a palpable lower abdominal mass. Vaginal symptoms include a mass protruding from the uterus into the vagina and abnormal vaginal bleeding. Testicular symptoms include a visible and palpable mass. Extremity symptoms include a visible and palpable mass.
Retinoblastoma	This is a malignant tumor of the retina that occurs early in life (6 weeks to preschool).	Pupil appears white or is described as a "cat's eye," because the red reflex is absent. The child eventually develops strabismus.

II. **NURSING PROCESS OVERVIEW FOR**
Children With Cancer

A. **Assessment**

1. **Health history**

   a. Elicit a description of symptoms including onset, duration, location, and precipitation. **Cardinal symptoms** of cancer in children include:

   (1) Unusual mass or swelling

   (2) Unexplained paleness and loss of energy

   (3) Sudden tendency to bruise or bleed

   (4) Persistent, localized pain or limping

   (5) Prolonged, unexplained fever or illness

   (6) Frequent headaches, often with vomiting

   (7) Sudden eye or vision changes

   (8) Excessive, rapid weight loss

    b. Explore prenatal, personal, and family history for **risk factors** for cancer.

        (1) Prenatal risk factors include exposure to ionizing radiation, maternal infections, medications, and substance use.

        (2) Personal risk factors include history of chromosomal abnormality, immune disorders, previous malignancy, exposure to ionizing radiation, previous health problems, medications, allergies, immunization status, nutritional status, exposures to toxic elements, and developmental history.

        (3) Family risk factors include a family history of cancer.

2. Physical examination

    a. **Vital signs**

        (1) Monitor temperature for elevation because fever may be an initial symptom.

        (2) Monitor and plot the child's weight; rapid weight loss is a sign of serious illness.

        (3) Blood pressure may be either low (sepsis) or elevated (kidney tumors/involvement, such as Wilms' or neuroblastoma).

    b. **Inspection**

        (1) Assess general appearance for listlessness or irritability.

        (2) Observe the skin for pallor, bruising, petechiae, or lesions.

        (3) Assess the eyes for unusual coloring; assess the pupils and extraocular muscles for abnormalities.

        (4) Assess the nose for signs of bleeding or drainage.

        (5) Inspect the mouth for bleeding and lesions.

        (6) Assess gait and symmetry of extremities.

        (7) Assess reflexes.

        (8) Assess for rectal and vaginal bleeding, redness, or drainage.

        (9) A cardinal sign of infection, purulent drainage/pus, may be absent in children with cancer (especially leukemia). Patients without functioning white blood cells (leukemia) are not able to produce pus. Redness may be the only sign of a potentially life-threatening infection.

    c. **Palpation**

        (1) Palpate the lymph nodes for enlargement.

        (2) Palpate the abdomen for tenderness, masses, and organomegaly. *Abdominal palpation is contradicted in Wilms' tumor because it may cause the tumor to rupture and spread.*

        (3) Palpate the extremities for tenderness and masses.

    d. **Auscultation**

        (1) Auscultate the lungs for abnormal breath sounds and adventitious sounds.

        (2) Auscultate the heart for murmurs.

3. Laboratory studies and diagnostic tests. (See Appendices A and B for normal findings and nursing considerations.)

    a. **Complete blood count (CBC)**, **urinalysis**, and **blood chemistries** are ordered to assess general health status. A 24-hour urinalysis is used to detect homovanillic acid, vanillylmandelic acid, and catecholamine in neuroblastoma.

    b. **Peripheral blood smears** are obtained to determine cell type and maturity.

    c. **Chest x-ray** is obtained on all children as a baseline or for diagnosis.

    d. **Ultrasound** is often used as a screening tool.

    e. A **bone scan** is a highly sensitive method of detecting bony lesions, but it does not discriminate between inflammation and malignancy.

    f. **Bone marrow aspiration** or **biopsy** is performed for definitive diagnosis of leukemia.

g. **Lumbar puncture** is performed to analyze cerebrospinal fluid (CSF) for leukemic cells, brain tumor cells, and other cancer cells that may metastasize to the spinal cord and brain.

h. **Imaging techniques (computed tomography [CT], ultrasonography, magnetic resonance imaging [MRI])** are used to detect solid tumors.

i. **Biopsies** are critical in determining the classification and stage of the cancer.

B. Nursing diagnoses

1. Risk for injury
2. Risk for infection
3. Risk for trauma
4. Risk for fluid volume deficit
5. Altered nutrition: less than body requirements
6. Altered oral mucous membranes
7. Pain
8. Risk for altered growth
9. Risk for altered development
10. Altered family processes
11. Anticipatory grief

C. Planning and outcome identification

1. The child will experience complete or partial remission from the disease.
2. The child will not experience an oncologic emergency.
3. The child will experience no to minimal infection.
4. The child will demonstrate no evidence of bleeding.
5. The child will remain adequately hydrated and experience minimal nausea and vomiting.
6. The child will receive adequate nutrition.
7. The child's oral mucous membranes will remain intact.
8. The child will be pain free.
9. The child will maintain appropriate growth and development.
10. The child and family will receive adequate support.
11. The child and family will cope with the possibility of death.

D. Implementation

1. **Assist in ensuring complete or partial remission from the disease by administering chemotherapy and by preventing, or minimizing, the complications of chemotherapy, radiation, and bone marrow transplant (BMT).**

   a. Administer chemotherapeutic agents, which may include those found in Drug Chart 19-1.

   (1) Follow guidelines and institutional policies for administration. *Some chemotherapeutic agents are vesicants (vincristine, doxorubicin) and can cause severe tissue damage if infiltration occurs. Chemotherapy should only be administered via a free-flowing intravenous (IV) line.*

   (2) Observe for signs of infiltration and irritation at the infusion site (eg, pain, stinging, swelling, or redness at the IV site). Immediately stop the infusion if infiltration occurs.

   (3) Observe the child for 20 minutes to note any signs of anaphylaxis (eg, cyanosis, severe urticaria, hypotension, or wheezing). Stop the infusion if a reaction is suspected.

   (4) Keep age-appropriate emergency equipment and medications nearby.

DRUG CHART 19-1   Medications Used for Children With Cancer

Classifications	Used for	Selected Interventions
Chemotherapeutic agents (general)	Treatment of neoplasms	Obtain accurate height and weight because dosages may be calculated on body surface areas.
		Always double check dosages with two nurses.
		Complete blood count (CBC) should be performed 24 hours before administration.
		Ensure patency of IV site before administration. Vesicants (agents that can produce blisters) should be administered through a fresh site if the site is already 24 hours old.
		Ensure needle placement and blood return if using plantable infusion device.
		If the child complains of burning at a patent peripheral site, slow down the IV and apply a cool cloth just above the site.
		Keep emergency medications and equipment readily available.
Alkalating agents		
mechlorethamine (Nitrogen Mustard)		Mechlorethamine is a vesicant and may cause discoloration of the veins.
cyclosphosphamide (Cytoxan)		Can cause severe nausea and vomiting
Other commonly used agents: ifosfamide (Ifos) melphalan (Alkeran) cisplatin (CDDP) carboplatin (Paraplatin)		Specific side effects include hemorrhagic cystitis, hyperpigmentation, and infertility.
		Cyclophosphamide can cause capillary leak syndrome. Force fluids to prevent cystitis.
Antimetabolites		
cytosine arabinoside (Ara-C)		Specific side effects include subclinical hepatitis and conjunctivitis
Other commonly used anti-metabolites include:		Use with caution in children with hepatic dysfunction
5-azacytidine (5-AzaC) and		A major specific side effect is neurotoxicity with intrathecal use. Drug must be mixed with a preservative-free diluent. Other major side effects are mucositis and photosensitivity.
mercaptopurine (6-MP)		
methotrexate (Folex PFS)		

(continued)

DRUG CHART 19-1   **Medications Used for Children With Cancer** (Continued)

Classifications	Used for	Selected Interventions
Plant alkaloids		
vincristine (Oncovin)		Vincristine is a vesicant.
VP-16 (Etopside)		A major specific side effect is neurotoxicity. Also monitor for ataxia, paresthesia, weakness, foot drop, hyporeflexia, and constipation.
vinblastine (Velban)		Specific side effects include hypotension with rapid infusion, bradycardia, neurotoxic effects, and anaphylaxis.
		Administer slowly IV with the child in a recumbent position.
Antibiotics		
doxorubicin (Adriamycin PFS) and daunorubicin (DaunoXome)	Doxorubicin has a cumulative lifetime dose that should not exceed 550 mg/m^2 (less with irradiation to the heart).	These drugs are vesicants. Observe for changes in heart rate and for heart failure.
bleomycin (BLM)		Inform the child and family that doxorubicin and daunorubicin routinely cause the urine to turn red or orange.
Enzymes		
L-asparaginase (Elspar)		Have emergency medications near the bedside because allergic reactions are possible.
		Monitor for side effects, which may include fever, nausea and vomiting, anorexia, weight loss, and arthralgia.
		Monitor for toxicity: liver toxicity, hyperglycemia, renal failure, and pancreatitis.
Nitrosourureas		Prevent extravasation; skin contact may cause brown spots.
carmustine (BCNU)	Used to treat brain tumors because they cross the blood–brain barrier.	
lomustine (CCNU)		Monitor for side effects, which may include severe nausea and vomiting, and alopecia.
Hormones		
Corticosteroids		Side effects include moon face, fluid retention, weight gain, mood changes, gastric irritation, and increased susceptibility to infection.
		Monitor weight.
		Decrease salt intake.
		Administer with an antacid.
		Observe for signs of infection.
		Test stools for occult blood.
		Monitor for hyperglycemia.

(continued)

DRUG CHART 19-1 Medications Used for Children With Cancer (Continued)

Classifications	Used for	Selected Interventions
Antiemetics	Minimize nausea associated with chemotherapy.	Administer 1–2 hours before chemotherapy, and around the clock.
ondansetron (Zofran)		Side effects include dizziness or drowsiness.
granisetron (Kytril)		Side effects include drowsiness, headache, diarrhea, or constipation.
Allopurinol (Lopurin)	Manage elevations in serum and urinary uric acid	Administer after meals.
		Force fluids.
		Check urine alkalinity.
		Monitor for side effects, which may include headache, drowsiness, nausea, vomiting, and diarrhea.
Granulocyte colony-stimulating factor (G-CSF)	To decrease the incidence of infection in patients with nonmyeloid malignancies receiving myelosuppressive chemotherapy.	Obtain a CBC prior to treatment and every 2 weeks during treatment.
		Do not give within 24 hours of chemotherapy.
		Store the medications in the refrigerator.
	To minimize neutropenia after bone marrow transplant	Monitor for side effects, which include nausea, vomiting, diarrhea, alopecia, or bone pain.

b. Monitor for specific chemotherapeutic side effects as well as general side effects.
   (1) Infection
   (2) Bleeding
   (3) Anemia
   (4) Nausea and vomiting
   (5) Altered nutrition
   (6) Mucosal ulceration
   (7) Alopecia
   (8) Other side effects (eg, diarrhea or constipation, pain, alterations in skin integrity, fluid and electrolyte imbalance, renal/hepatotoxicity, neurotoxicity, fatigue, pulmonary toxicity, cardiotoxicity, and ototoxicity [especially with carboplatin and cisplatin]).
c. Monitor for side effects of radiation therapy, which include those seen with administration of chemotherapy, and also dry or moist desquamation of the skin, dry mouth, sore throat, loss of taste, and parotitis. The acute untoward reactions from radiotherapy depend primarily on the area to be irradiated.
d. Monitor for complications of BMT.
   (1) BMT, when successful, destroys leukemic cells and replenishes the bone marrow with healthy cells.
   (2) There are two types of BMTs.
      (a) Allogenic (allo-BMT) refers to tissue from a histocompatible donor, usually a sibling (termed syngeneic if from twin) or an unrelated donor (UBMT).

(b) Autologous (auto-BMT) refers to tissue that is collected from the child's own tissue, frozen, and sometimes processed to remove undesired cells.

(3) Complications of BMT include:

    (a) Gastrointestinal (GI) problems such as nausea, vomiting, anorexia, watery diarrhea, and mucositis

    (b) Infections due to neutropenia

    (c) Hematologic problems such as anemia and bleeding

    (d) Veno-occlusive disease (VOD), manifested by sudden weight gain, jaundice, hepatomegaly, right upper quadrant pain, ascites, and encephalopathy

    (e) Interstitial pneumonia, characterized by fever, nasal flaring, tachypnea, dyspnea, nonproductive, dry cough, and hypoxia

    (f) Renal complications such as hypoproteinemia, hypovolemia, dehydration, and septic shock

    (g) Graft-versus-host disease (GVHD) manifested by a maculopapular rash, fever, jaundice, hypertension, infection, and hepatomegaly

    (h) Graft rejection or failure, manifested by fever, infection, and decreased blood count

    (i) Long-term effects (eg, growth hormone deficiency, cataracts, and pulmonary and cardiac toxicity)

2. Monitor for, and minimize, pediatric oncologic emergencies.

  a. Acute tumor lysis syndrome

    (1) Acute tumor lysis syndrome is characterized by an altered level of consciousness, including lethargy, nausea, vomiting, pruritus, flank pain, oliguria, and tetany.

    (2) It results from a rapid release of intracellular metabolites during the initial treatment of cancers, such as leukemia.

    (3) This syndrome causes hypercalcemia, hyperuricemia, hyperphosphatemia, and hyperkalemia.

    (4) Administer allopurinol to reduce uric acid formation, and exchange transfusions to reduce the metabolic consequences of massive tumor lysis.

  b. Hyperleukocytosis (white blood cell [WBC] count > 100,000/mm^3)

    (1) Assess for cyanosis, respiratory distress, altered level of consciousness, visual disturbances, ataxia, and delirium.

    (2) Hyperleukocytosis can lead to capillary obstruction, microinfarction, and organ dysfunction.

    (3) Assist with management, which includes rapid cytoreduction with chemotherapy, hydration, urinary alkalinization, and allopurinol. Leukophoresis or exchange transfusion may be warranted.

  c. Superior vena cava syndrome (SVCS)

    (1) Observe for cyanosis of face, neck, and upper torso; upper extremity edema, and distended neck veins.

    (2) SVCS results from compression of mediastinal structures, and is usually seen in children with space-occupying lesions, especially from Hodgkin's disease and non-Hodgkin's lymphoma.

3. Prevent infection.

  a. Assess the child for signs of infections, especially at the mouth, needle punctures, and irritated areas of the mucous membranes or skin. The risk for infection is significant in children at the nadir of chemotherapy when the WBC count is at its lowest, in children taking steroids, and in children after BMT.

b. Minimize the child's exposure to infected persons. Children after BMT are typically placed on strict isolation, which includes use of specially vented air.

c. Use strict, aseptic technique for all invasive procedures; use proper technique, including handwashing, for all other procedures.

d. Ensure that the child is up-to-date on inactivated immunizations. Do not administer live viruses to immunosuppressed children. Administer varicella-zoster immune globulin (VZIG) to children exposed to varicella (chickenpox).

e. Administer medications, which may include antibiotics and granulocyte colony-stimulating factor (GCSF).

f. Avoid exposure to live plants and flowers and uncooked fruits and vegetables, which may contain pathogens.

4. **Prevent trauma from bleeding and immobility**.

a. Monitor for signs of bleeding and impaired skin integrity. Observe for GI and genitourinary bleeding. Monitor hemoglobin, hematocrit, and platelet values regularly.

b. Minimize skin punctures for procedures such as intramuscular injections and venipunctures.

c. Avoid aspirin-containing compounds that can interfere with platelet function.

d. Minimize the risk of hemorrhagic cystitis by encouraging fluids and frequent voiding.

e. Move the child gently, pad the bedding, and use a pressure-relieving mattress.

f. Provide skin care, especially around the mouth and anus where ulcerations are likely to form.

g. Prevent rectal ulceration by keeping the area clean, using sitz baths, exposing excoriated areas to air, and applying protective barriers. Avoid taking rectal temperatures.

5. **Ensure adequate hydration**.

a. Monitor fluid intake and output (I&O).

b. Encourage frequent, small amounts of fluids.

c. Administer IV fluids.

6. **Encourage adequate nutrition**.

a. Allow foods the child wants and can tolerate.

b. Administer antiemetics around the clock to minimize nausea.

c. Encourage foods when the child appears hungry.

d. Make food appealing and create a pleasant atmosphere.

7. **Prevent mucosities**.

a. Monitor for signs of breakdown.

b. Provide mouth care. Use soft toothbrushes, frequently rinse the mouth, and apply local anesthetics to relieve pain, especially before eating.

c. Apply lip balm.

d. Avoid lemon-glycerin swabs and other irritants. Avoid hydrogen peroxide, which erodes tissue, and milk of magnesia, which is drying.

8. **Prevent pain**.

a. Minimize painful procedures whenever possible.

b. Administer analgesics on a preventive schedule and frequently assess their effectiveness.

c. Use nonpharmacologic pain relief measures.

9. **Foster healthy growth and development**

a. Allow the child to participate in self-care whenever possible.

b. Encourage age-appropriate activities that the child can manage.

c. Maintain the child's contact with school.

d. Assist the child in coping with body image disturbances, such as alopecia and weight gain or loss.
   (1) Reassure the child that hair loss is temporary; inform the child that new hair may have a different texture from the hair she lost.
   (2) Encourage the use of hats, scarves, and wigs.
   (3) Avoid use of hair chemicals, such as permanent wave solutions, when the hair grows back.
   (4) Assist the child in choosing apparel that will enhance positive aspects of appearance.

10. **Assist the family in coping with their child's disorder.**
    a. Encourage the child and family to verbalize their feelings. A child and her family need to adjust to living with the various phases of a life-threatening illness.
    b. Assist with coping skills. The child's reaction largely depends on her age, the information the child is given, and the physical impact of the disease on her energy level and coping skills.
    c. Teach the child and family to manage with the illness and its treatment, including the long-term consequences as described in Child and Family Teaching 19-1.

CHILD AND FAMILY TEACHING 19-1

Long-term Effects of Childhood Cancer

Instruct the child and family on the following possible long-term effects of cancer.

- **Cataracts.** Refer the child to an ophthalmologist and prepare for possible cataract surgery.
- **Hearing loss.** Refer the child to an audiologist and speech therapist; prepare for the possibility of wearing a hearing aid.
- **Pulmonary fibrosis.** Encourage flu vaccines and immediate care for respiratory infections; discourage smoking.
- **Cardiomyopathy, pericardial damage, early atherosclerosis, and ventricular arrhythmias.** Monitor cumulative chemotherapy dosages and refer the child to a cardiologist. Cardiac medications may be needed.
- **Chronic enteritis and cirrhosis.** Refer the child to a nutritionist because dietary modifications may be needed.
- **Chronic nephritis/cystitis.** Refer the child to a nephrologist, ensure hydration, and prepare the child for possible dialysis.
- **Scoliosis/kyphosis, facial asymmetry, or dental problems.** Refer the child to rehabilitation services and a dentist; encourage proper oral hygiene; instruct the child about avoiding contact sports.
- **Prolonged immunosuppression.** Encourage infection control measures, administer prophylactic antibiotics, monitor blood counts, and observe for signs of infection.
- **Ovary or testicular dysfunction.** Refer the child to an endocrinologist. Discuss replacement hormones. Adolescent boys may want to consider sperm banking before cancer treatment.
- **Hypothyroidism or hypothalamic dysfunction.** Refer the child to an endocrinologist and prepare the child for short stature.
- **Central nervous system disturbances, including leukoencephalopathy, peripheral neuropathy, and cognitive defects.** Monitor development and collaborate with family and school personnel to assist child in performing at optimum level.
- **Second malignancies.** Encourage the family to participate in ongoing follow-up care to monitor for possible secondary malignancies.

11. **Assist the child and family with the grieving process**.
  a. Provide consistent contact with the family to establish a trusting relationship.
  b. Assist the family in planning for the terminal stage of illness.
  c. Arrange for spiritual and other support.

E. **Outcome evaluation**
  1. The child experiences complete or partial remission from the disease.
  2. The child experiences no oncologic emergencies.
  3. The child experiences no infection.
  4. The child demonstrates no bleeding.
  5. The child remains adequately hydrated.
  6. The child is well nourished.
  7. The child's oral mucous membranes remain intact.
  8. The child is pain free.
  9. The child functions at the appropriate developmental level.
  10. The child and family cope with illness.
  11. The child and family cope with grief.

III. Leukemia

A. **Description**
  1. Leukemia is a proliferation of abnormal WBCs.
  2. Several different types of leukemia exist, and classification has become a complex process.
  3. The most common leukemia in children is acute lymphocytic leukemia (ALL), which is a proliferation of blast cells (immature lymphocytes). ALL is classified by form, structure, and morphology of the blast cells.
  4. Leukemia may be diagnosed at any age but has a peak onset between 3 and 5 years of age.

B. **Etiology**
  1. The etiology is unknown; a few cases in adults have been linked to environmental factors such as chemicals and radiation.
  2. Several genetic diseases have been associated with increased incidences of leukemia, including Down syndrome, Fanconi anemia, and Bloom syndrome.

C. **Pathophysiology**
  1. Malignant leukemia cells arise from precursor cells in blood-forming elements.
  2. These cells can accumulate and crowd out normal bone marrow elements, spill into peripheral blood, and eventually invade all body organs and tissues.
  3. Replacement of normal hematopoietic elements by leukemic cells results in bone marrow suppression, which is marked by a decreased production of red blood cells (RBCs), normal WBCs, and platelets.
  4. Bone marrow suppression results in anemia from deceased RBC production, predisposition to infection due to neutropenia, and bleeding tendencies due to thrombocytopenia. These put the child at risk of death from infection or hemorrhage.
  5. Infiltration of reticuloendothelial organs (eg, spleen, liver, and lymph glands) causes marked enlargement and, eventually, fibrosis.
  6. Leukemic infiltration of the CNS results in increased intracranial pressure (ICP) and other effects, depending on the specific areas involved.

7. Other possible sites of long-term infiltration include the kidneys, testes, prostate, ovaries, GI tract, and lungs.

8. The hypermetabolic leukemic cells eventually deprive all body cells of nutrients necessary for survival. Uncontrolled growth of leukemic cells can actually result in metabolic starvation.

D. Assessment findings

1. Clinical manifestations

a. Anemia from RBC suppression, which consists of fatigue, pallor, and tachycardia

b. Bleeding from platelet suppression, which includes petechiae, purpura, hematuria, epistaxis, and tarry stools

c. Immunosuppression from WBC suppression, which is manifested by fever, infection, and poor wound healing

d. Symptoms from reticuloendothelial involvement, which include hepatosplenomegaly (HSM), bone pain, and lymphadenopathy

e. CNS symptoms (if there is CNS metastasis), which include headache, meningeal irritation, and signs of increased ICP

f. General symptoms, which include weight loss, anorexia, and vomiting

2. Laboratory and diagnostic study findings

a. CBC may reveal normal, decreased, or increased WBC count with immature cells (blasts); decreased RBCs; and decreased platelets.

b. Bone marrow aspiration confirms the diagnosis by revealing extensive replacement of normal bone marrow elements by leukemic cells.

c. Lumbar puncture assesses abnormal cell migration to the CNS.

 E. Nursing management. Nursing management is completely covered in the nursing process overview for the child with cancer.

IV. Brain tumors

A. Description

1. Brain tumors are intracranial space-occupying lesions.

2. They are the most common childhood solid tumor and the second most common childhood cancer.

3. They are most commonly seen in children between 5 and 10 years old.

4. Tumors are classified according to histology and location.

a. Most tumors are gliomas, which originate from the glial cells (the supporting structural cells of the CNS).

b. Two-thirds of brain tumors are infratentorial (occur below the tentorium), which includes areas such as the cerebellum, fourth ventricle, and brain stem; one-third are supratentorial (occur above the tentorium).

5. Of the malignant tumors, astrocytomas are the most common, followed by medulloblastomas, brain stem gliomas, and ependymomas.

B. Etiology. The etiology is unknown, but various environmental factors have been associated with brain tumors, including industrial and chemical toxins and radiation exposure.

C. Pathophysiology

1. Tumors arise from anywhere in the cranium, glial cells, nerve cells, neuroepithelium, cranial nerves, blood vessels, pineal gland, and hypophysis.

2. Tumor or tumors enlarge and obstruct the circulation of CSF, resulting in increased ICP. As the tumor grows, it exerts pressure on nervous system components.

D. Assessment findings

1. Clinical manifestations

a. Characteristic findings usually are related to location of the tumor.

b. **The most common symptom is a headache.** It is typically described as intermittent and most common after the child wakes up. It may also be described as occurring with sneezing, coughing, and straining during a bowel movement.

c. Vomiting usually is projectile and occurs in the morning.

d. Other characteristic signs and symptoms include ataxia, hypotonia, and decreased reflexes.

e. Children may also display behavioral changes, changes in dexterity, weakness, spasticity, paralysis, and slurred speech.

f. Seizures, increased blood pressure, decreased pulse, and visual problems may also be seen.

2. Laboratory and diagnostic study findings

a. CT scan and an MRI may detect a lesion.

b. A lumbar puncture is performed to analyze cytology, glucose, protein, and enzymes. It usually is not done if the child has obstructive hydrocephalus or increased ICP.

E. Nursing management

1. Assess the child for symptoms of increased ICP (see Chap. 17).

2. Administer medications, which may include chemotherapeutic agents (see Drug Chart 19-1) and steroids.

3. Prepare the child and family for surgical removal of the tumor, including preoperative head shaving and postoperative bandaging, facial edema, and headache. Also prepare the child for the experience of the intensive care unit (ICU) and monitoring.

4. Provide postoperative care.

a. Monitor vital signs and neurologic status frequently during the first 24 to 48 hours after surgery.

b. Position the child to prevent pressure on the operative site.

c. Elevate the head to decrease edema and promote venous drainage from the cranial vault.

d. Provide eye care to prevent corneal irritation.

e. Monitor for cerebral edema and increased ICP.

f. Provide analgesia for headaches.

g. Observe for seizure activity; child may receive anticonvulsant medications.

h. Monitor incision for signs of infection.

5. Prepare the family for procedures and treatments, and for radiation and chemotherapy, if needed.

6. Assist the family in coping with their child's disorder.

7. Assist the family with the grieving process, if necessary.

V. Lymphomas

A. Description

1. Lymphomas are a group of neoplastic diseases that develop from the lymphoid and hemopoietic systems.

2. The two most common lymphomas seen in children are Hodgkin's disease and non-Hodgkin's lymphoma (NHL).

B. Etiology

1. The etiology of Hodgkin's disease is unknown, but studies suggest an infectious agent.
2. The etiology of NHL is unknown; however, there is a higher incidence in persons with HIV/AIDS, Epstein-Barr virus, and in persons whose immune systems were suppressed with medications.

C. Pathophysiology

1. Hodgkin's disease begins in a single lymph node or a group of lymph nodes. It is characterized by giant, multinucleated Reed-Sternburg cells. Humoral immunity remains normal, but cellular immunity is altered. Hodgkin's disease will spread from lymph nodes to nonlymph node sites such as the spleen, liver, bone, bone marrow, lungs, and mediastinum. The stages are as follows:
   a. In **stage I**, the disorder is limited to one lymph node area or only one extralymphatic site.
   b. In **stage II**, two or more lymph node areas on the same side of the diaphragm, or one additional extralymphatic site or organ, are involved.
   c. In **stage III**, lymph nodes on both sides of the diaphragm, or one extralymphatic site, spleen, or both, are involved.
   d. In **stage IV**, there are diffuse metastases throughout the body.
2. NHL begins with a proliferation of either B or T lymphocytes. The cells are either undifferentiated or poorly differentiated. Differentiation occurs earlier and more rapidly, and mediastinal involvement and invasion of meninges typically occur. The stages are as follows:
   a. In **stage I**, there is a single tumor at a single site.
   b. In **stage II**, there is a single tumor with regional involvement on the same side of the diaphragm.
   c. In **stage III**, there are tumors on both sides of the abdomen, or all tumors are primary thoracic, intra-abdominal, and paraspinal or epidural tumors.
   d. **Stage IV** is any stage I or II involvement combined with CNS or bone marrow involvement.

D. Assessment findings

1. **Clinical manifestations**
   a. **Hodgkin's lymphoma**
      (1) Hodgkin's lymphoma is characterized by painless enlargement of the lymph nodes. The most typical finding is enlarged, firm, nontender, mobile nodes in the supraclavicular area.
      (2) The "sentinel" node near the left clavicle may be the first to enlarge.
      (3) Other symptoms depend on the location and extent of involvement.
      (4) Systemic manifestations include fever, anorexia, nausea, weight loss, night sweats, and pruritus. These symptoms usually indicate advanced involvement.
   b. **NHL**
      (1) Manifestations depend on the site and extent of involvement.
      (2) Many characteristics are the same as those found in Hodgkin's disease.
      (3) Metastasis to the bone marrow or CNS may produce characteristics of leukemia.
2. **Laboratory and diagnostic study findings**
   a. **Hodgkin's lymphoma**
      (1) Lymph node biopsy confirms the diagnosis.

      (2) CBC, sedimentation rate, liver and thyroid tests, bone marrow biopsy, chest x-ray, and CT scans determine the extent of the disease.

      (3) A lymph angiogram may be used to visualize the lymphatic vessels to determine the presence of disease in various lymph node regions.

   b. **NHL**

      (1) Lymph node biopsy confirms the diagnosis.

      (2) Bone marrow aspiration, lumbar puncture, and CT scans of the lungs and GI tract are performed to assist in staging.

E. Nursing management. Nursing management is completely covered in the nursing process overview for the child with cancer.

VI. Wilms' tumor (nephroblastoma)

A. Description

  1. Wilms' tumor is a malignant neoplasm of the kidney. It is the most common intra-abdominal tumor in children, and the most curable solid tumor in children.

  2. Wilms' tumor occurs most often in young children but may occur in adolescents. The median age at diagnosis is between 2 and 3 years old.

  3. Usually it is unilateral and occurs with other abnormalities such as an absent iris or genitourinary problems.

B. Etiology

  1. The etiology is unknown.

  2. Siblings of children with Wilms' tumor have a higher risk of developing the disorder than the general population.

C. Pathophysiology

  1. The tumor originates from immature renoblast cells located in the renal parenchyma.

  2. It is well encapsulated in early stages but may later extend into lymph nodes and the renal vein or vena cava and metastasize to the lungs and other sites.

  3. Wilms' tumors are classified into five stages.

    a. In **stage I** the tumor is confined to one kidney.

    b. In **stage II** the tumor extends beyond kidney but can be resected.

    c. In **stage III** the tumor has residual nonhematogenous tumor cells confined to the abdomen.

    d. In **stage IV** the tumor is characterized by distant metastases involving lung, liver, bone, or brain.

    e. In **stage V** the tumor involves both kidneys.

D. Assessment findings

  1. Clinical manifestations

    a. The most common sign is an abdominal mass, usually discovered during a routine assessment or by the parents when bathing the child.

    b. Other characteristics may include fever, abdominal pain, hematuria, hypertension (due to secretion of excess renin from the tumor), and anorexia.

  2. Laboratory and diagnostic study findings

    a. Ultrasound or CT scan reveals a mass.

    b. Other studies may be performed if metastasis is suspected.

E. Nursing management

  1. Assess the child for hypertension.

2. **Do not palpate the abdomen**; doing so can rupture the encapsulated tumor *and cause dissemination of the disease to adjacent and distant sites.* Instruct parents to not palpate their child's abdomen.
3. **Administer medications**, which may include chemotherapeutic agents (see Drug Chart 19-1).
4. **Provide postoperative care**.
   a. Monitor bowel sounds and assess for signs and symptoms of intestinal obstruction resulting from abdominal surgery, vincristine-induced adynamic ileus, and radiation-induced edema.
   b. Help prevent infection by maintaining scrupulous handwashing and limiting the child's exposure to persons with infections. Monitor for evidence of infections.
   c. Help prevent postoperative pulmonary complications by providing frequent position changes and by encouraging coughing and deep-breathing exercises and ambulation.

STUDY QUESTIONS

1. Which of the following is the **most** common form of childhood cancer?
   (1) Lymphoma
   (2) Brain tumors
   (3) Leukemia
   (4) Osteosarcoma

2. A 4-year-old child with leukemia is admitted to the hospital because of pneumonia. Which of the following is the most likely cause of his current condition?
   (1) Anemia
   (2) Leukopenia
   (3) Thrombocytopenia
   (4) Eosinophilia

3. The nurse would prepare the parents of a child with suspected leukemia for which of the following tests that would confirm this diagnosis?
   (1) Lumbar puncture
   (2) Bone marrow aspiration
   (3) Complete blood count
   (4) Blood culture

4. Which of the following would be an appropriate nursing diagnosis for a child who is receiving chemotherapy?
   (1) Ineffective breathing pattern
   (2) Constipation
   (3) Altered skin integrity
   (4) Altered oral mucous membrane

5. When caring for a child with leukemia, which of the following goals should be considered as **primary**?
   (1) Meeting developmental needs
   (2) Promoting adequate nutrition
   (3) Preventing infection
   (4) Promoting diversional activities

6. Which of the following would the nurse expect to assess as the **most** common presenting manifestation of Wilms' tumor?
   (1) Hematuria
   (2) Pain on voiding
   (3) Nausea and vomiting
   (4) Abdominal mass

7. When caring for a child awaiting surgery for a Wilms' tumor, which of the following nursing actions would be **most** important?
   (1) Handling the child with care, particularly during bathing
   (2) Placing the child on low blood count precautions and isolation
   (3) Monitoring bowel sounds for vincristine-induced ileus
   (4) Placing the child in high Fowler position to facilitate breathing

8. Which of the following nursing interventions can help prevent or reduce nausea and vomiting during chemotherapy?
   (1) Providing a high-fiber diet prior to chemotherapy
   (2) Administering allopurinol 30 minutes before chemotherapy
   (3) Encouraging increased fluid intake before and during therapy
   (4) Administering antiemetic 30 minutes before chemotherapy

9. A 4-year-old boy is about to be discharged after undergoing surgery and follow-up treatment for a Wilms' tumor. Which of the following points would be a vital part of the teaching program for the child's parents?
   (1) Allowing him to resume activity, including contact sports
   (2) Monitoring for signs and symptoms of urinary tract infection
   (3) Making arrangements for a return visit in 6 months
   (4) Arranging for hospice care because Wilms' tumor is fatal

10. Which of the following is considered the most common assessment finding associated with a brain tumor in a child?
    (1) Projectile vomiting
    (2) Increased intracranial pressure
    (3) Headache
    (4) Diminished reflexes

ANSWER KEY

1. The answer is (3). Leukemia is the most common type of cancer in children, followed by brain tumors, lymphoma, and kidney tumors. Brain tumors are the second most common childhood cancer but they are the most common form of solid tumor cancer in childhood. Bone cancers account for 5% with osteosarcoma being the most common type.

2. The answer is (2). The decrease in functioning WBCs in leukemia causes the increased risk for infection in children with leukemia. Anemia would result in fatigue. Thrombocytopenia, decreased platelet count, would result in bleeding. An increased eosinophil count is not related to leukemia.

3. The answer is (2). A bone marrow aspiration is performed to confirm the diagnosis of leukemia through the examination of abnormal cells in the bone marrow. A lumbar puncture is performed to detect spread into the CNS, but it is not used to confirm the diagnosis. An abnormal CBC may suggest leukemia, but it is not used to confirm the diagnosis. A blood culture may be performed if infection is suspected.

4. The answer is (4). Chemotherapy destroys rapidly growing cells, including those in the GI tract, resulting in stomatitis, an inflammatory condition of the mouth. In general, there should not be an effect on the respiratory system related to chemotherapy. Because chemotherapy affects the GI tract, the child most likely would have diarrhea, not constipation. In general, skin integrity should not be affected by chemotherapy.

5. The answer is (3). The child is at high risk for infection due to immunosuppression from both the disease and the treatment, and infection is the leading cause of death in leukemia. Meeting developmental needs, promoting adequate nutrition, and promoting diversional activities are important goals. However, they are not the primary goal in caring for a child with leukemia.

6. The answer is (4). The most common sign of Wilms' tumor is a painless palpable mass, sometimes marked by an increase in abdominal girth. Gross hematuria is uncommon, although microscopic hematuria may be present. Pain on voiding is not associated with Wilms' tumor. Tumor encroachment should not cause abdominal obstruction and resulting nausea and vomiting.

7. The answer is (1). Handling the child carefully is essential to prevent rupture of an encapsulated tumor. The child usually does not undergo myelosuppression before surgery. In fact, the child may be suffering from polycythemia due to increased production of erythropoietin. Vincristine usually is administered postoperatively. Respiratory difficulty is not a common problem with Wilms' tumor.

8. The answer is (4). Antiemetics counteract nausea most effectively when given before administration of an agent that causes nausea. Antiemetics also work best when given on a continuous basis rather than as needed. A high-fiber diet has no effect on reducing nausea and vomiting. Allopurinol, a xanthine-oxidase inhibitor, is thought to prevent renal damage due to large releases of uric acid during chemotherapy; however, it has no antiemetic properties. High fluid intake during periods of nausea exaggerates the symptoms and may exacerbate vomiting.

9. The answer is (2). Urinary tract infections pose a threat to the remaining kidney. Therefore, the parents should be instructed to monitor the child for signs and symptoms of infection. Rough play and contact sports should be discouraged because of the residual effect of radiation to the abdomen and because the child needs to protect his lone kidney. Follow up at 6 months is too late; children receive chemotherapy for 6 to 15 months after surgery. Wilms' tumor is the most curable solid tumor of childhood; prognosis is usually favorable.

10. The answer is (3). In children with a brain tumor, the most common symptom is a headache. It is typically described as intermittent and most common after the child wakes up. It may also be described as occurring with sneezing, coughing, and straining during a bowel movement. Vomiting, which usually is projectile and occurs in the morning is not as common, but may be present. The tumor as it increases in size obstructs the circulation of CSF, resulting in increased ICP. Decreased reflexes are commonly reported in cerebellar tumors.

Comprehensive Test Questions

1. When assessing a child with a cleft palate, the nurse is aware that the child is at risk for more frequent episodes of otitis media due to which of the following?
   (1) Lowered resistance from malnutrition
   (2) Ineffective functioning of the eustachian tubes
   (3) Plugging of the eustachian tubes with food particles
   (4) Associated congenital defects of the middle ear

2. The nurse would expect that a healing would occur in 3-month-old with a fractured femur within which of the following?
   (1) 2 to 4 weeks
   (2) 4 to 6 weeks
   (3) 8 to 10 weeks
   (4) 10 to 16 weeks

3. Which of the following would be inappropriate when administering chemotherapy to a child?
   (1) Monitoring the child for both general and specific adverse effects
   (2) Observing the child for 10 minutes to note for signs of anaphylaxis
   (3) Administering medication through a free-flowing intravenous line
   (4) Assessing for signs of infusion infiltration and irritation

4. Which of the following disorders is characterized by a blue sclera and can result in pathologic fractures?
   (1) Osteomyelitis
   (2) Osteogenesis imperfecta
   (3) Osteosarcoma
   (4) Osteoarthritis

5. While assessing a child in a hip spica cast, which of the following assessment findings would alert the nurse to suspect a possible infection under the cast?

   (1) Cold toes
   (2) Absent pedal pulses
   (3) "Hot spots" on the cast
   (4) Cyanotic extremities

6. Which of the following actions would be included as the priority in the plan of care for a for a 3-month-old infant with a serum lead level of 90 mcg/dL?
   (1) Monitoring neurologic status due to possible encephalopathy
   (2) Initiating comfort measures to relieve bone pain
   (3) Teaching parents about lead sources to stop child's pica
   (4) Including dietary sources of iron to correct anemia

7. Which of the following adverse effects should the nurse be alert for in a child placed on lead chelation therapy with edetate calcium-disodium (CaNa2EDTA) and dimercaprol (BAL)?
   (1) Seizures
   (2) Muscular atrophy
   (3) Depression
   (4) Increased appetite

8. While performing a neurodevelopmental assessment on a 3-month-old infant, which of the following characteristics would be expected?
   (1) A strong Moro reflex
   (2) A strong parachute reflex
   (3) Rolling from front to back
   (4) Lifting of head and chest when prone

9. By the end of which of the following would the nurse most commonly expect a child's birth weight to triple?
   (1) 4 months
   (2) 7 months
   (3) 9 months
   (4) 12 months

10. Which of the following best describes parallel play between two toddlers?
(1) Sharing crayons to color separate pictures
(2) Playing a board game with a nurse
(3) Sitting near each other while playing with separate dolls
(4) Sharing their dolls with two different nurses

11. Which of the following is the best method for performing a physical examination on a toddler?
(1) From head to toe
(2) Distally to proximally
(3) From abdomen to toes, then to head
(4) From least to most intrusive

12. Which of the following would the school nurse check for when performing a screening examination on a 12-year-old girl?
(1) Hip dislocation
(2) Transient synovitis
(3) Scoliosis
(4) Tibial torsion

13. During the immediate postoperative period following surgery for a cleft lip repair, for which of the following complications should the nurses be alert?
(1) Bleeding and respiratory distress
(2) Scarring problems and infection
(3) Infection and respiratory distress
(4) Bleeding and suture line infection

14. Which of the following organisms is responsible for the development of rheumatic fever?
(1) Streptococcal pneumonia
(2) Haemophilus influenzae
(3) Group A β-hemolytic streptococcus
(4) Staphylococcus aureus

15. Which of the following would the nurse question if found on the plan of care for a child with rheumatic fever?
(1) Providing adequate rest periods
(2) Isolating the child to prevent disease transmission
(3) Ensuring compliance with medication therapy
(4) Providing adequate nutritional intake

16. For which of the following would the nurse assess in a child as early manifestations of plumbism?
(1) Diarrhea, blurred vision, and headache
(2) Dizziness, fever, and chills
(3) Anorexia, abdominal cramps, and vomiting
(4) Developmental delay, seizures, and coma

17. Which of the following acid–base disorders is most likely to develop secondary to diarrhea in a 6-month-old child?
(1) Metabolic acidosis
(2) Metabolic alkalosis
(3) Respiratory acidosis
(4) Respiratory alkalosis

18. Which of the following nursing interventions is a priority when caring for a 4-month-old with acute viral gastroenteritis?
(1) Initiating droplet precautions
(2) Obtaining daily weights
(3) Administering antiemetics
(4) Monitoring CBC results

19. Which of the following assessments would the nurse expect to note in an infant who has lost 11% of his body weight due to dehydration?
(1) Pallor
(2) Decreased pulse
(3) Bulging fontanelle
(4) Marked oliguria

20. Which of the following would the nurse identify as the initial priority for a child with acute lymphocytic leukemia?
(1) Instituting infection control precautions
(2) Encouraging adequate intake of iron-rich foods
(3) Assisting with coping with chronic illness
(4) Administering medications via IM injections

21. Which of the following demonstrates the nurse's understanding of the rationale for administering allopurinol to a child receiving chemotherapy?
(1) Prevention of acid formation
(2) Prevention of hyperuricemia
(3) Assistance in tumor disintegration
(4) Protection for liver function

22. Which of the following would the nurse expect to assess as the most common gastrointestinal complication associated with cystic fibrosis?
    (1) Meconium ileus
    (2) Ulcerative colitis
    (3) Rectal prolapse
    (4) Diverticulitis

23. At which of the following times would the nurse teach the parents of a child with cystic fibrosis to perform chest physical therapy?
    (1) Before meals and at bedtime
    (2) Immediately after meals
    (3) Immediately on arising
    (4) Never, because it is contraindicated

24. Which of the following statements by the parents of a child with cystic fibrosis (CF) indicates that the parents understand the teaching about the rationale for administering pancreatic enzymes (Pancrease)?
    (1) "The medication helps to soften the stools."
    (2) "The enzymes aid in the digestion of fats."
    (3) "This medication will prevent diabetes."
    (4) "The drug will help to treat the pneumonia."

25. Which of the following would the nurse keep in mind as a rationale for using a mist tent for the child with acute laryngotracheobronchitis?
    (1) Provide 100% oxygen
    (2) Liquefy secretions
    (3) Warm the respiratory tract
    (4) Provide reverse isolation

26. Which of the following must be monitored preoperatively before a child has a tonsillectomy and adenoidectomy?
    (1) Clotting times
    (2) Urinalysis
    (3) Serum electrolyte levels
    (4) White blood cell differential

27. Which of the following would the nurse anticipate as treatment when caring for a 2-month-old infant with developmental dysplasia of the hip?
    (1) Traction
    (2) Closed reduction

    (3) Abduction device
    (4) Surgical reduction

28. Which of the following information, when voiced by the mother, would indicate to the nurse that she understands home care instructions following the administration of a diphtheria, tetanus, and pertussis injection?
    (1) Measures to reduce fever
    (2) Need for dietary restrictions
    (3) Reasons for subsequent rash
    (4) Measures to control subsequent diarrhea

29. Which of the following actions by a community health nurse is most appropriate when noting multiple bruises and burns on the posterior trunk of an 18-month-old child during a home visit?
    (1) Report the child's condition to Protective Services immediately.
    (2) Schedule a follow-up visit to check for more bruises.
    (3) Notify the child's physician immediately.
    (4) Do nothing because this is a normal finding in a toddler.

30. Which of the following assessment findings would the nurse expect in a 6-week-old infant with pyloric stenosis?
    (1) Projectile vomiting
    (2) Choking cough after feedings
    (3) Currant jelly stools
    (4) Abdominal distention

31. Which of the following is **most** likely associated with a cerebrovascular accident (CVA) resulting from congenital heart disease?
    (1) Polycythemia
    (2) Cardiomyopathy
    (3) Endocarditis
    (4) Low blood pressure

32. Which of the following symptoms would the nurse expect to assess in a 9-month-old child with congenital heart disease who develops congestive heart failure?
    (1) Bradycardia and cyanosis
    (2) Dyspnea and bradycardia
    (3) Strong peripheral pulses and edema
    (4) Tachycardia and hepatomegaly

33. During hospitalization, which of the following fears would reflect a 4-year-old's intense psychosexual preoccupations?
(1) Loss of control
(2) Fear of the dark
(3) Fear of castration
(4) Fear of separation

34. Which of the following would be important to remember about the adult who commits child sexual abuse while assessing a child for possible sexual abuse?
(1) The abuser is usually a female person.
(2) The child knows the abuser.
(3) The abuser usually is addicted to drugs.
(4) The abuser exhibits a sociopathic personality.

35. Which of the following stages of separation anxiety are being exhibited by an 18-month-old girl who cries inconsolably when her mother leaves her to go to the admissions office?
(1) Protest
(2) Despair
(3) Detachment
(4) Denial

36. Which of the following is being used when the mother of a hospitalized child calls the student nurse and states, "You idiot, you have no idea how to care for my sick child!"?
(1) Displacement
(2) Projection
(3) Repression
(4) Psychosis

37. While performing a community assessment, which of the following would the community health nurse be aware of as the **most** overwhelming adverse influence on health in children?
(1) Race
(2) Customs
(3) Low socioeconomic status
(4) Genetic constitution

38. When caring for a child and family with a different cultural background, which of the following would be an appropriate goal?

(1) Striving to keep background from influencing health needs
(2) Discouraging continuation of cultural practices in the hospital
(3) Gently attempting to change family's cultural beliefs
(4) Adapting family's health needs to family's cultural practices as necessary.

39. Which of the following adolescents **most** likely would be allowed to give his or her own consent for examination and treatment?
(1) A 14-year-old with strep throat
(2) A 15-year-old requesting a school physical
(3) A 16-year-old with a sexually transmitted disease
(4) A 17-year-old with a broken arm

40. While caring for a premature infant, which of the following would the nurse anticipate as a possible complication of oxygen therapy?
(1) Bronchopulmonary dysplasia
(2) Necrotizing enterocolitis
(3) Congestive heart failure
(4) Meconium aspiration syndrome

41. In addition to ventricular septal defect, which of the following structural defects would the nurse also expect to be found in a child diagnosed with tetralogy of Fallot?
(1) Atrial septal defect
(2) Left ventricular failure
(3) Overriding aorta
(4) Aortic stenosis

42. When assessing the child with tetralogy of Fallot, which of the following positions would the nurse expect to see as a compensatory mechanism?
(1) Low Fowler's
(2) Prone
(3) Supine
(4) Squatting

43. Which of the following should the nurse expect to note as a frequent complication for a child with congenital heart disease?
(1) Susceptibility to respiratory infection
(2) Bleeding tendencies
(3) Frequent vomiting and diarrhea
(4) Seizure disorder

44. Which of the following would the nurse expect as a critical element in the plan of care for a child with thalassemia major?
(1) Oxygen therapy
(2) Adequate hydration
(3) Supplemental iron
(4) Frequent blood transfusions

45. Which of the following would the nurse expect to find in the history of a 9-year-old girl diagnosed with rheumatic fever?
(1) Treatment for strep throat 3 weeks ago.
(2) Congenital heart defect diagnosed at birth.
(3) Episode of chickenpox 1 month ago.
(4) Untreated fever and sore throat 2 weeks ago.

46. For which of the following reasons would the nurse expect to institute intravenous fluid therapy and nothing by mouth (NPO) status for an infant with bronchiolitis?
(1) Tachypnea
(2) Irritability
(3) Fever
(4) Tachycardia

47. Which of the following increases the risk of hemorrhage in a child 5 to 10 days following a tonsillectomy and adenoidectomy?
(1) Infection
(2) Tissue sloughing
(3) Retained secretions
(4) Tissue vascularity

48. Which of the following blood study results would the nurse expect as **most** likely when caring for the child with iron deficiency anemia?
(1) Increased hemoglobin
(2) Normal hematocrit
(3) Decreased mean corpuscular volume (MCV)
(4) Normal total iron-binding capacity (TIBC)

49. When assessing a child with a possible Wilms' tumor, which of the following would the nurse expect as the **most** common symptom early in the disease?
(1) Abdominal pain
(2) Frank hematuria
(3) Hypertension
(4) Abdominal mass

50. When obtaining a history from a parent, which of the following statements **best** describes primary enuresis in a child?
(1) "He never attained dryness."
(2) "She was once bladder trained for a year."
(3) "He is dry only during the day."
(4) "She is usually incontinent during the day."

51. Which of the following would the nurse expect to administer intranasally to treat enuresis?
(1) Imipramine (Tofranil)
(2) Amoxicillin (Amoxil)
(3) Pseudoephedrine (Sudafed)
(4) Desmopressin (DDAVP)

52. Which of the following is appropriate when administering ribavirin (Virazole) for a child with severe bronchiolitis?
(1) Give the medication by deep intramuscular injection.
(2) Administer the medication directly into the mist tent.
(3) Monitor the child's vital signs every 1 to 2 hours.
(4) Administer the medication orally with milk.

53. Which of the following would the nurse do **first** for a 3-year-old boy who arrives in the emergency room with a temperature of 105 degrees, inspiratory stridor, and restlessness, who is leaning forward and drooling?
(1) Auscultate his lungs and place him in a mist tent.
(2) Have him lie down and rest after encouraging fluids.
(3) Examine his throat and perform a throat culture.
(4) Notify the physician immediately and prepare for intubation.

54. Which of the following is inappropriate when caring for a child receiving an aminoglycoside?
(1) Assessing the child's hearing
(2) Increasing the child's fluid intake
(3) Assessing kidney functioning
(4) Administering the drug with food

55. Which of the following antibiotics would be contraindicated for use in a 5-year-old boy because of his age?
(1) Tetracycline
(2) Erythromycin
(3) Penicillin
(4) Amoxicillin

56. Which of the following would the nurse identify as the **most** common problem requiring close monitoring for a child with thalassemia being given a blood transfusion?
(1) Iron toxicity
(2) Hemolytic reaction
(3) Fluid overload
(4) Sickle cell crisis

57. At which of the following frequencies would the nurse expect to administer analgesia to an adolescent in sickle cell crisis?
(1) Highly infrequently to avoid addiction
(2) Once a day at bedtime
(3) As needed, as prescribed
(4) Rarely because of severe depression

58. In which of the following would the nurse avoid using aspirin, rectal temperatures, and intramuscular injections?
(1) Iron deficiency anemia
(2) Idiopathic thrombocytopenic purpura
(3) Sickle cell anemia
(4) Thalassemia

59. Which of the following should the nurse suspect in a child with hemophilia who complains of a sudden, severe headache, vomits, and exhibits confusion and lethargy.
(1) Intracranial bleeding
(2) Factor reaction
(3) Psychogenic stress
(4) Acquired immunodeficiency syndrome (AIDS)

60. Which of the following statements by an adolescent with sickle cell anemia would indicate the need for additional teaching about the disease?
(1) "I need to perform aerobic exercise frequently."
(2) "I need to avoid others who may have an infection."

(3) "I need to eat a well-balanced diet."
(4) "I might experience some transient bed-wetting."

61. For which of the following conditions would the nurse expect that genetic counseling for the child and family would be inappropriate?
(1) Sickle cell anemia
(2) Thalassemia
(3) Hemophilia
(4) Idiopathic thrombocytopenic purpura

62. Which of the following would the nurse need to keep in mind as a predisposing factor when formulating a teaching plan for a child with a urinary tract infection?
(1) A shorter urethra in females
(2) Frequent emptying of the bladder
(3) Increased fluid intake
(4) Ingestion of acidic juices

63. When obtaining a history, which of the following is the **most** likely cause of acute glomerulonephritis in a child?
(1) Impaired reabsorption of bicarbonate ions
(2) An antecedent streptococcal infection
(3) Gross inability to concentrate urine
(4) Vesicoureteral reflux

64. Which of the following clinical manifestations would the nurse expect to note in a child with nephrotic syndrome?
(1) Hematuria and bacteriuria
(2) Massive proteinuria and edema
(3) Gross hematuria and fever
(4) Hypertension and weight loss

65. During the acute phase of post-streptococcal glomerulonephritis, which of the following diagnostic test results would the nurse expect to find?
(1) Negative protein in the urine
(2) Decreased serum creatinine
(3) Decreased urine specific gravity
(4) Elevated erythrocyte sedimentation rate

66. Which of the following is the **primary** objective when caring for a child with nephrotic syndrome?
(1) Reducing excretion of urinary protein
(2) Encouraging a low-protein diet
(3) Controlling the development of hematuria
(4) Encouraging normal development

67. Which of the following would the nurse expect to assess **most** commonly in a school-aged child with a possible brain tumor?
(1) Ataxia and seizures
(2) Poor fine and gross motor control
(3) Fever and irritability
(4) Headache and vomiting

68. Which of the following would the nurse **most** likely suspect after assessing "raccoon eyes" and a "battle sign" in a 10-year-old who fell and injured his head?
(1) Linear skull fracture
(2) Basilar skull fracture
(3) Epidural hematoma
(4) Subdural hematoma

69. Which of the following is the **most** likely cause of noncommunicating hydrocephalus?
(1) Developmental malformation
(2) Bacterial meningitis
(3) Prenatal infection
(4) Birth trauma

70. Which of the following phrases best describes the pathophysiology of communicating hydrocephalus?
(1) Precursor of spina bifida occulta
(2) Obstruction of cerebrospinal fluid flow in ventricular system
(3) Impaired absorption of cerebrospinal fluid in arachnoid space
(4) Cystic formation of the cerebral hemisphere

71. While preparing to teach a group of child-bearing-age women about healthy pregnancies, the nurse is aware that which of the following prenatal maternal disorders may significantly influence the development of myelomeningocele?
(1) Iron deficiency anemia
(2) Protein-losing enteropathy
(3) Folic acid deficiency
(4) Diabetes insipidus

72. Which of the following clinical manifestations is **most** characteristic of spastic cerebral palsy?
(1) Athetosis
(2) Dyskinesia
(3) Wide-based gait
(4) Hypertonicity

73. Which of the following manifestations would cause the nurse to suspect rubeola?
(1) Koplik's spots
(2) Occipital adenopathy
(3) Vesicular rash
(4) Parotid swelling

74. At which of the following would the nurse teach the parents of a child with varicella that the disease is no longer communicable?
(1) When crusts form
(2) In 2 to 3 weeks
(3) As soon as rash appears
(4) During the prodromal phase

75. Which of the following is the **most** dangerous complication of rubella?
(1) Arthralgia
(2) Pyrexia
(3) Purpura
(4) Teratogenic effects

76. Which of the following would the nurse expect to be ordered to confirm a 2-month-old infant's diagnosis of HIV infection?
(1) ELISA
(2) Western blot
(3) HIV viral assay
(4) CD4 count

77. Which of the following is characterized by a whitish-gray membrane adherent to the tonsils?
(1) Pertussis
(2) Diphtheria
(3) Poliomyelitis
(4) Kawasaki's disease

78. Which of the following is a contraindication for a child to receive MMR vaccine?
(1) Previous anaphylactic reaction to eggs
(2) Presence of HIV disease
(3) Concurrent administration of DTP
(4) Use of immunoglobulins 1 year ago

79. When evaluating the teaching given to the parents of a child with cerebral palsy, which of the following manifestations, if stated by the parents, indicates the need for additional teaching?
(1) Delayed gross motor development
(2) Decreased cognitive functioning
(3) Abnormal muscle performance
(4) Altered muscle tone

80. Which of the following is characteristic of a preschooler with mild mental retardation?

(1) Slow to feed self

(2) Lack of speech

(3) Marked motor delays

(4) Gait disability

81. Which of the following assessment findings would lead the nurse to suspect Down syndrome in an infant?

(1) Small tongue

(2) Transverse palmar crease

(3) Large nose

(4) Restricted joint movement

82. For which of the following is Gower's sign a prominent characteristic in the early stages?

(1) Cerebral palsy

(2) Spina bifida

(3) Muscular dystrophy

(4) Down syndrome

83. Which of the following statements is true about the administering immunizations to a child with HIV/AIDS?

(1) MMR is contraindicated.

(2) The child should receive TIPV.

(3) All immunizations are given as scheduled.

(4) The child should not receive any immunizations.

84. In which of the following would the nurse assess unilateral or bilateral parotid enlargement?

(1) Diphtheria

(2) Poliomyelitis

(3) Mumps

(4) Pertussis

85. Which of the following nursing diagnoses takes priority for a child who has just had a fresh hip spica cast applied?

(1) Risk for infection

(2) Risk for injury

(3) Risk for impaired skin integrity

(4) Altered tissue perfusion

86. Which of the following instructions would be **best** to assist parents in preventing rheumatic fever?

(1) Avoid all exposure to strep infections.

(2) Treat all sore throats with antibiotics.

(3) Learn the early signs and symptoms of rheumatic fever.

(4) Use prescribed treatment for streptococcal infections.

87. Which of the following would be the nurse's **best** response to a mother who asks the nurse what to do when her toddler cries and clings to her as she attempts to leave the hospital?

(1) "Don't worry, he'll stop crying as soon as you leave."

(2) "It's probably better if you didn't visit that often."

(3) "I'll stay with him while you leave."

(4) "Try to sneak away while he is playing."

88. Which of the following should the nurse do first for a 15-year-old boy with a full leg cast who is screaming in unrelenting pain and exhibiting right foot pallor signifying compartment syndrome?

(1) Medicate him with acetaminophen.

(2) Notify the physician immediately.

(3) Release the traction.

(4) Monitor him every 5 minutes.

89. Which of the following instructions would the nurse include in the parent teaching plan for a child placed in a Pavlik harness for bilateral developmental dysplasia of the hip?

(1) Removing the harness during baths

(2) Turning the child a maximum of three times a day

(3) Having the child lie primarily on the affected side

(4) Checking the child's skin for areas of breakdown

90. To which of the following immunizations is the nurse referring when alerting the mother of a toddler about the possibility of a rash, pruritus, low-grade fever, and arthralgia?

(1) DTaP

(2) MMR

(3) VZV

(4) HIB

91. At which of the following ages would the nurse expect to administer the varicella zoster vaccine to child?

(1) At birth

(2) 2 months

(3) 6 months

(4) 12 months

92. Which of the following interventions would be included in the plan of care for a child with juvenile rheumatoid arthritis to relieve the pain of swollen and tender joints?

(1) Increasing range of motion exercises

(2) Applying cold compresses

(3) Using warm tub baths

(4) Administering corticosteroids

93. Which of the following would the nurse do to decrease the pruritus associated with eczema?

(1) Keep the child's skin dry

(2) Use wool clothing on child

(3) Bathe child in oatmeal solution

(4) Avoid the use of topical steroids

94. Which of the following would the nurse suspect when a child develops a maculopapular rash, fever, jaundice, hypertension, and hepatomegaly following a bone marrow transplant (BMT)?

(1) Graft-versus-host disease

(2) Interstitial pneumonia

(3) Veno-occlusive disease

(4) Graft rejection

95. Which of the following would the nurse monitor to evaluate the effectiveness of allopurinol for the child receiving chemotherapy?

(1) Episodes of nausea and vomiting

(2) Serum white blood cell count

(3) Evidence of fluid retention and weight gain

(4) Serum and urinary uric acid

96. Which of the following would the nurse suspect when an adolescent has enlargement of the "sentinel" node (the node near the left clavicle)?

(1) Hodgkin's disease

(2) Leukemia

(3) Osteogenic sarcoma

(4) Nephroblastoma

97. Which of the following adverse effects would the nurse include when teaching parents about growth hormone (GH) administration?

(1) Increased blood glucose

(2) Palpitations

(3) Cushingoid appearance

(4) Hypotension

98. Which of the following assessments would indicate to the nurse that bronchodilator therapy is effectively treating the child's asthma?

(1) Dyspnea

(2) Improved breath sounds

(3) Increased wheezing

(4) Pallor

99. Which of the following would the nurse suspect when the mother reports that her infant is passing currant jelly-like stools?

(1) Tracheoesophageal fistula

(2) Intussusception

(3) Pyloric stenosis

(4) Celiac disease

100. When discussing normal infant growth and development with parents, which of the following toys would the nurse suggest as most appropriate for an 8-month-old?

(1) Push-pull toys

(2) Rattle

(3) Large blocks

(4) Mobile

101. Which of the following aspects of psychosocial development is necessary for the nurse to keep in mind when providing care for the preschool child?

(1) The child can use complex reasoning to think out situations.

(2) Fear of body mutilation is a common preschool fear.

(3) The child engages in competitive types of play.

(4) Immediate gratification is necessary to develop initiative.

Comprehensive Test Answers

1. The answer is (2). Because of the structural defect, children with cleft palate may have ineffective functioning of their eustachian tubes creating frequent bouts of otitis media. Most children with cleft palate remain well-nourished and maintain adequate nutrition through the use of proper feeding techniques. Food particles do not pass through the cleft and into the eustachian tubes. There is no association between cleft palate and congenital ear deformities.

2. The answer is (1). For a 3-month-old, a fractured femur would heal within 2 to 4 weeks. Children tend to heal in 4 to 6 weeks, adolescents tend to heal in 8 to 10 weeks, and adults tend to heal in 10 to 16 weeks.

3. The answer is (2). When administering chemotherapy, the nurse should observe for an anaphylactic reaction for 20 minutes and stop the medication if one is suspected. Chemotherapy is associated with both general and specific adverse effects. Therefore close monitoring for them is important. IV care measures, such as administering drugs through a free-flowing IV and assessing for signs if infiltration and irritation, are critically important when administering chemotherapy. Some agents are vesicants and can cause severe tissue damage if infiltration occurs.

4. The answer is (2). Osteogenesis imperfecta is a congenital disorder that results in pathologic fractures and is usually characterized by blue sclerae. Osteomyelitis is an infection of the bone. Osteogenesis imperfecta is a cancer of the bone that may result in a fracture but is not associated with blue sclerae. Osteoarthritis is a degenerative disorder.

5. The answer is (3). Hot spots on the cast, areas of warmth that radiate from inflamed tissue below the cast, usually signify infection. Cold toes, absent pulses, and cyanosis may all indicate neurovascular compromise.

6. The answer is (1). A lead level greater than 70 mcg/dL is indicative of possible lead encephalopathy. Therefore, the child's neurologic status must be carefully monitored. Bone pain is unusual in lead poisoning. Teaching the parents how to decrease or stop pica to stop lead ingestion and including iron-rich foods to decrease anemia are important but they are not the priority at this time.

7. The answer is (1). A major adverse effect of therapy with edathamil calcium-disodium (CaNa2EDTA) and dimercaprol (BAL) is seizures. Muscle atrophy, depression, and increased appetite are not associated with these drugs.

8. The answer is (4). A 3-month-old infant should be able to lift the head and chest when prone. The Moro reflex typically diminishes or subsides by 3 months. The parachute reflex appears at 9 months. Rolling from front to back usually is accomplished at about 5 months.

9. The answer is (4). A child's birth weight usually triples by 12 months and doubles by 4 months. No specific birth weight parameters are established for 7 or 9 months.

10. The answer is (3). Toddlers engaging in parallel play will play near each other, but not with each other. Thus, when two toddlers sit near each other but play with separate dolls, they are exhibiting parallel play. Sharing crayons, playing a board game with a nurse, or sharing dolls with two different nurses are all examples of cooperative play.

11. The answer is (4). When examining a toddler or any small child, the best way to perform the exam is from least to most intrusive. Starting at the head or abdomen is intrusive and should be avoided. Proceeding from distal to proximal is inappropriate at any age.

12. The answer is (3). Idiopathic scoliosis is most likely to occur in adolescent females during their growth spurt. Congenital hip dysplasia and tibial torsion are usually noted in infancy. Transient synovitis usually is seen in preschoolers.

13. The answer is (1). Postoperative bleeding and respiratory distress, secondary to anesthesia or edema, are the primary complications in a child immediately after cleft lip repair. Scarring and infection are likely to occur later in the postoperative course. Infection, including suture line infection, most likely would occur later.

14. The answer is (3). Rheumatic fever results as a delayed reaction to inadequately treated group A β-hemolytic streptococcal infection. Streptococcal pneumonia does not result in rheumatic fever. Haemophilus influenzae, depending on strain, is responsible for illnesses such as otitis media, epiglottitis, and meningitis. Staphylococcus aureus is responsible for a number of pyrogenic infections, but it does not result in rheumatic fever.

15. The answer is (2). Rheumatic fever is not contagious and therefore does not require isolation. Therefore, the nurse should question the need for isolation. The child will need adequate rest periods, especially if carditis is present. Adherence to medication therapy is needed to promote recovery and to prevent relapse of streptococcal infection. Adequate nutrition is needed to promote recovery.

16. The answer is (3). Anorexia, abdominal cramps, and vomiting are all early signs of plumbism, another name for lead poisoning. Plumbism may present with constipation. However, blurred vision and headache typically are later signs, usually associated with encephalopathy. Dizziness also may be a later sign associated with encephalopathy, but fever and chills are not associated with lead poisoning. Mild developmental and behavioral changes may be noted in early plumbism. However, seizures and coma accompany encephalopathy.

17. The answer is (1). Since a 6-month-old has an immature homeostasis-regulating system, metabolic acidosis would be most likely, resulting from a loss of base such that would occur in diarrhea. Metabolic alkalosis, produced by a gain in base or a loss of acid, would most likely result from vomiting. Respiratory acidosis results from diminished or inadequate pulmonary ventilation, leading to an elevated Pco_2 level. Respiratory alkalosis results from an increase in the rate and depth of respiration leading to a decreased Pco_2 level.

18. The answer is (2). Because an infant is at high risk for fluid imbalance secondary to a greater percentage of water as body weight, monitoring daily weights is crucial for assessing the infant's hydration status. Standard precautions would be used. Droplet precautions are indicated for infections transmitted through coughing, sneezing, or talking, or procedures involving contact with the conjunctivae or mucous membranes of the nose or mouth. A 4-month-old usually is too young for antiemetics. Monitoring the CBC, more specifically the hematocrit, would be helpful to monitor the infant's hydration status, but it is not the primary method or priority action.

19. The answer is (4). A loss of greater than 10% of body weight indicates severe diarrhea. Thus the nurse would expect marked oliguria to occur. Pallor would be noted in mild dehydration, loss of less than 5% of body weight. As the child becomes more dehydrated and approaches hypovolemic shock, the pulse would increase. Also, the fontanelle becomes depressed, not bulging, with dehydration.

20. The answer is (1). Acute lymphocytic leukemia (ALL) causes leukopenia, resulting in immunosuppression and increasing the risk of infection, a leading cause of death in children with ALL. Therefore, the initial priority nursing intervention would be to institute infection control precautions to decrease the risk of infection. Iron-rich foods help with anemia, but dietary iron is not an initial intervention. The prognosis of ALL usually is good. However, later on, the nurse may need to assist the child and family with coping since death and dying may still be an issue in need of discussion. Injections should be discouraged, owing to increased risk from bleeding due to thrombocytopenia.

21. The answer is (2). With chemotherapy, cell breakdown leads to hyperuricemia. Allopurinol is given in conjunction with chemotherapy to prevent kidney damage due to this hyperuricemia. Allopurinol does not prevent acid formation nor does it aid in tumor disintegration. It also does not protect the liver. In fact, allopurinol may actually alter liver function study results.

22. The answer is (3). Rectal prolapse is the most common GI complication in cystic fibrosis. Meconium ileus, seen at birth, is the earliest manifestation of cystic fibrosis. There is no association between cystic fibrosis and ulcerative colitis. Diverticulitis is not the most common GI complication in cystic fibrosis.

23. The answer is (1). Chest physical therapy, consisting of chest percussion and postural drainage, should be given before meals to increase the ease of eating and also before sleep to promote adequate rest. Chest physical therapy should be avoided after meals because it may induce vomiting. Many children with CF cough spontaneously on awakening and do not require chest physical therapy at this time. Chest physiotherapy is a crucial component in the treatment of CF and should be performed to improve the child's respiratory function.

24. The answer is (2). Children with CF have thickened secretions that inhibit the release of pancreatic fat-digesting enzymes. Therefore, pancreatic enzyme supplements, such as Pancrease, aid fat digestion. Pancrease is not given to soften stools. Chidren with CF may have loose fatty stools from malabsorption. Pancrease does not prevent diabetes mellitus. It is an enzyme supplement, not an anti-infective agent. It has no effect on pneumonia.

25. The answer is (2). Acute laryngotracheobronchitis is characterized by inflammation and narrowing of the laryngeal and tracheal areas, causing profound airway edema, possibly leading to obstruction and seriously compromised ventilation. A mist tent administers moisturized air that raises atmospheric humidity and aids in thinning secretions. As a result, respirations are eased and hypoxia is alleviated. Usually, an oxygen level greater than 40% is avoided. The mist tent cools and soothes the respiratory tract. Although the tent does provide some restriction of movement and isolation, this is not its purpose in this case.

26. The answer is (1). The tonsils and adenoids are highly vascular tissues. Thus prior to surgery, clotting and also bleeding times must be monitored to reduce the risk of possible hemorrhage. A urinalysis and a differential blood count are often done preoperatively, and in some cases, may be required. However, they are not the most important. Serum electrolyte levels are seldom needed unless there are complicating factors.

27. The answer is (3). When treating the newborn or infant up to 6 months of age, an abduction device, such as the Pavlik harness, is commonly used. This device centers the femoral head into the acetabulum in an attitude of flexion and deepens the acetabulum by pressure. The device is worn until the hip joint is clinically and radiographically stable. For the infant 6 to 18 months of age, traction is used for gradual reduction, followed by closed reduction with cast immobilization until the joint is stable. Older children often require surgical reduction.

28. The answer is (1). The pertussis component may result in fever and the tetanus component may result in injection soreness. Therefore, the mother's verbalization of information about measures to reduce fever indicates understanding. No dietary restrictions are necessary after this injection is given. A subsequent rash is more likely to be seen 5 to 10 days after receiving the MMR vaccine, not the diphtheria, pertussis, and tetanus vaccine. Diarrhea is not associated with this vaccine.

29. The answer is (1). Multiple bruises and burns on a toddler are signs of child abuse. Therefore, the nurse is responsible for reporting the case to Protective Services immediately to protect the child from further harm. Scheduling a follow-up visit is inappropriate because additional harm may come to the child if the nurse waits for further assessment data. Although the nurse should notify the physician, the goal is to initiate measures to protect the child's safety. Notifying the physician immediately does not initiate the removal of the child from harm nor does it absolve the nurse from responsibility. Multiple bruises and burns are not normal toddler injuries.

30. The answer is (1). Projectile vomiting is a key indicator of pyloric stenosis, a narrowing of the pyloric sphincter at the outlet of the stomach. Choking cough after feedings usually is seen in tracheoesophageal fistula. Currant jelly stools are indicative of intussusception. Abdominal distention is not usually noted in pyloric stenosis, but a pyloric "olive" may be palpated.

31. The answer is (1). The child with congenital heart disease develops polycythemia resulting from an inadequate mechanism to compensate for decreased oxygen saturation. Thus, the resultant increase in red blood cells may lead to clumping and emboli formation and subsequently, CVA. Cardiomyopathy usually is not directly associated with emboli formation. Endocarditis may develop from infection. CVAs are more likely to be associated with high blood pressure.

32. The answer is (4). In the first 3 years of life, congestive heart failure is primarily the result of congenital heart disease. Tachycardia and hepatomegaly are manifestations of congestive heart failure. Although cyanosis and dyspnea may be present, the child would have tachycardia, not bradycardia. The child may exhibit weight gain from edema, but peripheral pulses would be weak, not strong.

33. The answer is (3). The preschool period is a time when children are preoccupied with their genitalia and the time of the oedipal conflict. Thus, during hospitalization, fear of castration would reflect this psychosexual preoccupation. A fear of loss of control is noted more often in toddlers. Preschoolers do have fear of the dark, but this is not related to psychosexual preoccupations. Fear of separation may be noted in preschoolers, but it is seen more often in toddlers and it is not related to psychosexual preoccupations.

34. The answer is (2). Anyone can be the abuser, including siblings and mothers. However, the abuser is typically a male that the child knows. Perpetrators may have substance abuse or personality disorder problems, but this is not always the case.

35. The answer is (1). The child's crying signifies the stage of protest. The toddler verbally cries for parents, verbally or physically attacks others, attempts to find parents, clings to parents, and is inconsolable. The second stage, despair, is evidenced by the toddler being disinterested in environment and play, exhibiting passivity, depression, and loss of appetite. The third stage, detachment or denial, is manifested as the toddler makes a superficial adjustment and shows apparent interest, but remains detached. This phase usually occurs after prolonged separation and is rarely seen in hospitalized children.

36. The answer is (2). The mother is using projection, the defense mechanism used when a person attributes his or her own undesirable traits to another. Displacement is the transfer of emotion onto an unrelated object, such as when the mother would kick a chair or bang the door shut. Repression is the submerging of painful ideas into the unconscious. Psychosis is a state of being out of touch with reality.

37. The answer is (3). The most overwhelming adverse influence on health in children is low socioeconomic status. Race, customs, and genetic constitution also may be factors influencing a child's health, but they are not the most influential factors.

38. The answer is (4). When caring for a family with a different cultural background, the nurse should adapt health care needs to cultural practices as necessary. Cultural influences are always present and any practices should be allowed when possible. The nurse should not attempt to change a family's sociocultural beliefs.

39. The answer is (3). In most states, adolescents with sexually transmitted diseases can be evaluated and treated by their own consent. In most states, nonemergent medical interventions such as treatment for a strep throat, fractured arm, or school physical require parental consent for a minor unless the minor is emancipated.

40. The answer is (1). Bronchopulmonary dysplasia usually results in low-birth-weight infants who are mechanically ventilated and receive high concentrations of oxygen. Necrotizing enterocolitis is an acute inflammatory bowel disorder that usually is seen in low-birth-weight infants, but its cause is unknown. Congestive heart failure usually results secondarily to congenital heart disease. Meconium aspiration syndrome usually results from some form of intrauterine stress.

41. The answer is (3). Tetralogy of Fallot consists of pulmonic stenosis, ventricular septal defect, overriding aorta, and hypertrophy of the right ventricle. There is failure of the right, not left, ventricle and pulmonic, not aortic, stenosis.

42. The answer is (4). The child with tetralogy of Fallot may assume a squatting position to decrease venous return of poorly oxygenated blood from the lower extremities and to increase systemic vascular resistance, which increases pulmonary blood flow and eases respiratory effort. Low Fowler's, prone, and supine positioning do not alleviate this problem and therefore would not be used as compensation.

43. The answer is (1). Children with congenital heart disease are more prone to respiratory infections. Bleeding tendencies, frequent vomiting and diarrhea, and seizure disorders are not associated with congenital heart disease.

44. The answer is (4). Because thalassemia major involves faulty hemoglobin, therapy with frequent blood transfusions is crucial. Oxygen therapy is not the primary treatment modality. Adequate hydration is important, but it is more crucial in children with sickle cell anemia. Supplemental iron is contraindicated in children with thalassemia because iron toxicity would develop.

45. The answer is (4). Rheumatic fever results from inadequately treated infections from group A β-hemolytic streptococci. Rheumatic fever should not develop if the child has been adequately treated. Children with congenital heart disease are prone to endocarditis, not rheumatic fever. There is no association between chickenpox and rheumatic fever.

46. The answer is (1). Bronchiolitis involves inflammation of the bronchioles with tenacious mucus causing varying obstruction, leading to air trapping and hyperinflation. As the illness progresses, respiratory distress increases with tachypnea, air hunger, and retraction. Children with tachypnea may be unable to suck and may aspirate. Therefore, the child may be placed on intravenous fluids and NPO. Irritability alone does not interfere with fluid intake. The presence of fever may require IV fluids, but the child would not need to be NPO. Tachycardia alone does not interfere with fluid intake.

47. The answer is (2). Hemorrhage may occur 5 to 10 days after a tonsil and adenoidectomy from tissue sloughing that occurs with healing. Infection usually is not related to bleeding. Secretions do not cause bleeding. Tissue vascularity most likely causes bleeding immediately postoperatively.

48. The answer is (3). For the child with iron deficiency anemia, the blood study results most likely would reveal decreased mean corpuscular volume (MCV), which demonstrates microcytic anemia, decreased hemoglobin, decreased hematocrit, and an elevated total iron-binding capacity.

49. The answer is (4). The most common presenting sign in Wilms' tumor initially is an abdominal mass. Abdominal pain and hypertension may be noted as later signs. Microscopic hematuria may be present. However, frank hematuria is rarely seen.

50. The answer is (1). Children with primary enuresis have never attained dryness. Children who have previously been bladder trained and then develop enuresis have secondary enuresis. Dryness during the day, nocturesis, does not specifically denote primary enuresis. Daytime incontinence is not a sign of enuresis.

51. The answer is (4). Desmopressin (DDAVP) is the nasal spray used to treat enuresis. The drug acts to reduce urinary output. Imipramine is an oral antidepressant that may be used for enuresis. Amoxicillin is an antibiotic that may be used for a urinary tract infection. Pseudoephedrine is a decongestant and is unrelated to treatment for enuresis.

52. The answer is (3). Ribavirin may cause hypotension; therefore, vital signs, including blood pressure, must be monitored frequently. Ribavirin is administered as an aerosol through a small particle aerosol generator. It is not placed directly into the mist tent reservoir. Since the drug is administered by an aerosol device, it does not need to be given with milk.

53. The answer is (4). The child is exhibiting classic signs of epiglottitis, always a pediatric emergency. The physician must be notified immediately and the nurse must be prepared for an emergency intubation or tracheostomy. Further assessment with auscultating lungs and placing the child in a mist tent wastes valuable time. The situation is a possible life-threatening emergency. Having the child lie down would cause additional distress and may result in respiratory arrest. Throat examination may result in laryngospasm that could be fatal.

54. The answer is (4). Most aminoglycosides are administered either IM or IV. Therefore, administering the drugs with food is inappropriate. Aminoglycosides are ototoxic and renal toxic. Thus, assessing the child's hearing, increasing fluid intake, and assessing kidney function are important to prevent these possible complications of drug therapy.

55. The answer is (1). Tetracycline may cause dental and bone problems in children under age 9 and therefore should be avoided in children under the age of 9. Erythromycin, penicillin, and amoxicillin are not contraindicated in this age group.

56. The answer is (1). The most common problem associated with blood transfusion being given to treat thalassemia is iron overload or toxicity. Hemolytic transfusion reactions and fluid overload are possible, but they are not the most common. Sickle cell crisis is not associated with blood transfusion therapy and thalassemia.

57. The answer is (3). Sickle cell crisis is extremely painful and adolescents should be medicated as needed, as ordered. Addiction is not a priority issue in this case. Bedtime-only medication is highly inadequate. Children in sickle cell crisis need to be medicated for pain, even if depression is present, because pain may increase depression.

58. The answer is (2). Idiopathic thrombocytopenic purpura results in decreased numbers of platelets. Thus, the child is at risk for excessive bleeding. Any medications, such as aspirin, which has anti-platelet properties, or treatments that may increase the risk of bleeding such as rectal temperatures, which could traumatize the rectal mucosa, or IM injections should be avoided. Since iron deficiency anemia, sickle cell anemia, and thalassemia are not associated with an increased risk for bleeding, it would not be necessary to avoid these measures.

59. The answer is (1). The child with hemophilia is at risk for bleeding. The sudden severe headache and vomiting, in combination with confusion and lethargy, strongly suggest intracranial bleeding. These symptoms are not associated with a factor reaction. Psychogenic stress would not be manifested with sudden onset of such signs and symptoms. Although some of these symptoms may be noted in AIDS, the onset would not be as abrupt.

60. The answer is (1). Frequent aerobic exercise increases tissue oxygen demand and may cause sickling. Children should avoid overexertion to promote tissue oxygenation. Children with sickle cell anemia may go into sickle cell crisis when they develop infections. Therefore, they should avoid contact with infected persons. A well-balanced diet will help the child to remain as healthy as possible. Children with sickle cell anemia are prone to bed-wetting.

61. The answer is (4). Idiopathic thrombocytopenic purpura is not a genetic disorder. Therefore, genetic counseling would not be indicated. Genetic counseling, however, would be indicated with sickle cell anemia, an autosomal recessive disorder, thalassemia major, an autosomal recessive disorder, and hemophilia, usually an X-linked disorder.

62. The answer is (1). In females, the urethra is shorter than in males. This decreases the distance for organisms to travel, thereby increasing the chance of the child developing a urinary tract infection. Frequent emptying of the bladder would help to decrease urinary tract infections by avoiding sphincter stress. Increased fluid intake enables the bladder to be cleared more frequently, thus helping to prevent urinary tract infections. The intake of acidic juices helps to keep the urine pH acidic and thus decrease the chance of flora development.

63. The answer is (2). AGN usually is associated with an antecedent infection, most commonly streptococcus. No relationship between AGN and impaired reabsorption of bicarbonate ions exists. The gross inability to concentrate urine usually is a sign of diabetes insipidus. Vesicoureteral reflux is not associated with AGN.

64. The answer is (2). Nephrotic syndrome is a complex condition characterized by proteinuria, hypoalbuminemia, hyperlipidemia, altered immunity, and edema. Typically, manifestations include massive proteinuria and edema ranging from periorbital, pedal, and pretibial edema to generalized edema. Hematuria, including gross hematuria, and bacteriuria usually are not noted. Typically the child is afebrile unless the child develops an infection. The blood pressure is either normal or slightly decreased.

65. The answer is (4). An elevated erythrocyte sedimentation rate is typically seen in the child with post-streptococcal glomerulonephritis. Additional diagnostic test findings include red blood cells, white blood cells, casts and protein in the urine, possibly an increase in the urine specific gravity, and elevated BUN and creatinine levels.

66. The answer is (1). In this condition, membrane permeability to protein is increased, resulting in the leakage of proteins through the glomerular membrane. Thus, the primary objective when caring for a child with nephrotic syndrome is reducing the excretion of urinary protein. Typically, the diet is high in protein and calories without added salt. With nephrotic syndrome, there is no hematuria. Normal development should be encouraged for any child experiencing any disorder. Thus, this would be a secondary objective.

67. The answer is (4). The most common symptoms of brain tumors in children are headache and vomiting. Ataxia and seizures are late signs and are not noted in all children. Poor fine and gross motor control may develop, but this is not typical. Whether or not a fever occurs depends on location of the tumor.

68. The answer is (2). "Raccoon eyes" and "battle sign" (bruising behind the ear from bleeding into the mastoid sinus) are classic signs of a basilar skull fracture. Linear skull fractures usually do not trigger any symptoms. An epidural hematoma is characterized by rapid deterioration, including headache, seizures, coma, and brain herniation. A subdural hematoma is characterized by developing agitation, lethargy, headache, and drowsiness within the first 48 hours of a head injury.

69. The answer is (1). The most common cause of noncommunicating hydrocephalus, obstruction to the flow of cerebrospinal fluid through the ventricular system, is developmental malformation. Other causes include neoplasms, infection, such as meningitis or pre-natal infections, and trauma, such as birth trauma.

70. The answer is (3). A communicating hydrocephalus refers to a condition caused by impaired absorption of cerebrospinal fluid within the arachnoid space. Hydrocephalus is not a precursor of neural tube defects, such as spina bifida occulta, but they may occur together. In fact, hydrocephalus occurring within the first 2 years of life often is the result of developmental defects such as spina bifida. A noncommunicating hydrocephalus results from an obstruction in cerebrospinal fluid flow within the ventricles. Cystic formation of the cerebral hemispheres is incompatible with life.

71. The answer is (3). Folic acid deficiency has been associated with the development of neural tube defects, such as anencephaly, encephalocele, and spina bifida, including spina bifida occulta, meningocele, and myelomingocele. The development of these defects is not associated with iron deficiency anemia, protein-losing enteropathy, or diabetes insipidus.

72. The answer is (4). For the child with spastic CP, the most common type, hypertonicity with poor control of posture, balance, and coordination is seen. Athetosis, worm-like movements, and dyskinesia, abnormal involuntary movements that disappear in sleep and increase in stress, are associated with dyskinetic CP. A wide-based gait is associated with ataxic CP.

73. The answer is (1). Koplik's spots are seen in rubeola, or measles. Occipital adenopathy occurs in rubella, or German measles. A vesicular rash may be seen in herpes. Parotid swelling is noted in mumps.

74. The answer is (1). The nurse would teach the parents that varicella is no longer contagious or communicable when crusts form on the lesions. Two to 3 weeks is not specific enough because no information is presented to state when the child contracted the disease. Two to 3 weeks is typically the incubation period during which time the disease is contagious. The child will still be contagious when the rash appears and during the prodromal phase.

75. The answer is (4). The most dangerous complication of rubella is its teratogenic effects on the fetus. Arthralgia and fever may occur, but they usually are mild and self-limiting. Purpura does not develop with rubella.

76. The answer is (3). The most likely test to be ordered to confirm HIV infection in an infant is an HIV virus assay. A positive virologic test (culture or DNA or RNA polymerase chain reaction) indicates possible infection and should be confirmed by a second virologic test. The ELISA and Western blot tests are not helpful because the child still has maternal antibodies present in his or her system. A CD4 count will not be used for confirmation, but will be needed for assessing immune status and progression of the disease.

77. The answer is (2). A whitish-gray membrane adherent to the tonsils is characteristic of diphtheria. A whooping-like cough is characteristic of pertussis. Paralysis is characteristic of poliomyelitis. Involvement of the skin, conjunctivae, and mucous membranes is characteristic of Kawasaki's disease.

78. The answer is (1). Because the MMR vaccine is cultivated in eggs, it is contraindicated in children who have had a previous serious allergic reaction to eggs. Children with HIV disease may receive an MMR vaccination. There is no contraindication for the concurrent administration of DTP. If the child has received immunoglobulins, waiting a period of 3 to 4 months is necessary prior to giving an MMR vaccine.

79. The answer is (2). Children with CP exhibit varying manifestations of the disorder. However, decreased cognitive functioning is not noted in all children with CP. In fact, it is very possible to have CP without cognitive impairment. Delayed gross motor development, abnormal muscle performance, and altered muscle tone are associated with CP.

80. The answer is (1). Mild mental retardation refers to developmental disability involving an IQ of 50 to 70. Typically, the child is not noted as being retarded, but exhibits slowness in performing tasks, such as self-feeding, walking, and talking. Little or no speech, marked motor delays, and gait disabilities would be seen in more severe forms of mental retardation.

81. The answer is (2). Down syndrome is characterized by the following: a transverse palmar crease (simian crease), separated sagittal suture, oblique palpebral fissures, small nose, depressed nasal bridge, high-arched palate, excess and lax skin, wide spacing and plantar crease between the second and big toes, hyperextensible and lax joints, large protruding tongue, and muscle weakness.

82. The answer is (3). Gower's sign refers to the child rolling over, kneeling, and pressing his or her hands against the ankles, shins, knees, and thighs in a climbing action to rise from a supine to a standing position. It is a characteristic finding with muscular dystrophy. Gower's sign is not seen with cerebral palsy, spina bifida, or Down syndrome.

83. The answer is (2). Children with HIV disease should not receive the live polio vaccine (TOPV). Therefore, the child is given the inactivated form (TIPV). Children with HIV do receive MMR. Since TIPV is used instead of TOPV, children with HIV do not receive all immunizations as scheduled. However, all children, including those with HIV/AIDS, need to be immunized.

84. The answer is (3). Unilateral or bilateral parotid swelling is noted in mumps, also known as parotitis. Diphtheria is characterized by a whitish-gray membrane on the tonsils. Poliomyelitis is characterized by paralysis. Pertussis is characterized by a whooping cough.

85. The answer is (4). Because of the increased risk for neurovascular complications related to cast application, altered tissue perfusion is the priority nursing diagnosis for a child in a new spica cast. Risk for infection, injury, and impaired skin integrity also may be appropriate, but not immediately after application of the cast. These nursing diagnoses may be more appropriate after the cast has been on for a while.

86. The answer is (4). Rheumatic fever can best be prevented by using prescribed treatment for streptococcal infections, specifically administering antibiotics as ordered with completion of treatment for the specified number of days. It is almost impossible to avoid contact with all streptococcal infections. Treating all sore throats with antibiotics is inappropriate because not all sore throats are caused by streptococcal infection. A rapid strep test or a culture must be obtained for verification. Learning to identify the early signs of a disease, although important, is not a prevention strategy.

87. The answer is (3). The toddler is exhibiting manifestations of separation anxiety. Staying with a toddler who is experiencing separation anxiety is an appropriate intervention for both the child and the parent. Doing so offers reassurance and feelings of security for both.

The child will not stop crying when the mother leaves. Visiting should be encouraged, not discouraged. Parents should never sneak away because doing so could injure the child's sense of trust.

88. The answer is (2). Compartment syndrome is an emergent situation and the physician needs to be notified immediately so that interventions can be initiated to relieve the increasing pressure and restore circulation. Acetaminophen (Tylenol) will be ineffective since the pain is related to the increasing pressure and tissue ischemia. The cast, not traction, is being used in this situation for immobilization, so releasing the traction would be inappropriate. In this situation, specific action, not continued monitoring, is indicated.

89. The answer is (4). A Pavlik harness is a device that maintains the legs in abduction through the use of straps. Thus, parents need instruction to check the child's skin, especially around the areas of the straps, for breakdown and irritation. Since the harness is to be used continuously, it should not be removed for bathing. Sponge baths are required until the harness is no longer needed. The child needs to be turned frequently, at least every 4 hours. Less frequent turning or maintaining one position may increase the risk for skin breakdown.

90. The answer is (2). Rash, pruritus, low-grade fever, and arthralgia are possible with the rubella component of MMR. DTaP may cause redness and tenderness at the injection site and fever. These effects range from mild to severe, and may include seizures. VZV may cause transient fever and edema and redness at the injection site. HIB may lead to possible discomfort and low-grade fever.

91. The answer is (4). The varicella zoster vaccine (VZV) is a live vaccine given after age 12 months. The first dose of hepatitis B vaccine is given at birth to 2 months, then at 1 to 4 months, and then again at 6 to 18 months. DtaP is routinely given at 2, 4, 6, and 15 to 18 months and a booster at 4 to 6 years.

92. The answer is (3). Moist heat relieves pain and stiffness, and the best way to deliver it is to submerge the child in warm water tub baths. Increased exercise can aggravate pain. Cold compresses can increase stiffness. Corticosteroids are reserved for severe problems or life-threatening complications.

93. The answer is (3). Oatmeal solution relieves itching. Skin should be kept moist because dryness aggravates itching. Wool clothing irritates sensitive skin. Rather, loose cotton clothing is preferred. Topical steroids commonly are used to treat eczema.

94. The answer is (1). Following a BMT, evidence of a maculopapular rash, fever, jaundice, hypertension, and hepatomegaly suggest graft-versus-host disease. Interstitial pneumonia would be manifested by fever, nasal flaring, tachypnea, cough, and hypoxia. Veno-occlusive disease would be evidenced by sudden weight gain, jaundice, hepatomegaly, right upper quadrant pain, and encephalopathy. Graft rejection would be manifested by fever, infection, and decreased blood count.

95. The answer is (4). Allopurinol is used to manage uric acid elevation secondary to chemotherapy. The nurse would monitor serum and urinary uric acid levels. Assessing the episodes of nausea and vomiting would be done when antiemetics such as ondansetron are administered to relieve nausea and vomiting associated with chemotherapy. When granulocyte colony stimulating factor (GCSF) is used to manage neutropenia after bone marrow transplant, the nurse would monitor the child's white blood cell count. If the child was receiving corticosteroids, the nurse would monitor the child for signs of fluid retention and weight gain.

96. The answer is (1). Enlargement of the sentinel node is often the first sign of Hodgkin's disease. This adenopathy is not specific to leukemia. A painful swelling on a long bone is a sign of osteogenic sarcoma. A firm, palpable, nontender abdominal mass is usually noted in nephroblastoma.

97. The answer is (1). With growth hormone administration, increased blood glucose levels may occur. Palpitations are a possible effect of thyroid hormone administration. This a is side effect of GH. Cushingoid appearance results from corticosteroid therapy. Hypotension occurs with administration of glucagon.

98. The answer is (2). Bronchodilator therapy is effective when the nurse would auscultate improved breath sounds, indicating that the airways are opening and air is moving in and out more freely. Evidence of dyspnea, increased wheezing, or pallor would suggest that the child is still experiencing respiratory distress, and possibly a worsening of his condition.

99. The answer is (2). Intussusception is an invagination or telescoping of one portion of the intestine into an adjacent portion, causing obstruction. If the obstruction continues, the child typically passes currant jelly-like stools, which contain blood and mucus. Tracheoesophageal fistula is usually evidenced by choking after feedings. Pyloric stenosis is associated with projectile vomiting. Celiac disease leads to impaired fat absorption manifested by steatorrhea and exceedingly foul-smelling stools.

100. The answer is (3). Because the 8-month-old is refining his gross motor skills, being able to sit unsupported and also improving his fine motor skills, probably capable of making hand-to-hand transfers, large blocks would be the most appropriate toy selection. Push–pull toys would be more appropriate for the 10- to 12-month-old as he or she begins to cruise the environment. Rattles and mobiles are more appropriate for infants in the 1 to 3 month age range. Mobiles pose a danger to older infants because of possible strangulation.

101. The answer is (2). During the preschool period, the child has mastered a sense of autonomy and goes on to master a sense of initiative. During this period, the child commonly experiences more fears than at any other time. One common fear is fear of body mutilation, especially associated with painful experiences. The preschool child uses simple, not complex, reasoning, engages in associative, not competitive, play (interactive and cooperative play with sharing), and is able to tolerate longer periods of delayed gratification.

Bibliography

Ahern, J., & Grey, M. (1996). New developments in treating children with insulin-dependent diabetes mellitus. *Journal of Pediatric Health Care, 10*(4), 161–166.

American Academy of Pediatrics Committee on Children with Disabilities. (1998). Managed care and children with special needs: A subject review. *Pediatrics, 102*(3), 657–660.

American Psychiatric Association. (1994). *Diagnostic and statistical manual of mental disorders* (4th ed.). Washington, DC: Author.

Ashwill, J., & Droske, S. (1997). *Nursing care of children: Principles and practice.* Philadelphia: W. B. Saunders.

Bakarat, et al. (1995). Management of fatal illness and death in children. *Pediatric Review, 16*(11), 419–423.

Bickley, L. (1999). *Bates guide to physical examination and history taking* (7th ed.). Philadelphia: Lippincott Williams & Wilkins.

Bowden, V., Dickey, S., & Greenberg, C. (1998). *Children and their families: The continuum of care.* Philadelphia: W. B. Saunders.

Bowden, V., Dickey, S., & Greenberg, C. (1999). CDC publishes ACIP rotavirus recommendations. *Infectious Diseases in Children, 12*(5), 25–27.

Cohen, A. (1999). Choosing the best strategies to prevent iron deficiency. *Journal of the American Medical Association, 281*(23), 414.

Danjani, A. (1997). Prevention of bacterial endocarditis: recommendations by the American Heart Association. *Journal of the American Medical Association, 277,* 1794–1801.

Elder, J. S., Peters, C. A., Arant, B. S. Jr., Ewalt, D. H., Hawtrey, C. E., Hurwitz, R. S., Parrott, T. S., Snyder, H. M. 3rd, Weiss, R. A., Woolf, S. H., & Hasselblad, V. (1997). Pediatric Vesicoureteral Reflux Guidelines Panel summary report on management of primary vesicoureteral reflux in children. *Journal of Urology, 157*(5), 1846–1851.

Feigin, R., & Perlman, E. (1998). Bacterial meningitis beyond the neonatal period. In R. D. Feigin & J. D. Cherry (Eds.). *Textbook of pediatric infectious diseases* (4th ed.). Philadelphia: W. B. Saunders.

Fonkalsrud, E., Ashcraft, K., Coran, A., Ellis, D., Grosfeld, J., Tunell, W., & Weber, T. (1998). Surgical treatment of gastroesophageal reflux in children: A combined-hospital study of 7467 patients. *Pediatrics, 101*(3), 419–422.

Fox, J. (1997). *Primary health care of children.* St. Louis: Mosby.

Garfinkel, B., Carlson, G., & Weller, E. (1990). *Psychiatric disorders in children and adolescents.* Philadelphia: W. B. Saunders.

Gildea, J. (1998). Human parvovirus B19: Flushed in the face though healthy (fifth disease and more). *Pediatric Nursing, 24*(4), 325–332.

Hart, J. (1996). Pediatric gastroesophageal reflux. *American Family Physician, 54*(8), 2463–2472.

Hartley, B., & Fuller, C. (1997). Juvenile arthritis: A nursing perspective. *Journal of Pediatric Nursing, 12*(2), 100–109.

Fisher, A., & Vessey, J. (1998). Preventing lead poisoning and its consequences. *Pediatric Nursing, 24*(4), 348.

Fischbach, F. (1997). *A manual of laboratory and diagnostic tests* (5th ed.). Philadelphia: Lippincott-Raven.

Friebert, S., & Shurin, S. (1998). ALL: Treatment and beyond. *Contemporary Pediatrics, 15*(3), 39–56.

Hoffman, G. (1998). New AAP recommendations for blood lead screening in children. *American Family Physician, 8,* 862.

Karch, A. (2000). *2000 Lippincott's nursing drug guide.* Philadelphia: Lippincott Williams & Wilkins.

Kuis, W., et al. (1997). How painful is juvenile chronic arthritis? *Archives of Diseases of Children, 77*(5), 451–453.

Kunin, C. (1997). Urinary tract infections in children. In B. O'Donell & S. Koff (Eds.). *Pediatric urology.* Oxford: Butterworth-Heinemann.

Morrow, J., & Kelsey, K. (1998). Folic acid for prevention of neural tube defects: Pediatric anticipatory guidance. *Journal of Pediatric Health Care, 12*(2), 55–59.

Muscari, M. (1998). Assessment of infants, children, and adolescents. In J. Weber & J. Kelley (Eds.). *Health assessment in nursing* (Chap. 22). Philadelphia: Lippincott-Raven.

National Asthma Education and Prevention Program. (1997). *Expert panel report II: Guidelines for the diagnosis and management of asthma.* Bethesda, MD: National Heart, Lung, and Blood Institute.

Nesbitt, M., Hill, M., & Peterson, N. (1997). A comprehensive pediatric bereavement program: the patterns of your life. *Critical Care Nursing, 20*(2), 48.

North American Nursing Diagnosis Association. (1999). *NANDA diagnoses: Definitions and classification 1999-2000.* Philadelphia: Author.

Noll, R., Garstein, M., Vannatta, J., Bukowki, W., & Davies, W. (1999). Social, emotional, and behavioral functioning of children with cancer. *Pediatrics, 103,* 71.

O'Connell, K. (1996). Attention deficit hyperactivity disorder. *Pediatric Nursing, 2,* 1.

Pillitteri, A. (1999). *Maternal and child health nursing* (2nd ed.). Philadelphia: Lippincott Williams & Wilkins.

Riddel, J., & Moon, M. (1996). Children with HIV becoming adolescents: Caring for long-term survivors. *Pediatric Nursing, 22*(3), 220–225.

Robertson, R., & Cone, J. (1996). Burn injuries: A guide to assessment, proven management approaches. *Pediatrics, 36*(9), 1873–1879.

Saenz, L., Beebe, R., & Triplett, D. (1999). Caring for infants with congenital heart disease and their families. *American Family Physician, 59*(7), 1857.

Schulman, D., & Bercu, B. (1998). Growth hormone therapy: An update. *Contemporary Pediatrics, 15*(8), 95–110.

Siberry, G., & Iannone, R. (2000). *The Harriet Lane handbook* (15th ed.). St. Louis: Mosby.

Stephenson, M. (1999). Pediatricians have choices for treatment, diagnosis of UTIs. *Infectious Diseases in Children, 12*(1), 36.

Walsh, K., Magnusson, M., & Napoli, L. (1999). Asthma clinical pathway: An interdisciplinary approach to implementation in the inpatient setting. *Pediatric Nursing, 25*(1), 79.

Westmoreland, D. (1999). Critical congenital cardiac defects in the newborn. *Journal of Perinatal and Neonatal Nursing, 2,* 7.

Woestman, R., Perkin, R., Serna, T., Stralen, D., & Knierim, D. (1998). *Journal of Pediatric Health Care, 12*(12), 288–298.

Wong, D. L. (1999). *Whaley and Wong's nursing care of infants and children* (6th ed.). St. Louis: Mosby.

Working Group on Antiretroviral Therapy and Medical Management of HIV-Infected Children. (1998). Guidelines for the use of antiretroviral agents in pediatric HIV infection. *www.medscape.com/govmt/CDC/MMRW/1998/04.98/MMWR-p.../pnt-MMWR-phiv.htm.*

Zickler, C., Morrow, J., & Bull, M. (1998). Infants with Down syndrome: A look at temperament. *Journal of Pediatric Health Care, 12*(3), 111–117.

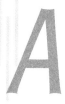
A Normal Laboratory Study Values

COMPLETE BLOOD COUNT

TEST	NORMAL VALUE
Leukocyte (White Blood Cell)	×1000 cells/mm³ (μL)
Birth	9.0–30.0
24 hours	9.4–34.0
1 month	5.0–19.5
1–3 years	6.0–17.5
4–7 years	5.5–15.5
8–13 years	4.5–13.5
Adult	4.5–11.0
Neutrophils Bands	3–5% (total WBC count)
Segs	54–62%
Lymphocytes	25–33%
Monocytes	3–7%
Eosinophils	1–3%
Basophils	0–0.75%
Erythrocytes (Red Blood Cells)	
Cord	3.9–5.5 million/mm³
1–3 days	4.0–6.6 million/mm³
1 week	3.9–6.3 million/mm³
2 weeks	3.6–6.2 million/mm³
1 month	3.0–5.4 million/mm³
2 months	2.7–4.9 million/mm³
3–6 months	3.1–4.5 million/mm³
0.5–2 years	3.7–5.3 million/mm³
2–6 years	3.9–5.3 million/mm³
6–12 years	4.0–5.2 million/mm³
12–18 years (male)	4.5–5.3 million/mm³
12–18 years (female)	4.1–5.1 million/mm³
Hemoglobin	
1–3 days	14.5–22.5 g/dL
2 months	9.0–14.0 g/dL
6–12 years	11.5–15.5 g/dL

(continued)

COMPLETE BLOOD COUNT (Continued)

TEST	NORMAL VALUE
12–18 years (male)	13.0–16.0 g/dL
12–18 years (female)	12.0–16.0 g/dL
Hematocrit	
1 day	48–69%
2 days	48–75%
3 days	44–72%
2 months	28–42%
6–12 years	35–45%
12–18 years (male)	37–49%
12–18 years (female)	36–46%
Mean Corpuscular Volume (MCV)	
1–3 days	95–121 μm^3
0.5–2 years	70–86 μm^3
6–12 years	77–95 μm^3
12–18 years (male)	78–98 μm^3
12–18 years (female)	78–102 μm^3
Mean Corpuscular Hemoglobin (MCH)	
Birth	31–37 pg/cell
1–3 days	31–37 pg/cell
1 week–1 month	28–40 pg/cell
2 months	26–34 pg/cell
3–6 months	25–35 pg/cell
0.5–2 years	23–31 pg/cell
2–6 years	24–30 pg/cell
6–12 years	25–33 pg/cell
12–18 years	25–35 pg/cell
Mean Corpuscular Hemoglobin Concentration (MCHC)	
Birth	30–36 g Hg/dL RBC
1–3 days	29–37 g Hg/dL RBC
1–2 weeks	28–38 g Hg/dL RBC
1–2 months	29–37 g Hg/dL RBC
3 months–2 years	30–36 g Hg/dL RBC
2–18 years	31–37 g Hg/dL RBC
Reticulocyte Count	
Infants	2–5% of RBCs
Children	0.5–4% of RBCs
12–18 years (male)	0.5–1% of RBCs
12–18 years (female)	0.5–2.5% of RBCs
Platelet Count	
Birth–1 week	84,000–478,000/mm^3
Thereafter	150,000–400,000/mm^3

ERYTHROCYTE SEDIMENTATION RATE (ESR)

TEST	NORMAL VALUE
Westergren	
Child	0–10 mm/hour
Adult (male)	0–15 mm/hour
Adult (female)	0–20 mm/hour
Wintrobe	
Child	0–13 mm/hour
Adult (male)	0–9 mm/hour
Adult (female)	0–20 mm/hour

BLOOD CHEMISTRIES

TEST	NORMAL VALUE
Amylase	
1–19 years	35–127 IU/L
Blood Urea Nitrogen (BUN)	
Newborn	3–12 mg/dL
Infant/Child	5–18 mg/dL
Thereafter	7–18 mg/dL
Calcium (total)	
Child	9.2–11.0 mg/dL
Carbon Dioxide, Total; (CO_2)	
Newborn	13–22 mEq/L
Infant/Child	20–28 mEq/L
Thereafter	23–30 mEq/L
Chloride	
Newborn	98–113 mEq/dL
Thereafter	98–107 mEq/dL
Cholesterol	
0–4 years (male)	114–203 mg/dL
0–4 years (female)	112–200 mg/dL
5–9 years (male)	121–203 mg/dL
5–9 years (female)	126–205 mg/dL
10–14 years (male)	119–202 mg/dL
10–14 years (female)	124–201 mg/dL
15–19 years (male)	113–197 mg/dL
15–19 years (female)	119–200 mg/dL
Creatinine	
Newborn	0.3–1.0 mg/dL
Infant	0.2–0.4 mg/dL

(continued)

BLOOD CHEMISTRIES (Continued)

TEST	NORMAL VALUE
Child	0.3–0.7 mg/dL
Adolescent	0.5–1.0 mg/dL
Creatinine Kinase (CK, CPK)	
Newborn	68–580 U/L
6–11 years (male)	56–185 U/L
12–18 years (male)	35–185 U/L
≥19 years (male)	38–174 U/L
6–7 years (female)	50–145 U/L
8–14 years (female)	35–145 U/L
15–18 years (female)	20–100 U/L
≥19 years (female)	96–140 U/L
Glucose	
1 day	40–60 mg/dL
After 1 day	50–90 mg/dL
Child	60–100 mg/dL
Adult	70–105 mg/dL
Magnesium	
Newborn	1.2–1.8 mEq/L
Adult	1.3–2.1 mEq/L
Phosphate	
0–5 days	4.8–8.2 mg/dL
1–3 years	3.8–6.5 mg/dL
4–11 years	3.7–5.6 mg/dL
12–15 years	2.9–5.4 mg/dL
16–19 years	2.7–4.7 mg/dL
Potassium	
Newborn	3.0–6.0 mEq/L
Infant	3.5–5.5 mEq/L
Child	3.5–5.0 mEq/L
Thereafter	3.5–5.0 mEq/L
Sodium	
Newborn	136–146 mEq/L
Infant	139–146 mEq/L
Child	138–145 mEq/L
Thereafter	136–146 mEq/L

THYROID FUNCTION TESTS (TFTs)

TEST	NORMAL VALUE
Triiodothyronine (T_3)	
Child	90–240 ng/dL
Adult	120–195 ng/dL
Total Thyroxine (T_4)	
1–3 days	8.2–19.9 μg/dL
1 week	6.0–15.9 μg/dL
1–12 months	6.1–14.9 μg/dL
1–3 years	6.8–13.5 μg/dL
3–10 years	5.5–12.8 μg/dL
Thereafter	4.2–13.0 μg/dL
Free Thyroxine (FT_4)	0.8–2.4 ng/dL
Thyroid-Stimulating Hormone (TSH)	
Newborn	3–20 μIU/L
Adult	0.5–6 mIU/L

LIVER FUNCTION TESTS (LFTs)

TEST	NORMAL VALUE
Alkaline Phosphatase	
Infant	73–266 IU/L
Child	57–150 IU/L
Adolescent	57–258 IU/L
Bilirubin	
Newborn	1.5–12.0 mg/dL
Total	0.2–1.0 mg/dL
Conjugated	0.0–0.2 mg/dL
Indirected Conjugated	0.2–0.8 mg/dL
Lactate Dehydrogenase (LDH)	90–200 IU/L
Aspartate Transaminase (AST) formerly Glutamic-Oxaloacetic Transaminase (SGOT)	5–40 μ/mL
Glutamate Pyruvate Transaminase (SGPT)	5–35 IU/L

IRON-RELATED TESTS

TEST	NORMAL VALUE
Iron	
Newborn	100–250 µg/dL
Infant	40–100 µg/dL
Child	50–120 µg/dL
Thereafter (male)	50–160 µg/dL
Thereafter (female)	40–150 µg/dL
Total Iron-Binding Capacity (TIBC)	240–250 µg/dL
Transferrin	240–480 mg/dL

COAGULATION STUDIES

TEST	NORMAL VALUE
Partial Thromboplastin Time (PTT)	16–25 seconds
Prothrombin Time (PT)	10–15 seconds
Bleeding Time	Forearm (Ivy method): 2–9.5 minutes Earlobe (Duke method): <8 minutes

GLUCOSE TOLERANCE TEST (GTT)

TEST	NORMAL VALUE
GTT Dosages:	
Child: 1.75 g/kg of ideal body weight up to maximum of 75 g	Fasting: 70–105 mg/dL
Adult: 75 g	60 min: 120–170 mg/dL
	90 min: 100–140 mg/dL
	120 min: 70–120 mg/dL

ARTERIAL BLOOD GASES (ABGs)

TEST	NORMAL VALUES
pH	Newborn: 7.11–7.36
	Child: 7.39
	Adult: 7.35–7.45
Pao_2	Newborn: 45–95 mm Hg
	Child: 96 mm Hg
	Adult: 90–100 mm Hg
$Paco_2$	Newborn: 27–40 mm Hg
	Child: 37 mm Hg
	Adult: 35–45 mm Hg
HCO_3	Newborn: 20 mEq/L
	Child: 22 mEq/L
	Adult: 22–26 mEq/L
Base Excess	Child: +/−3
	Adult: +/−2

OTHER COMMONLY ORDERED BLOOD TESTS

TEST	NORMAL VALUES
Antistreptolysin O Titer (ASO)	<166 Todd units
Antinuclear Antibody (ANA)	Negative
	If the test is positive, the serum will be titered, and a pattern will be reported.
C-Reactive Protein (CRP)	
2–12 years	67–1800 ng/mL or <0.8 mg/dL
Mono Test; Heterophile Antibody; Epstein-Barr Virus (EBV)	Negative titer <1:80
Rheumatoid Factor (RF)	0–69 IU/mL

ROUTINE URINALYSIS

TEST	NORMAL VALUE
Color	Pale yellow to amber
Turbidity	Clear to slightly hazy
Specific Gravity	1.015–1.025
pH	4.5–8.0
Glucose	Negative
Ketones	Negative
Blood	Negative
Protein	Negative
Bilirubin	Negative
Urobilinogen	0.1–1.0
Nitrate for Bacteria	Negative
Leukocyte Esterase	Negative
Casts	Occasional hyaline casts
Red Blood Cells	Negative or rare
Crystals	**Acid Urine:** Amorphous urates Uric acid Calcium oxalate Sodium acid Urates **Alkaline Urine:** Amorphous phosphates Calcium phosphate Ammonium biurate Triple phosphate Calcium carbonate
White Blood Cells	Negative or rare
Epithelial Cells	Few

CEREBRAL SPINAL FLUID (LUMBAR PUNCTURE) BY COMMON PEDIATRIC DIAGNOSES

DISORDER	PRESSURE (MM H_2O)	APPEARANCE	LEUKOCYTES	PROTEIN
Normal	<180	Clear	0–5 lymphocytes	15–35

B Nursing Considerations for Laboratory and Diagnostic Studies

TEST	NURSING CONSIDERATIONS
Arterial blood gases	Maintain pressure at the site for approximately 5 minutes to prevent bleeding and hematoma formation.
Angiography	May require sedation. After test, monitor the child for complications, which may include arterial/vascular occlusion, venous thrombus, air embolism, coronary arterial injection, myocardial stain, and myocardial perforation.
Arthrography	Prepare the child for local or general anesthesia. After procedure, monitor for bleeding and infection. Use an ice bag to reduce swelling.
Arthroscopy	Check for iodine allergies. Prepare for local anesthesia. Encourage joint rest for 12 hours after procedure. Compression dressing may reduce swelling.

Blood studies
  Complete blood count (CBC)
  Erythrocyte sedimentation rate (ESR)
	No special considerations

Blood urea nitrogen (BUN)	No special considerations
Bone scans	Young children may require sedation. Encourage fluids to rid the body of radioactive contrast. Encourage the child to void if the pelvic bones are to be visualized.
Cardiac catheterization	Requires precatheterization teaching. May require sedation. After catheterization, monitor the insertion site for bleeding, and monitor the circulatory status of the affected extremity.
Computed tomography (CT) scan	Sedation is usually required for infants and young children. Keep infant and child NPO before the examination. Assess for iodine allergies if a contrast is required. Be aware that the equipment may cause claustrophobia.
Creatinine	No special considerations are necessary unless creatinine clearance is ordered. Creatinine clearance requires 24-hour urine collection, which is refrigerated as retrieved.
Cultures	Obtain all cultures before starting antibiotics.
Cystoscopy	Requires anesthesia, preoperative preparation, and postoperative care.
Echocardiography	May require sedation because the child must be still for about 45 minutes.

(continued)

TEST	NURSING CONSIDERATIONS
Echoencephalography	No specific preparation is required, but the child must remain still.
Electrocardiogram (ECG)	No special considerations are necessary.
Electroencephalography (EEG)	The child's hair should be clean. No caffeine or stimulants should be used before the test. Sedation may be required for young children.
Intravenous pyelography (IVP)	This test is contraindicated if the child has an iodine or shellfish allergy. Bowel preparation is required. Increase fluids after this test.
Joint aspiration fluid	Prepare for local anesthesia. Use pain management techniques after procedure.
Lower GI endoscopic procedures	Keep the child NPO before the procedure. The procedure requires conscious sedation or general anesthesia. Vital signs and oxygen saturation should be monitored during the procedure. Bowel preparation may be required.
Lumbar puncture	Use proper positioning during the test. Monitor the child during the test for signs of distress. The child may need to lie flat after the procedure.
Magnetic resonance imaging (MRI)	Sedation is usually required. Keep the child NPO before the examination. Tell the child that his head will have to be restrained.
Nuclear brain scan	The child will need an IV.
Pulse oximetry	Choose appropriate sensor for the child's size. Place the sensor with the light source directly opposite the photodetector. Be aware of potential errors in reading, which include abnormal hemoglobin, poor peripheral perfusion, and motion artifact.
Radiographs	Inquire about the pregnancy status of female adolescents.
Radiographic imaging—upper GI series, barium enema	The child is usually kept NPO before the procedure. Children who are unwilling or unable to drink contrast medium may require nasogastric tube insertion. Barium enema may require a bowel preparation.
Renal biopsy	Children are typically kept NPO because sedation is usually required.
Renal scan (radioisotope renogram)	Be aware that this test should not be scheduled within 24 hours of IVP. Radiation exposure is minimal.
Stool tests	Collect fresh stool in appropriate containers.
Transesophageal pacing/echocardiography	This test may require sedation.
Ultrasonography	No special considerations are necessary.
Upper GI endoscopic procedures	Keep the child NPO before the procedure. This procedure requires conscious sedation or general anesthesia. Vital signs and oxygen saturation should be monitored during the procedure.
Urinalysis	Clean the perineal area of children in diapers before obtaining specimens.
Urine culture and sensitivity	Obtain a clean-catch, or, if ordered, catheterized specimen.
Urine toxicology	Toxicology specimens may require specific collection methods.

(continued)

TEST	NURSING CONSIDERATIONS
Urodynamics	Prepare the child for externally placed perineal electrodes, and for possible catheterization or the need to void on command.
Voiding cystourethrography (VCU)	Be aware that VCU should not be performed in the presence of urinary tract infection.

Index

Note: Page numbers followed by *f* refer to figures; those followed by *t* refer to tables; and those followed by *b* refer to boxed material.

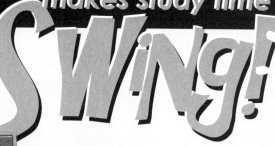

Lippincott's Review Series CD-ROMs provide a convenient way to assess readiness for academic tests and licensure exams. One hundred carefully selected, multiple-choice questions are provided for study and simulated testing. In Study Mode, correct and incorrect feedback with rationale is provided following each question. In Test Mode, questions are scored with feedback available for review at the conclusion of the test.

System Requirements

Windows 95 or higher
486/66 Processor or higher
16 MB RAM
6 MB Free Hard Disk Space
CD-ROM Drive
640 x 480 Color Monitor or higher
256 Colors or higher

Installation

Insert the CD-ROM into your CD-ROM drive.
Click on the **Start** button, and then click **Run**.
At the command line, type **D:\setup.exe**. (Note: The letter D represents the CD-ROM drive. If your drive is designated by a different letter, use your drive letter instead.)
Click **OK**.
Follow the online instructions.

Technical Support

If you experience difficulty viewing the text, it may be the result of the color settings on your system. Should you need assistance or you have any questions regarding the use or content of this CD-ROM, please contact our Technical Support department by telephone at **800-638-3030** or **410-528-4532**, by fax at 410-528-4422, or by email at techsupp@LWW.com. Technical Support is available from 8:30 am to 5:00 pm (EST), Monday through Friday.